COVENANTS
inspiring the soul of healing

Revised Edition

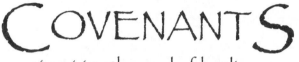

COVENANTS
inspiring the soul of healing

GLENNA M. CROOKS

Covenant Matters Press • Fort Washington, PA

To my Father and Mother
For my Children

The deplorable events of September 11, 2001 brought the world's violence to the American doorstep. Responses to the tragedies of the day have offered healing comfort to those here who were affected. Most Americans, though changed by the experience, have now returned to lives of relative peace and security.

Millions around the world cannot say that. Their tragedies have not faded into memory. They are harmed by violence and poverty each day, in ways we, thankfully, cannot imagine.

The Medical Missionaries of Mary, as described in the mission statement of this group of women, work "... in a world deeply and violently divided." They "... go to people of different cultures, where human needs are greatest... to embrace holistic healing and to work for reconciliation, justice, and peace." They engage in their work of healing in war-torn areas, despite air raids and landmines, and in places where millions have been displaced from their homes, thousands have been maimed, and too many are buried in mass, unmarked graves.

The proceeds from this book are being donated to this group of healers. Doing this is a part of the covenant I have made to help others heal. It is a privilege to be able to assist in these healing activities. By their example, may these healers lead others to do likewise.

Contents

Foreword to the Revised Edition

The American system of health and healthcare is currently trapped—trapped into delivering inadequate results and rising costs. In response to the rising costs, the system is becoming increasingly more bureaucratic and more impersonal. Whether you are a patient or provider trapped in a public sector or private sector bureaucracy makes no difference; you are still trapped—in rules and regulations based on the wrong model and the wrong principles.

The outcome in human terms is staggering. The Institute of Medicine (IOM) estimates between 44,000 and 98,000 Americans die in hospitals from medical errors each year. There are 2,000,000 hospital-induced illnesses and 1,500,000 long-term care-induced illnesses each year. As a result, the institution gives you a disease and then charges you for curing it. Hospital infections are now the fourth leading cause of death in the United States. But it does not stop there. The number of people who die prematurely from chronic conditions is staggering. If the disease conditions were properly managed (including self-management by patients) these people would have lived longer and healthier lives. Diabetes, obesity, heart disease, violence—the implications are enormous, both in costs and quality of life, and the current system has no ability to respond or manage it with the seriousness and proportion that it deserves. In response to these challenges the focus is on more rules, more laws, more regulators, and, as a consequence, there is more alienation, more providers retiring in frustration, even less time between the doctor and patient. The downward spiral continues.

Clearly something has to change, and that change has to be profound.

You will never think about the process of health and healthcare in quite the same way after you read *Covenants: Inspiring the Soul of Healing.* Glenna Crooks has the courage to go totally outside the usual modern, secular, micromanaged, reductionist efforts of rules and systems, and instead asks profound questions based on thousands of years of healing history.

In my own work, I will use again and again her simple but profound insight into the decline of "healing" and "healer" in our health language. In moving from "healer" to "provider" we made a huge leap towards depersonalization and alienation. Glenna focuses powerfully on the invisible dimensions of being human—both individually and as communities. She has the courage to raise openly the question of divine relationship and the notion that people must be seen within contexts larger than dollars and cents or solely rational administrative rules and science.

If we return to a world of healers and healing, we embrace a moral sense in our health system which, increasingly, is being driven out by commercialization and by bureaucratization. A health company that sells you goods or services, whether or not it is best for you, solely because of profit motives is clearly an alienating and dehumanizing force. A bureaucrat (government, insurance company, or employer) who defines your health needs in terms of rules and regulations without regard to consequences or your uniqueness is an alienating and depersonalizing force. A doctor, nurse or hospital administrator who sees you as another opportunity for profit or loss is an alienating and depersonalizing force.

Glenna Crooks captures these trends—too many of which are weakening our modern system—with her simple but profound treatment of healers and a community of healing. Think of yourself as a healer—or as a company involved in healing—and the entirety of your decision process is different than when you were only a profit—or cost—center. Everyone at the Center for Medicare and Medicaid Services (CMS) should read this book—and then rethink Medicare and Medicaid. For that matter, all employer purchasers and everyone in insurance companies should read this book. Finally, the providers—hospital workers, doctors, nurses, pharmacists—should read this book. If we can return to a healer´s approach, all our decisions will be better. In this book, Glenna captures the heart of the moral imperative that makes health different from any other activity in our society. Health is inherently moral, and healing inherently has a human dimension that transcends both the bureaucratic or commercial rules that today trap us in self-destructive patterns that cost lives and raise costs.

A moral activity implies a relationship which goes "both ways", and Glenna begins a discussion which must now become central to healing our health system. People must have a key—and decisive—role in their own health. The individual person has an obligation—she calls this a "covenant"—to the healer to accept responsibility for a share of their own health. This part of the relationship between the healer and the healed is what is missing in American health policy today. Diabetes, heart disease, alcoholism, and other chronic conditions can best be addressed within a true healer-healed covenant with better outcomes and dramatically lower costs. However, in each case a key part of the opportunity rests on the shoulders of the patient. Unless patients accept obligations toward their own health, it is impossible to control chronic conditions or achieve optimum outcomes. A passive, ignorant, unempowered patient model is a model that produces the worst outcomes at the highest costs. Glenna understands this principle and outlines the covenant between healer and patient that can begin to unlock the potential for better care with better outcomes at lower costs.

Finally, *Covenants* outlines the importance of community involvement at local, national and global levels. We know instinctively that an AIDS epidemic in the third world is important to us. We know instinctively that a sick side of town is important to us, even if it is the other side of town. We know instinctively that an outbreak of diabetes among teenagers in the American southwest matters to us, even if we do not live in that region. In this book, Glenna explains why, and shows us the underlying moral framework of community covenants that instinctively lead us to this understanding and should, now, spur us on to act to create global change.

Our health system is a mess because the fundamental principles are wrong. *Covenants* gives us some powerful intellectual tools to begin to think through the right tools. It is a major contribution to the unavoidable debate about replacing the current system with a much better, much more humane, and ultimately less expensive and more responsive system of healing in which the provider, the patient and the community work together within a covenant of mutual obligation.

Newt Gingrich
Washington, D.C.

Foreword to the First Edition

Every now and then a book comes along that is a breath of fresh air. This is such a book. Dr. Glenna Crooks presents a new model for thinking about health care for at least the next hundred years. Her novel concept of health care as a covenant relationship opens up new possibilities that enable us to escape the fixations and entrapments of the current health care marketplace.

Ironically, the idea of covenant relationships is not a new thought for humanity. It is an old idea and reaches far back into human history. What is new, however, is Dr. Crooks' application of covenant relationships to modern healers, patients, and communities.

A covenant, unlike a contract, has a sacred or moral dimension. This is precisely the dimension I find missing in much of health care discussion today, whether that discussion takes place in public policy circles or in the boardrooms of health care institutions. Somehow, legal and business concerns have displaced the more central issues of moral obligation and social consciousness.

Today, there is very little going on in the modern health care arena that inspires anyone. Physicians are dispirited. Many health care organizations totter on the brink of financial disaster. Public health policy is a vacuum. Patients are angry and confused. Third-party payers are targets of public dissatisfaction. Somehow the healing, renewing spirit of the health enterprise has escaped our industry. What Dr. Crooks does so well in this book is lead us through our current labyrinth into the clear light of day.

I hope this book challenges your thinking as it challenged mine. There is simply no easy way out of our present morass. We can't expect a better future by simply doing more of what we are doing now. Increased capital dollars, better reimbursement, renewed consumer efforts, more and better legislation simply won't do it. A new mindset is required that embodies purpose and meaning, spells out mutual obligations and views the healing enterprise as a spiritual calling. This is what Glenna Crooks offers us in this book. Providing health care will always be a business, but it must also be more than a business.

When you read this book, you will have a better sense of the history of the healing enterprise as it developed through the centuries. Better yet, you will gain a vision of how health care could be in our new century. It offers a prescription for a positive future. The author's background in government, public policy, and consulting enables her to remain grounded as she explores the reaches of philosophy, ethics, morality and spirituality. It is not a rambling philosophic essay. It is a focused prescription for building a better health care system.

As a futurist, I am always interested in new visions of health care. I run across many of them. What is usually lacking in these visions is any sense that they could easily become future realities. This is why I am pleased with this book. Dr. Crooks tells us how to manifest her vision. Doctors, patients, hospitals, legislatures, third-party payers, and communities must think in terms of the mutual obligations that bind them to one another. These mutual obligations are sacred covenants that transcend single-party interests and rise above simple legal contract. The covenant mentality is a change of consciousness.

To make the covenant relationship work, everyone is required to make significant changes. Not only providers must change, patients must assume responsibility for their own health behaviors. Patients are as important a part of the healing covenant as the physicians who treat them. We all like to find a single "bad actor" upon whom to blame our system troubles. It is rather sobering to discover there is no single guilty party in the health care marketplace. We have collectively gotten ourselves into this untenable situation, and we must collectively work ourselves out of it. There is bound to be resistance to this discovery. We are quick to point out the need for someone else to reform. We are slower to volunteer ourselves for change. Even communities do not escape covenant responsibilities. They exert a profound effect upon the health or sickness of their members.

I especially enjoyed Chapter 11 where the author reviews people and sites already practicing the new covenants. Patch Adams, Gil Bashe, Griffin Hospital, Cooperative Health Clinic, Celebration Health, Florida Health System, the Accelerating Community Transformation project, and many others lead the way by demonstrating new covenant relationships. Their successes validate the new model. What Dr. Crooks is talking about is not only possible, it is highly desirable.

But before I tell you more about this great book—why don't you read it? Don't skip the Epilogue. It may be the chapter that launches you into a new covenant relationship with physicians, patients, and community.

Leland Kaiser, Ph.D.
Brighton, Colorado

Preface to the Revised Edition

We live in a privileged nation, with abundant resources and opportunities to shape a better health future for all people—not just in our own country, but in other countries as well. Our discoveries touch the world. Our communications inform the world. Our health care knowledge reaches out to those beyond our borders. Our government is designed to be responsive. Our public health and clinical care systems are designed to protect us from the ravages of disease that are all too common in many part of the world.

Most people in the world cannot say that. They do not share in the abundance we have come to expect and believe we deserve. They do not have the safe food or sanitary systems that support life, nurture health, and create prosperity. We bemoan the weaknesses of the best health care system in the world by day, and by evening tend our manicured lawns with water that is safer and more pure than that consumed by most of the world's population.

Recently, violent terrorist attacks on September 11, 2001 radically altered our lives. We became more aware of the world beyond our own borders. We also watched as so many of the strengths and weaknesses of our health care system became clearer. Charles Inlander, president of the People's Medical Society, enumerated the strengths better than anyone else. He noted how, within minutes of the first World Trade Center crash, emergency responders and medical professionals arrived on the scene to help, selflessly—some of them giving their lives in attempts to save others. Hundreds of other people arrived at the various disaster sites of the day without even being asked. Hospital staffs stood nearly at attention, waiting for the patients they hoped to serve, crushed when so few arrived because the death toll was so staggering. Pharmacists came to airports and hotels to distribute medicines to stranded travelers; mental health professionals visited information centers, businesses, and schools—and no one asked for an insurance card.[1]

Our weaknesses also became even more apparent. As the weeks and months passed since those sentinel events we saw the limits to our internal homeland security and preparedness and we calculated the costs of other such threats looming on the horizon. We also recognized that these attacks were distracting us from pressing policy discussions of the day concerning Medicare reform and the needs of the elderly for a pharmaceutical drug benefit. This intensified as we confronted the evaporation of the budget surplus intended to fund new health care programs and as we realized that terrorists could employ not only airplanes and other weapons, but also biological organisms to accomplish their aims. As a nation we confronted what the experts already knew: that it was past time to examine the frayed edges of a public health system that could not prevent or protect us from diseases that could cross our borders.

Yes, on September 10, 2001, we as a nation were not satisfied with the health care services we had. We wanted more and better care. We demanded ever-new advances in research. We were worried about how we would pay for what we received and we believed that the prices we paid were too high. We had not taken to the streets in protest, but we had gone to court and to Congress seeking changes in the practice of medicine and the operations of health care businesses. As a result, important policy, political, and business decisions were pending resolution. These decisions might well have shaped the future of our own health and that of other nations. The problems we were attempting to solve were now ripening as we entered this new millennium. They had been evolving over at least the past 50 years and were maturing with the baby boomers, whose aging would stress our creative and financial resources for decades to come. When the sun set on September 10, we anticipated another day to address these issues, largely with the confidence that we would succeed—somehow. But at sunrise the next day, events outside the control of America's health care experts radically altered the nature of these challenges. It was important, before the attack, to consider what we, as a nation, expected from our healers, our healing enterprises, and our selves. Since the attack, it has become critical.

How much of our total personal and national resources will we choose to spend on health care? How will we spend it? What public health measures will we fund and how much are we willing to invest in order to prevent the new diseases we now know about and fear? How will we allocate our human and financial capital between personal health care interests and societal health concerns? Who will have the greatest influence on those decisions? What role will patients play? Who should fill the important leadership roles in making these decisions—clinicians, policymakers, or patients? Will government take a larger role in providing health care products and services in order to secure the nation and ease the public's fears? In the future, what choices will patients be allowed to make as consumers of health care services? What are the "right" choices? Will we as individuals change our lifestyles to support better health, or will we expect medical care to save us from our bad habits as well as from the acts of terrorists? Will we continue to expect society to pay for all of our care, or will we assume a larger share voluntarily, and gladly? Will more of us participate in the public debates in health care to reach real solutions, or will we leave it to lobbyists and Congress to resolve the issues in special interests, polls, and partisan political rancor? Will we engage each other in reasoned discussions, or will we make the other party the scapegoat for national health care problems? Will our encounters with and new awareness of serious diseases encourage us to better examine the state of the world's health, or will we attempt to be even more isolationist than in our past? Will we use our knowledge to help heal the world? Or will we continue to allow disease to spread unchecked and reach our own shores?

These questions are directed at those in health care businesses and in the policy, political, and regulatory agencies that shape health care markets today. But they are not only for those select few that hold such power. Rather, these are questions for each individual who practices prevention or needs health care services and for each individual who delivers those services—for each patient and for each healer. In other words, these questions are for all of us. They are especially pertinent because our founding fathers gave us the gift of freedom, and we, as citizens, have important roles to play within this democracy. This is true whether we work within the healing professions, whether we are individuals who depend on and use those services, or whether we are active within our workplaces, local communities, or the nation in shaping policy. We are participants in the politics that are increasingly central to decision making in health care. These questions are timely because this new post-attack era will show Americans just how interrelated we are with each other and the rest of the world, and just how vulnerable we can be to diseases—those that come our way accidentally as well as those that infect us deliberately. These are the questions that will determine our future and that provide the framework for this book.

This book is neither a theoretical text for economists and political scientists, nor is it a treatise for ethicists or theologians. My apologies to each of them if my observations fall short of doing justice to their own analytic disciplines. This book is not intended for academic discourse, but for public dialogue—new public dialogue about the health of the world from the perspective of those living in the United States and working within our democracy and health care system. It is not intended as a scholarly analysis of all the health care issues of the day, nor can it fully represent the perspectives of those living outside the U.S., even in the developed nations like our own. That would be impossible. It is, instead, intended as an initial, practical exploration of selected pivotal issues for those interested in understanding the important system changes and public policies of tomorrow's health care. It is not a guide for clinicians and health systems executives, though I suspect that they may be among the largest number of readers.

There is no way that this book can chart the course for the changes that I believe are necessary for the future. They are too numerous, and only those who are parties to the covenants proposed here can accomplish that task. This book invites those parties to enter into the dialogue, to expand on the issues discussed here, and to address the many questions that the book enumerates. The book addresses a subset of the issues that will define the future of our health and our healing systems. It considers a few of the important international issues with roots in what we, in this nation, can offer to others. It proposes that, as privileged Americans, we would do well to examine our own attitudes—as individuals, patients, healers, and communities—about those neighbors who reside outside this country.

This book is not intended to tinker at the margins of new health care proposals or tinker with the margins of health care companies. It is not intended to demonstrate how to close our borders or our minds to problems that do not immediately appear to be ours. Nor will it shield us from the consequences of our under-investment in public health or our former health isolationist perspectives. It is, instead, intended to open our eyes and radically challenge the nature of the relationships that are the foundations of health and health care in the world today. I will not offer specific solutions or propose changes I believe will "fix" health care—save one. It is my contention that if health care is to be healed, everyone involved in the healing enterprises, from the healers themselves to individual people and communities, must enter into new and reinvigorated covenant relationships—here and elsewhere. If Americans are to be healthy, we must look inward at ourselves, but also outward beyond our borders to the challenges awaiting us in other parts of the world.

It is important to say here that this book is not intended to be a criticism of any individual, organization, policy, administration, or political party. There is no need to change the names to protect the innocent because, in my view, there are no guilty parties—or innocent ones, for that matter. Hunting rascals is entertaining, but it is not productive when the goals are healing and change. In addition, creating conflicts is costly and repairing the damage from conflict is even more expensive. As individuals and as groups we have "muddled through" the science and art of healing hand-in-hand with each other and with our global, national, and state governments to arrive at where we are today. No individual, regardless of how talented and committed—and I have seen some of the best in action—can undertake the magnitude of all the changes required at all levels and at all times. "It's the system." If it is a confused mess, then we are all responsible. We created too many expedient solutions to health care problems and these "solutions" have caused other problems. In Washington, we called that a "bad idea whose time has come." There are too many of these ideas, whose unintended consequences have confronted us with larger problems.

Creating good ideas, and making the changes required to shape a positive future in health care, must start with individuals before they need the formal systems of care we have built for the sick. It also requires addressing the encounters between individual patients and physicians, and so this book questions the nature of those dynamics and proposes new relationships. Change will also occur in community settings, and so it deals with community concerns and imperatives. Change will require the actions of

Congress and the White House (as well as state legislatures and governors' offices). Thus, this book also addresses the policy and political tenor of the day. Few challenges have greater immediacy and reach into the heart of the nation more than health. Yet there are no obvious solutions to these problems, and the political venues for finding solutions are increasingly bankrupt.

There was a time when I thought the solution was in the pursuit of good public policy. If everyone participated in this democracy, I was confident that our collective effort would yield workable solutions to the health care challenges of the day. After all, I had been facilitating public policies in health care for nearly twenty years—as a Reagan administration health policy advisor, as a policy executive for a Fortune 50 company, and as a consultant to health care firms. I had flirted with politics, had been asked to run for Congress, and had advised candidates on health care issues. I had no particular training in political science. Like most Americans in these positions—whether in government, in organizations, in think tanks, or as activists—I learned about policy and politics by doing. It was not difficult. Policy and politics are embedded in our cultural fabric. They are a part of the national way of life. We teach them to our children, and we encourage their practice in schools and scouts. If "Potomac Fever" could infect my blood, certainly anyone could fall prey to a similar fate. I began my own campaign to spread the disease. I was the "Typhoid Mary" of public policy. I took it everywhere.

I have enjoyed public policy since the bug first bit me in graduate school, but I began to study it seriously in 1984. I was invited to participate in a meeting among ethicists and academics, government representatives from many nations, theologians from the world's religions, and experts from the clinical and scientific disciplines of medicine and public health in Athens, Greece. The group was charged to explore how ethical and religious values affected health policy decisions.[2] My directives as an appointee in the

Reagan administration were to describe how health policy decisions were made in the United States and to represent the American experience in case studies of infant mortality, organ transplantation, and care of the dying. In preparing for the meeting, I began my examination of health policy. It continues and evolves even today.

So, how did we make policy in the United States? What drives our decisions to address a public policy issue? How do we deal with issues? Who makes the decisions? When do they make those decisions? Trade associations, patient disease groups, and graduate students came to Washington to learn the ropes and to ask how it was done. My colleagues could explain what legislative button to push or regulatory string to pull, but I had no simple, clear way to describe policymaking. On visits home, my father would ask, "Now, just what is it that you do in Washington?" I never knew quite where to begin my answer.

Approaching the study of policy the way a sociologist, anthropologist, or psychologist approaches the study of a new group, a new culture, or a new patient was useful. What emerged was a deceptively simple paradigm of policy as a consensus-building process with cultural, constitutional, and legal roots. This paradigm was embraced readily by my international colleagues at the meeting in Athens—particularly by Europeans—as an accurate representation of their own decision making, and it became a central thread in the conference discussions. In subsequent work in countries around the world, this simple observation has been validated. Along the way, I engaged in a similar study of politics. I saw how conflicts created in politics balanced the consensus developed in policy. The two—policy and politics—danced together. When consensus moved too quickly or too slowly, or when it did not deliver satisfactory results, conflict stimulated the corrective change. Over the long run, policy and politics delivered the goods. They also protected the liberty and freedom desired by the founders of the nation, and that fact was central to understanding the dilemmas of health care. Democracy, after all, was not created to be efficient; it was created to preserve liberty. As a result, pressing problems worsen while political forces balance power and different, but valid, interests. Individual freedoms impede efficient ways to reduce health care costs. In the 1970s and 1980s this meant that health care costs and tobacco-related deaths increased as tobacco farmers, companies, and civil libertarians argued for economics of the industry and social rights of smokers. It was not until the late 1990s that slow, incremental steps would make health and the cost of illness preeminent goals. Policy and politics eventually took incremental steps in the right direction. To achieve the desired outcome we needed more—and better—public policies. Or so I thought.

In 1995, believing that public policy was the essential core competency of any important player in health care, I founded Strategic Health Policy International, Inc. Working with business and government clients, I continued to see how policy and politics were the domain of every successful company, government agency, and health care executive. Through the earliest years of our work we remained optimistic that the policy and political processes that are so embedded in this nation's character would be fully capable of resolving the many issues in modern health care. I believed that conflicts in priorities for research, allocation of health care resources, assurances of quality in care, and access to care would all sort themselves out in the policy centers of the nation and the states. I believed that if our clients and all of their stakeholders participated in government policymaking, then collective needs would be identified and successfully addressed—slowly, to be sure, but successfully.

Increasingly, I came to believe that I was wrong. There were all-too-disturbing trends in health care and government. Patients were no longer "patient." They were increasingly fearful and felt vulnerable within a system intended to be protective and healing. As a result, they were angry and were taking their empowered search for healing to alternative healers and to active politicians. Healers were frustrated as well. Many felt they could not provide the care they trained years to provide. At a time when we were on the brink of extraordinary science and clinical practice technologies, healers were unable to respond to any but the most emergent needs during shorter and shorter office visits, clocked to monitor productivity like some assembly-line factory. Most businesses that comprise health care were engaged in near-term commercial survival tactics, struggling to make investments for the future. Investors were walking away from these formerly profitable operations as regulations and litigation became a greater threat. Policy advocates, who came to Washington in droves to craft the Clinton administration's health care reform, replaced policy analysts. Single-interest health care politics were driving single-interest health care policies. Pressures were building to a blowing point. Bad policy created in eleventh-hour, highly politicized debates has become more the rule than the exception. And then, planes smashed lives and buildings; bacteria shattered the nation's public health security. Experts who had for years been unable to convince the nation to prepare better for such disasters were now under fire themselves for inadequate national public health security systems. At a time when the enemy should have been defined as terrorism and disease, it was characterized instead as the very experts and companies who, for years, had been warning us this day would come. We turned our anger inward at each other, not just outward toward the known and unknown enemies who so changed our lives.

The anger was pervasive. Peace was difficult to find. In addition to understanding how policy and politics—consensus and conflict—work in health care, I began to search for the underlying causes of the anger and conflicts and to wonder if there could be a new path to peace. I had been searching for ways to advise clients about how to succeed in increasingly chaotic markets and contentious milieus.

Each of them was engaging the important dilemmas in health care. At times, the costs of doing "the right thing" seemed insurmountable and the opportunities, nonexistent. I saw good projects and good products fail because the marketplace was too hostile for straight talk, honest relationships, and reasoned dialogue. I saw extraordinary discoveries, heroic healing, and global philanthropy criticized. I saw dead capital—particularly in human energy and resources—everywhere. The most talented among us could not use the full range of their skills. There was too little time to care for patients, too few funds for researchers investigating viable disease targets, and too few leaders willing to risk being the next target of national frustration. Something was horribly wrong and terrorism was making it worse.

I came to believe that the key to dealing with these challenges lies in understanding the breakdown in the relationships among the important parties to healing—the healer, the individual, and the community. This relationship is based on core values of every society in recorded history. When healing was the prerogative of the primitive shaman or village wise woman, and when it was institutionalized by the Greeks, who framed our own traditions in medicine, the nature of the healing relationship was that of a covenant. Not a contract, a covenant. Medical ethicists, in particular William May, Robert Veatch, and Edward Pelligrino, had laid the foundation for exploring the notions of covenant. I believed they were onto something.

Covenant defined a relationship, a commitment, and an identity for the parties beyond the more common contracts of health care today. Covenant could very well be the seed of the solution. Covenant establishes that a relationship has sacred origins, that no one party benefits to the detriment of the other, that the parties are changed by entering into it, and that the parties are mutually interrelated in the venture—be it in marrying, governing, or healing. If notions of covenant were embedded in the earliest healing systems, should modern systems of health care be built on anything less? Should modern health care settle for less? And was it being asked to do that? Could that be the nature of the problem? Had government bureaucrats, third-party payers, corporate providers of health care, and even policymakers forgotten that they, too, were healers? Did they even know that they were healers? Have they broken an ancient and sacred covenant, perhaps without realizing that they are a party to it? Has modern era medicine created so many contracts that we have all lost sight of covenant on the way to the legal department?

Most people today would assert that healers have broken the covenant, that they have "fallen out" of the covenant in a spate of self-interest and greed. Frankly, that is too easy an answer, and it's not true. I am inclined to hold healers accountable, because they are so privileged and powerful—particularly by virtue of the knowledge they have gained through the research and education provided to them, in part, through societal funding. But others are also accountable. Each individual or patient and entire communities, as well, are responsible for keeping the covenant. This is only possible, however, if they realize that they, too, are parties to it. In my view, they are. We are. We are all parties to the covenant.

The foundation of the healer-patient relationship was, at the outset, a one-to-one, person-to-person encounter. It quickly evolved into more complex systems of care involving communities, however, particularly as communities recognized the nature of public health and later as they organized to pay for care and healers organized to deliver it. Groups of healers refined their skills, investigated their art, and formed guilds. They promised their communities that they would provide quality care in ethical ways. Communities responded by providing healers with privileges and protections and laid down expectations for individuals to practice healthy behaviors.

An ancient tribal healer could anticipate that patients would act within the covenant and the community would build sanctions for those who did not. Patients were expected to follow the prescribed directives of the healing and would reciprocate the healer's skills and sacrifices with payments and respect for the healing arts. Today's healers can have no such expectation. Compliance with even the simplest of medical regimens is quite low. Ancient communities, particularly the Hebrews as we can see from the records they left behind, could count on the collective efforts of the group to practice and enforce good public health for the benefit of each individual and for the community as a whole. Today's patients can have no such assurances about their communities. Healers of millennia past would recognize the limits of healing power, and their patients would do likewise. Today's patients sue for bad results, and courts reach into deep pockets to compensate plaintiffs.

Ancient tribal and community healers may have confronted epidemics of disease and, in some cases, even primitive bioterrorism as diseases were used to inflict genocide on conquered people. In most situations, however, the healer of old could count on the limits of the disease itself, or the limits of the sick person to carry it, to stem the tide of disease either within the community or between that community and some other group. Today's healers have no such assurance. In ancient times, even a healthy individual could not have circumnavigated the globe in a lifetime. Today, in less than a day, any one of our six billion neighbors can board a plane and arrive in our country, if not at our doors—even if they are critically ill. New diseases, unknown to or unrecognized by today's American healers, can penetrate the most sophisticated border controls. It hardly matters whether they come from some isolated part of the world with an innocent traveler or from some terrorist laboratory, their impact is the same. These dynamics create new technical challenges for us. They also create new relationship challenges for us as well. Thankfully, the ancients left us with a roadmap for creating and sustaining relationships that will help us, even today, in the midst of such trying times.

This book will discuss the historical, sacred origins of healing and covenant roadmaps in more depth. It will begin to unravel the nature of the multiple covenants that exist in our health care relationships today. It will point to a new set of covenants that will recognize more mature, reciprocal relationships. And it will address the toughest question about covenants today: What is the role and responsibility of each player—healer, individual and community—within the covenant? It will suggest that covenants cross borders and include all healers, all nations, and all people.

This is a practical book intended to stimulate a creative, new, positive, and global public discussion to answer the questions posed here. It is for everyone involved in the practice of caring for others and for everyone receiving that care. In other words, it is for all of us. It is intended to end the debate and begin a dialogue. It is intended to rewire the hard-wired conflicts between people, between communities, and among those who are the essential parties to good health. It is intended to disarm our hair-triggered willingness to shoot the enemy on the other side of whatever table we share as we work to see that we are able to live healthy and productive lives. It is intended to declare that there is no enemy but disease and only if we work together can we conquer it effectively and humanely. It is intended to bring peace to those caught in primal screams and tantrums as they confront the restrictions of managed care—restrictions we collectively and deliberately built into today's practice of medicine. It is intended to suggest that compassion and caring cannot occur without attention to the very real disease problems of others around the world. This is a look "back" at the origins of our health care system, and it is a look "forward" to its potential. It is a look "in" at ourselves, as Americans, and "out" towards the rest of the world.

Can our health care system change? Can it become a center for the more comprehensive healing that patients now want it to be? Can it be a satisfying place to work? Can it continue to be a vibrant source of new knowledge and life-enhancing discoveries? Can it heal the world? In my opinion, absolutely! But the potential in health care can only be realized if we cease our endless conflicts and work together. I don't claim to have all the answers to the many pressing questions in health care today and particularly to those related to costs. Costs, in my view, are not the cause of our problems, but in larger part a reflection of them. I don't claim to have exhausted every possible solution to the world's health and healing challenges or to have cata-logued even a small number of the most important ones in this updated edition. Although I've worked around the world, I admit to a biased, limited, American perspective. I do not believe that this book proposes perfect solutions. For too long, the perfect has been the enemy of the good in health care policy. If we can "only" do "good," we will have done better than we might otherwise without such an attempt. I do believe, however, that returning to our roots in the sacredness of healing and in the nature of covenants will move us closer to finding more of the right answers.

My conviction about covenants is deeper now, as I write this new edition, than when I first tackled the exploration of the concept several years ago. As I travel and speak with healers across the country—and around the world—I see how covenant resonates with their values. Their intention is to heal. Covenant enables that and returns them to the soul of their work. If I had any doubt, one audience, in particu-lar, would have resolved my concerns. On August 1, 2001, I was the wrap-up speaker at a conference focusing on resistant pathogens and the problems that could ensue for the American hemisphere from emerging diseases. I opened with these remarks: "We began this session stating that our goal was better health outcomes. I would like to propose a bigger goal: world peace and prosperity—for everyone, not just in this hemisphere, but throughout the entire globe. Peace and prosperity will not be possible if we fear our neighbors for the pathogens they may harbor in a handshake. These will not be possible if we spend our money treating diseases that we could have prevented. These will not be possible if we are burying our loved ones precisely at the time when they are the most economically productive in their lives, or, when they are very young or very old and not enriching our economies, but enriching our hearts." The reaction was stunning. People cried. Afterwards, they came to touch me and to tell me how I had touched them. It was then that I realized how weary we all are of working our best to shave another cent from the health care dollar and how much we all wanted a higher purpose for our work.

The Latin Americans in that audience helped me see that if, as Americans, we address not only our own challenges, but those of the developing world, we will make the greatest strides possible in securing a better future for those we serve now and for those generations to come. I feel so strongly about this that all the income related to my writings is being donated to projects to improve the health of women and children in developing nations. This contribution is small compared to the tireless work of healers in those countries and small compared to the needs of those vulnerable people. If we act in new ways to create covenants and to heal the world, and not just our own, I think we can make even more substantial strides—toward healing not only the patients, healers, and communities here, but also those around the world. If we can do that, we will have healed health care. If we heal health care, might we also take some steps towards world peace? What better time is there than now?

Introduction

Breakdown of the Covenant

When the first edition of this book was written, it addressed the American landscape as the nation approached the new millennium. That time provided us with an opportunity to look back and reflect on the past with gratitude, to observe the present with optimism, and to imagine the future with hope. I believed, at that time, that if we as Americans could come to understand the past and the present and not limit ourselves to the health care structures built to "fit" old needs, we would be more capable of crafting a better health care future for everyone. I believed that if we could understand the paths we walked to arrive at today's health care systems, we would be better able to choose whether to stay on those paths or to venture off them for new ones. I felt it was likely that after our analysis, we would want to do some of both.

When health care companies and healing professionals prepared for the millennium rollover, they, too, assessed the past, the present, and the future. They examined their own goals, aspirations, and programs to determine which of many choices they would make about what they would continue and what they would transform. They considered the decisions that they, their patients, customers, or government regulators would most likely be required to make. Doing this, they identified the principal challenges as being demographics, technology, demands, and resource limits. They observed how the population was aging and how older people required more health care. They noted that technology was advancing as well. There was not only more of it, but technological solutions were increasingly sophisticated and costly. The public was demanding more access to better care. Patients were more informed about their options and more capable than ever of placing demands on their employers, providers, and legislators. As health experts, they recognized that resources were scarce. There never seemed to be enough people, time, and capital to meet the needs created by these merging trends.

This dilemma attracted media coverage. The promises of science, the new demands for care, the interests of the elderly, and the hostility of patients became front-page news. Health care became good copy. Trial lawyers noticed as well. In the wake of tobacco industry settlements, for instance, litigation loomed as a new tactic to bring the industry to the table—if not to its knees—to force changes in health care delivery practices.

Health care also became good politics. The stunning failures of catastrophic health care and health care reform were no longer echoing in the Nation's Capital, but the din from clashes over health care reached Capitol Hill once again—as if on cue for millennium election campaigns. A season of campaign rancor, rascal hunting, and eleventh-hour election-driven political compromises began again. As the nation entered the new century, it risked taking steps away from productive dialogue and toward the demise of a healthy society as it gridlocked in conflict.

Then, as millennium babies turned toddlers, disaster struck the nation. Stunned, Americans watched as terrorism invaded their lives, homes, and news on September 11, 2001. Diplomatic and military responses to securing domestic and international security began in earnest. Suddenly, what had been simple decisions to travel, to work, to shop, or to attend school were considered thoughtfully, as people contemplated possible new risks to health and safety. The needs of the nation for health security— including public health security, disaster relief, hospital capacity, and protection from bioterrorism—loomed large in the national consciousness.

How would health care respond? Could healers cope?

Both were already steeped in conflict. Both were being crushed with increasing demands for more access and better quality care, and all at cheaper rates. How would healers now meet new health care needs as we confronted national security threats? How would healers address not only the fall-out from a particular attack, but the plans and preparations for possible new ones? Would the presence of an external threat draw us together and cause us to re-invest in health care security needs, or had past disputes so poisoned our own wells of cooperation that we would be unable to chart a better, forward course? These became the critical questions in the months following the attacks on the World Trade Center and Pentagon buildings.

This was the reality: America's health care system was already weakened and stressed when the nation asked it to rise up and serve it at heroic levels in the wake of the attacks. How had it become weak? What was the nature of that stress? How did the wealthiest nation in the world arrive at such a critical and unprepared juncture? How did healing become such a contentious enterprise? What had happened to the healer's covenant? Had the covenant been broken? How could so many people, working for a positive end and with so many resources, fail? How, even with an infusion of medical expertise into the staff and membership of the Congress, did things seem to get worse even as science brought us more knowledge and technology brought us more possibility? How could the United States become such an advanced, industrialized nation with so many of its people—including its working people—uninsured? How could we ignore the pressing issues of the poor around the world and the arrival of "their" diseases on "our" doorstep? How could we leave our national door open to the threats of diseases crossing our borders as easily as those who could—intentionally or unintentionally—carry them?

In the wake of new threats to health, all eyes are focused on governments, at both national and state levels.

Insurance companies suspended the usual health care utilization controls and encouraged mental health services to help with the emotional responses to the disaster, but more help was clearly needed and government seemed the place to turn. Was this always the case? Is government the best leader for the health care challenges we would face? Preventing bioterrorism or protecting us from it with vaccines and antibiotics (when it happens) seems a government responsibility, but is there also a role for the private sector and individuals? Is the government capable of taking on the international issues that terrorism would draw us into, while it also addresses all the domestic issues we face in health care today? How would government address threats from abroad, some of which extend beyond health care, and also resolve disputes at home about patients' rights and health care benefits? How could government continue to micromanage health care companies as it confronted the immediate crises left in the wake of terrorism? Were the domestic challenges we were facing at the time being left to smolder, only to erupt later into a new health budget crisis as Medicare reform and drug benefits evaporated with the budget surplus that could have supported them? Are we headed for an even greater domestic crisis as we seek to address the global ones? Can it be averted? Who and what in this nation will be at risk if health care fails? What will be the consequences for the world if American health care does fail?

Traditionally, business and policy analysts have focused on the specific aspects of health care: demographics, technology, demands and resource limits. Without a doubt, they will reassess their analyses in light of the changed world and our heightened awareness of national needs. However, while each of those driving forces of change is important, I believe that it is the relationship between those forces and the players in health care that is the key to understanding and managing the enabling and restraining forces we will encounter in the future. Without delving into the nature of the interrelationships, we cannot appreciate the complexity of the changes that are required to address even more complex dilemmas and debates.

We face these questions today for four reasons. First, health care players paid too little attention to government as it emerged as a potent force in national health care planning, management, and payment. Welcome investment soon became micromanagement. Second, the traditional covenant, between healers and those in their care, broke down—on both sides—and was replaced with contracts. Instead of building on the empowering process of democracy and the solid foundation of covenant, we abandoned both. Third, the nation developed an antipathy to profit within the health care sector. This was very much at odds with our otherwise capitalist culture and our needs as a society for investors willing to risk capital to improve heath care knowledge and systems. Fourth, we failed to understand the inter-relatedness of health and disease across national borders. We did not recognize that diseases from other parts of the world could arrive in our land— accidentally or intentionally—and that the resources we had developed to safeguard our own health should be used to protect ourselves by protecting others as well.

Let's begin by addressing the issue of government involvement in health care ventures. To be sure, trade associations and professional societies representing the major providers of health care traditionally addressed the workings of government at their national meetings, in their houses of delegates, and in the corridors of Congress. But those activities were the turf of a few leadership-inclined members, staff, and lobbyists. Usually, they were the policy and political wonks of their own associations—they ran committees and ran for office. National or state policy and politics were an extension of their own personal inclination to be leaders.

In general, the health care practitioners and business executives who were members of health care professional societies and trade associations left policymaking to those individuals while they built their practices and followed their business plans. They appeared in Washington and state capitals only when necessary and contributed to political action committees and campaigns if asked. But for the most part, they traded dealings on the Hill for the next deal on the street—whether Main Street or Wall Street. Few of them envisioned a future where the relationship between government and their own health care enterprises would be so contentious as it has become at the turn of the millennium. Such an outcome was difficult to predict in the halcyon days of health care growth.

During the 1950s and 1960s, improving access to health care was the principal driver of national health policy. As a result, the resources available for health care increased substantially. The federal government influenced the health care industry in two critical ways. The Congress passed the Hill Burton Act in the late 1940s to build hospital capacity and it increased the budget for the National Institutes of Health (NIH), to provide more research and research training capacity. In the 1950s and early 1960s, institutional budgets grew 15% to 18% annually at a time when the United States' Gross Domestic Product (GDP) grew 5% to 9% annually.[1]

In the 1970s, Medicare coverage for the elderly and a demand for quality improvements in care increased investments in the health care infrastructure. National expenditures grew from $73.2 billion in 1970 to $247.3 billion in 1980. As a result, health costs emerged as a national public policy issue in the United States in the early 1980s and continued into the 1990s, as the total resources devoted to health care continued to grow at rates exceeding the GDP. Increases ranged from 4.4% to 11.6% annually during the past two decades, always at higher rates than the annual percent change within the GDP.[2]

Because health care was a fast-growing sector of the economy, it was a builder's dream and an entrepreneur's playground. Whether the business was biomedical research, services, or bricks and mortar facilities, the opportunities for growth seemed unlimited. Health services employment was a great example of this growth, nearly doubling as it rose from $5.3 million in 1980 to $9.7 million in 1997.[3]

Research and development expenditures in the public and private sectors grew from $12 billion in 1984 to $42 billion in 1995.[4] At the same time, investments in biomedical research were paying off. Of the more than 3,000 prescription pharmaceuticals and 300,000 over-the-counter medicines on the market at the turn of the millennium, most were produced since the 1960s. New technologies and pharmacotherapeutics saved lives and improved them. Organ transplants, cardiac bypass surgery, and fetal medicine became commonplace. New generations of medicines eliminated side effects and cured diseases that previously went untreated or were managed only through surgical solutions and long periods of convalescence. The polio epidemic and childhood diseases gave way to new vaccines and the appreciation for the prevention of disease.

Not only were health care businesses disengaged from government during this era, patients were largely uninvolved as well. A few politically-inclined individuals addressed their special needs through legislation—creating programs for kidney dialysis, rare diseases, transplants, and HIV/AIDS—but the average "citizen patient" did not join groups, speak out at town meetings, or foster single-issue campaigns to make health care demands. In those decades of growth, patients' needs for access and quality were identified and met without substantial need for broad-based citizen action and coalitions. At the same time, patients became more knowledgeable and insistent about the care they would receive. News stories communicated the miracles of modern medicine and drove demand, while employer-based health care insurance paid the bills for workers and retirees alike. More often than not, patients could count on two things: American medicine would have a solution to their next health problem, and they would be insulated from the cost of the care.

But there were problems looming on the horizon. As the capacity to treat diseases improved and demand for treatment grew, so too, did the population of patients who would require care.[5] Public health improvements and health care services increased the average life span in the United States from 68.2 years in 1950 to 76 years in 1996. The population of elderly began to grow at over one million per year, currently representing about 12% of the population and spending nearly one-third of all health care expenditures.[6] Baby boomers started their own families, and birth rates began to rise. As they turned 50, the baby boomers joined the ranks of the "elderly" and became eligible for membership in the first major consumer group with definitive health care interests: the American Association of Retired Persons (AARP). AARP soon became the largest membership organization in the country, representing more than 33 million people over the age of 50.[7] In addition to providing health care products and services, AARP had lobbyists and leaders who were active, engaged spokespersons for many issues—with health care key among them. Employers began offering long-term care insurance policies for workers and their parents. The era of the young-old, the middle-old, and the old-old was launched. New centenarians were becoming old news.

Congress attempted to resolve some of the burden for the cost of health care by shifting the risks to managed care organizations. Promoted in the 1980s as a creative solution to the increasing costs of care and the "perverse" incentives in fee-for-service, cost-plus reimbursement, Congress enacted legislation to provide managed care organizations with marketplace opportunities. By the late 1990s, on the heels of managed care's penetration into the private and state Medicaid markets, Congress created Medicare+Choice for seniors in Medicare. This national option for care within the Medicare program soon became a national nightmare. Created in 1997 and implemented in 1999, 40 million elderly and disabled (about 15% of all beneficiaries) chose to enroll in Medicare+Choice, which absorbed the unforeseen consequences of a stalemate in a Bipartisan Commission's attempt to save Medicare from insolvency, rising drug costs, and anti-managed-care sentiment. The Health Care Financing Administration (HCFA), later re-named the Centers for Medicare and Medicaid Services (CMS), tinkered with Medicare+Choice, creating havoc when it penalized the very efficiencies HMOs were created to achieve. Managed care programs were forced to reconsider their business plans and by the start of the year 2002, a majority of the managed care plans attempting to serve Medicare under this option had either terminated, or dramatically reduced, their plans. Some, but not all, Medicare enrollees were able to find alternative sources of care.

In the final decade of the twentieth century, health care had become a payer's nightmare with no end in sight to the problems of unrestrained growth in spending, demand for services, and opportunities for treatments. Per capita expenditures for health care rose from $141 in 1960 to $3,759 in 1996[8], as patients had access to increasingly sophisticated diagnostic technologies and surgical interventions. Employers sought to control their portion of the costs by reducing the share of health bills they would cover, driving some families to insure only the breadwinner, but not the nonworking spouse or children. New ranks of workers joined the ranks of the formerly unemployed and uninsured. These newly uninsured were young workers. Many were employed in information-era companies, in small companies, and in part-time and nonunion jobs. The ranks of the uninsured grew to more than 40 million. Although the number would fall in subsequent government projections, it would not fall far or for long, as the economy suffered in the wake of terrorist attacks. Substantial insurance reform was needed, but seemed to be neither a national priority nor a budget possibility. This was not good news, as stem cell debates and health cost control projections peaked just as another shot was fired in the biotechnology and genomic revolutions. While the hope of science aimed to heal hearts in many ways, this would not happen without damage to wallets.

On the eve of the twenty-first century, health care was poised to reap the rewards of past decades of investments. But at the same time, tremendous pressures had built up in health care delivery and financing systems. These issues have captured the attention of the general public, which seems ready to make some collective decisions about what changes are needed. And what will their decision be? Demand more care for more people, at less cost to patients and payers? Demand more accountability from health care providers, especially those profit-making enterprises financed by Wall Street? Health care expenditures had increased over one trillion dollars in a decade, with only a 1%–2% increase in healthy, quality years of life for Americans.[9] Something was surely amiss. Providers became "the problem." Controlling providers became "the solution."

Now squarely encamped in the twenty-first century, what is the likely future? Beginning in 1993, much to the relief of payers, health care spending leveled out at 13.6% of GDP and remained there until 1996. The projections for spending to increase to 16.6% of GDP by the year 2007 did not contemplate the impact of terrorism, which even after a few short weeks was mounting a growing price tag.[10] The aged population will continue to grow. Scientists will become more productive in their discoveries. Consumers will demand more—and better quality—service, but at less cost relative to the intensity of care they receive. Consumers will continue to demand choice, whether or not they are required to pay for it, or, more accurately, especially if they are required to pay for it.

Public and private payers will feel the pinch, and continual cost increases will be challenged. Payers will continue to blame managed care, which will in turn blame its suppliers and physician contractors. If history prevails, as managed care companies eliminate utilization controls, additional increases in services and attendant increases in costs will be common. In that event, the idyllic days of growth, consumer satisfaction, and unlimited opportunity will be replaced by increasing, unremitting, and intractable conflict. Employers will be hit hardest and will pass the blows on to employees. Demanding baby boomers will vote with legislative agendas to secure their rights and will vote with their feet to leave managed care plans that do not meet the demands to do it all—quickly and cheaply. Consumers will pay out-of-pocket, but only for those alternative and complementary services they value. They will not pay for the traditional clinical care to the degree they can union-negotiate or advocacy-legislate mandatory coverage.

These challenges do not end with the simple need to balance demand and expenditure controls; they are increased by a seismic shift of power and presence among payers and providers. In 1980, private sector payers accounted for 75% of health care expenditures, the federal government accounted for 12%, and the states accounted for 13%. In 2000, the states continue to contribute 13% of all health care dollars, but private-payer spending has shrunk to 50% of expenditures and the federal portion has risen proportionately to 37%.[11] One-third of the private market has become public as the health care market share shifted with the aging population and newly covered groups. As the principal payers of health care, state and federal governments have been forced to become increasingly involved in the regulation of the health care market and increasingly active in seeking public support—through taxes and other means—to meet their responsibilities. President Johnson, in the Medicare debate with the American Medical Association (AMA), reassured physicians that nothing would change in the practice of medicine, except that the government would be paying the bills. As many predicted and physicians and others have since learned, the power to pay is the power to build or to destroy. Government, as a very powerful buyer, has profound influence over the practice of medicine and the operation of health care businesses. Government is also a regulator of other buyers, acting through the tax codes, appropriations, regulations, and oversight authority, and, thus, affects the buying of the private sector and even the states. As a result, the federal government is a much bigger influence than its 37% market share implies.

A similar shift occurred for providers. In 1980, physician-driven health care was the norm. Nearly all physicians practiced in solo or group practice arrangements and were responsible for controlling much of health care expenditures. By the end of 1996, 88% of physicians had at least one managed care contract.[12]

Decisions were no longer solely those of the individual practitioner, but often were directed by groups of physicians serving on committees. The committees were charged with directing the practice patterns of those in the group. It mattered little that many physicians continued to practice within their own offices. They were now in contractual relationships with large, business-oriented organizations, which made them responsible for the dual mission of caring for the health of the patient and the health of the corporate bottom line.

Almost imperceptibly, the relationships between healers and patients began to change. There had long been a covenant between healer and patient. That covenant had ancient historical roots and was about to undergo radical change. The nature of the healer and the nature of the patient were no longer the same as when the covenant was established.

George Merck, founder of what is now Merck & Co., said, "Medicine is for the people. It is not for the profits."[13]

His corporation adopted a culture in which profit was expected only if the medicines it developed had value to people. As health care companies prospered in the 1980s and 1990s this was a difficult ethic for newcomers to embrace. Investors—not healers—flooded the healing enterprise. Managed care entrepreneurs mastered the art of buying and selling "insured lives," negotiating tough contracts with providers, squeezing the easy, excess capacity out of local health care systems, and selling off their companies before the longer-term results would be suffered. They did not build a lasting infrastructure to manage the care. They shook the foundations of care in many communities, leaving a trail of angry patients and providers in their wake.

Even in those health care companies with longer-term visions and health care missions, few people viewed themselves as healers. "Healer" was a term rarely used in the vernacular and, if it was, it was associated with "alternatives" that had little credibility in the maturing business enterprise of health care. And, if "healer" was perceived as an appropriate term for those in clinical care, it would certainly not have been applied to those who supported the delivery of that care. The growing number of those who worked in health care, but without any direct access to patients, rarely, if ever, viewed themselves in healing roles. They had fresh MBAs and marketing or financing missions to fulfill, not healing aspirations to accomplish. Those who staffed and managed the corporations providing and paying for health care did not see the connection to the healing of the "covered lives" in their care and in their own responsibilities. Insurance clerks, government bureaucrats, congressional staff, and others did not engage in covenantal ethics and practice. Patients were too remote from the daily activities of their job descriptions and professional responsibilities. Gradually, those who did not even know about—much less ascribe to—a covenant were making important health care decisions.

At the same time, employers paying for health care swept employees into group insurance plans bent on controlling costs. Employers, as paying corporations, negotiated service contracts with provider corporations. Relationships between healers and patients were then increasingly determined by employment contracts. Individual healer prerogatives and patient expectations, demands and rights were no longer central as large bureaucracies began to manage care and money. Some patients suffered as a result, particularly if they lost or changed their jobs and were no longer parties to the negotiated contract. Whether they actually suffered or not, most patients feared they could suffer if these bureaucracies went unchecked. Everyone felt at risk, but for different aspects of health. Managed care and their physician contractors appeared at risk for costs. Patients feared being at risk for abandonment at a time of need. Corporations feared the risks of increasing premiums and government mandates. Congress feared voter rage from a failure to control managed care and its doctors. Fear had come full circle.

If the increasing health care payment pressures faced by government had not created demands for a renewed political debate, the public certainly would have. In fact, the public was about to do that. More empowered, knowledgeable consumers—many of them middle-class baby-boomers who were suffering for the first time from the gap between demand and receipt of health care—started to take matters into their own hands. They held health care providers accountable in the only way they felt they could: they maneuvered onto the health policy and political scene. They demanded change in legislatures and they held government representatives accountable as well, making health care a new, more highly visible issue in electoral politics.

These empowered consumers have arrived and demanded a seat at the negotiating table at a vulnerable time for health care in America. Despite the wealth of opportunity and promises of health care for the future, political rhetoric dominates the debate. Despite the imperative that health care professionals pool their talents and agendas for the good of the nation, selfish interests prevail. Despite the quest for private capital to fund the next generation of technologies and system improvements, regulatory zeal and legislative threats create hostile investment climates. Despite the need for public-private collaboration in areas of research, development and health care services, governments and private concerns view each other with hostility and mistrust. Despite the cry for leadership, few emerge from the limited self-interests of their restrictive economic incentives and personal roles. Those who do are overwhelmed by the immensity of the task of reshaping health care in some rational, but not rationed, way. Is this our future?

Congress addressed the issues more forthrightly than did the professions. Charged with raising the funds and finding new ways to pay for the care—such as requiring employers and the states to ante up for some programs—Congress had to engage the public in a discussion of what and how the money would be spent.   There were politics, pork barreling, and conflicts to be sure, but at least there was a clear, established process to address those conflicts: the policy and political forums at the national and state levels. As campaigns progressed, the candidates touted their plans. Back in Washington and in state capitals, the legislatures debated and voted on proposals. They passed patient-protective legislation that added to health care costs. The constituency took note. Patients applauded. Managed care, in an attempt to forestall even more legislation, stepped out from between patients and physicians. The press kept score on the evening news.

Health care professionals in the clinical arena were less successful in dealing with these issues. Historically, they had come to feel that they were in competition with each other for limited health care resources. Increasingly, health care professionals lost in those competitive ventures to forces outside health care that grew to control health resources. They did not have a forum to engage patients in a dialogue about the transition to corporate medicine. The relationships of corporate medicine were with corporate America, not with patients who were the employees of those corporations. Employers in corporate America initially acted in the interests of patients and provided generous benefits to attract and retain a workforce. But as health costs grew, the concerns of corporate America shifted. The enhancements to benefit plans institutionalized in the Nixon wage and price freeze era now translated into lower earnings-per-share returns for shareholders and higher costs of goods to customers. Corporations had no choice but to shift some costs of care to employees and some dependent coverage was terminated altogether. By the year 2001, even major employers were reducing coverage and requiring larger employee contributions for care. Polaroid is dropping coverage altogether.

This left the individual healer and individual patient feeling they had little recourse, few alternatives, and no power in their relationships with each other. They certainly, by now, felt they had no covenant. The system may not yet have been broken, but the covenant was crumbling fast. Other players crowded into exam rooms and surgical suites. Peer review and formulary committees, payer clerks, government bureaucrats, and investors all had a stake in the process of healing. Some of them actually selected which healer the patient could use. Others controlled which types of diagnostic and healing technologies the healer could use and how often they could use them. Others monitored the encounter after the fact and declared deviations from the norm "fraud." Still others held the healer responsible if the patient failed to follow prescribed advice and did not recover.

The healers, principally physicians, articulated their frustrations the earliest. Some of them, inappropriately, complained to patients during office visits and exams. At times like that, it was difficult to tell who was the patient and who was the healer. Physicians and health care executives needed therapy as much as patients did—not for a physical illness, but for the emotional stress of losing control of their practices. They suffered from the stresses inherent in the growing inability to fulfill the covenant to which they had sworn a sacred oath and were committed personally and professionally. Hospital executives left their positions in record numbers under the stresses. Physicians' economic health took a beating as well, but the uncertainties of contracting were even more significant. Many were left unsure of whether to duck or to run from the next blow. Managed care took a bite out of physician earnings and raised the costs of doing business. Eventually patients complained as well.

Lacking a way to have meaningful discussions to resolve these complaints in the health care, employment, or community sectors, each side turned to the government as the only readily available forum to resolve the conflicts. Each of the players was, after all, a citizen of a state and the nation. Whether or not legislatures were inclined to micromanage health care, they were being called upon to do so.

The concerns were popular even when the problems were not clear. The problems were clear even when the solutions were not. Driven by public concerns and political opportunism, legislators embraced the debates with a fury. By the end of the 1990s, legislators introduced over 40,000 health care bills annually into the legislatures across the country. Litigators joined in, too. Patients went to court to pursue their rights to experimental therapies, access to specialist providers, and timely access to care for their conditions. Where patients did not have the right to sue corporate health care providers, legislation enabled them to do so. Failing to achieve those rights nationally, attorneys took up the cudgel and sued for-profit HMOs under racketeering theories, hoping to force investors to drive changes in managed care business practices. Not being in the business of forcing social change of this magnitude, investors behaved predictably: they took their risk capital elsewhere and will stay away until the investment climate is more favorable for returns. The managed care sector was thus affected, as was pharmaceuticals in the early Clinton years when investors fled that sector as price controls loomed large and corporate returns seemed at risk. In the midst of these challenges, is it any wonder that too many of us lost sight of the value of public health and the importance of developing an infrastructure to support health and healing improvements?

We arrived at the twenty-first century with clear challenges and nearly at a point of crisis. The needs of society to educate its youth, rebuild its cities, explore outer space, and maintain peace at home and abroad competed with desires for more and better care of its own health. Employers are no longer a secure source of health coverage, and tax-funded Medicare and Medicaid programs no longer provide the safety net of decades past. Future generations have not yet staked their claim in the policy arena, and the global internet is creating a whole new set of challenges, opportunities, and players in healing and health care. In writing the first edition of this book in 1999, I said, "These influences are so powerful and moving so fast that it is likely that forces outside, rather than inside, health care will have the greatest influence in shaping the future in which the young will live and the older will retire." On September 11, that outside influence was felt in a very tangible way. Before the attacks that day, the American public listed education, the economy, jobs, health care, taxes, and social security as the most important issues. A month following the attacks, terrorism, war/defense, economy/jobs, education, and health care were the new set of priorities. Within health care, before the attack the major concerns were the cost of care, the lack of coverage, and the cost of drugs. After the attacks, the cost of care was the first priority of consumers interviewed, but health care problems resulting from terrorism were number two.[14] Hospitals felt the impact as well. Those in New York lost an estimated $370 million within the first six weeks, and as hospitals prepared for terrorism nationwide the price tag was estimated in the $10 billion range.[15]

This walk down memory lane can cause pessimism about the future. But it need not. Medical science is poised to reap the benefits of decades of research and deliver on the promises of a biogenetic revolution. New therapeutics will be so stunning in their magnitude that they will challenge the frontiers of our visions about the possible. New practice relationships are emerging between patients and healers, including cash-only practices, pharmacist-led clinical care, and entrepreneurs capitalizing on the needs of the nation for diversity and choice. In addition, health care may yet emerge as one of the nation's most recognized assets. Charles Morris, a writer/observer/analyst, offers a contrarian view to those who fear scarcity, by pointing to the abundance of health care today.[16] According to Morris, and I agree with him, health care is a remarkably productive industry. It is a highly scientific, technological, and productive sector. It is a clean, "green" sector, which pays high wages, most of which stay in the United States. Its hospitals and physicians care for people all over the world. Its schools train clinicians for the rest of the world. Its pharmaceutical sector is one of the few remaining industries in the United States with a favorable balance of trade. Its research enterprise is the best on the globe. Busloads of Americans may be crossing the border to take advantage of exchange rates and price controls in other countries to buy the medicines discovered and developed here. But, there are busloads and planeloads of foreign nationals coming here for the diagnostics and therapeutics that are not offered at any price in other countries. A similar point at the individual level received front-page coverage in the

Wall Street Journal recently. Life spans have increased and quality of life has improved. At a cost, certainly, but costs that many people judge to be worth the investments. Individual people are better off.[17] Perhaps that is also why economists assessing the post-September 11 economic slump predicted that the health care sector may be the growth leader of the recovery. They note the returns from investments in health in the last half-century, the desire of consumers for good health, and the infusion of funds to fight bioterrorism.[18]

As a society, will we craft twenty-first century health care based on scarcity or on abundance? Will we choose to be generous in our funding of care for ourselves and for the poor? If not, then why not? What are the ethics and values of our nation? How much do we want to spend on the necessities and the luxuries of life? How much do we want to spend on health care? And on which health care goods and services? Will we insulate people from the financial consequences of personal choices that drive health care costs? Will we choose to allow people the personal freedom to engage in health-risky behaviors at the cost of higher health care expenditures? Who will make those decisions, and how will they decide? Which decisions will be made by individuals? Which decisions will be made by physicians and patients, and which will be made by communities, corporations, and governments? Which players will be at the table when those decisions are made? How will terrorism affect the course of our personal and public health systems?

None of these decisions will be easy. A crisis can be averted, but only with a substantial change in perspective about the nature of health care. Health care is a personal, one-on-one, intimate relationship between a healer and a patient. Health care is also a collective, public relationship between communities, and between the individual and the community in which he lives, works, and travels. Increasingly, our lifestyles demand that we view these relationships not as local or national, but as global. Health care is also a covenant that is crumbling before our eyes, but it can be repaired, reinstated, and reinvigorated. This can happen within the intimate relationships of healing and in public settings. It can happen between individual healers and patients, and between nations. Doing so will require shifting our perspectives. If we can move from contract towards covenant, from fears of scarcity to promises of abundance, from blame shifting to personal responsibility, from rascal hunting to collective problem solving, and from conflict to consensus, we might do it. If a new dialogue—not an escalating debate—is created, we can address the more fundamental questions of how we collectively, as a nation and a world, will approach the healing needs and opportunities of the new era.

Acknowledgments

It is a pleasure to recognize so many people who contributed to the conception and birth of these thoughts and words. The first is Edward N. Brandt Jr., M.D., Ph.D., who, as Assistant Secretary for Health, steered the nation through some tough times in health care during the 1980s era of HIV, Tylenol poisonings, and block grants, and likewise this junior policy wonk through the transition from Indiana to Washington and global health care. Because of his skill and trust, I had the rarest of opportunities to see leadership from the inside and learn from the best and most thoughtful physician I have ever met. He cared for the nation the way we would all like to be cared for by a healer.

Next are Robert Ingram, who recruited me to Merck & Co. in 1988, and P. Roy Vagelos, M.D., who, as Chairman, is likewise trusted. When I first arrived, Roy admitted that he did not understand policy but knew it was important. I think he came to appreciate its value; under his leadership policy attention expanded and gained influence in Merck's business operations. Bob and Roy showed me global business operations in what was the best health care enterprise of its day. Bob brought his own style of covenant commitment to his role in representing the company in Washington and was the very model of covenant-in-action in the policy and political worlds. Like Ed, Roy cared for patients from a distance, but his caring was no less valuable than if he had tended to them personally. He brought them biomedical discoveries and healed millions of patients around the world. My experiences with these gentlemen shaped certain pro-government and pro-industry biases that will, no doubt, show through this writing. I say this without apology because my respect for them is well deserved.

I am indebted to an outstanding group of medical ethicists, especially William May. His writings on covenants in health care provide the underpinnings for my own. While our views are somewhat different, I believe they are not inconsistent. We share the same plate of spaghetti—I unravel it a bit differently. He knows ethics and theology; I know health care, policy, and politics. I hope he will forgive any less than scholarly treatment of his life's work and will see how his studies have provided a foundation for these extensions into new interpretations of today's health care challenges. As a freshman at Indiana University I was a student of Professor May and enjoyed crossing paths with him again as I pursued the topics here.

I know about politics because Thomas R. Donnelly taught me the live-ammunition, hands-on course and provided the cover when I needed it. I am also grateful to a number of other people. My clients have presented me with their challenges, allowed me to think about their problems, and search for policy solutions. Laudy Robinson ran the business so that I could write. Sister Maura O'Donohue, M.D., Sharon Sokoloff, Marty Wasserman, M.D., J.D., Jack Meyer, Ph.D., Malvise Scott, Brian Crawford, Eugene Smith, John Eichert, Carsten Bischoff, and Jodie Klein reviewed early drafts and provided helpful reactions and encouragement. The Marisches kept me supplied with surprises during a summer writing sabbatical. I am indebted to those who read and commented on the first edition and to Robert F. Williams, III, Ibrahim Al-Zakwani, Arlene Lee, and Debra Notturno Bayley for their research assistance in preparing the second edition. This book offers an important, global perspective I might not have pursued but for the swift kick from Doc Childre. Thanks, Doc, for that all-night discussion and for sharing your heart. I love you. Deborah Thornton provided not only precision editing, but helpful words of encouragement along the way in both editions.

Nancy Zatzman prepared the publication formats and cheered me on all the way. Chris McRobbie translated covenants into a stunning visual image and his illustration was prescient. Drawn in the summer months before the World Trade Towers crumbled under the weight of terror, Chris saw the primacy of relationships over structure. His portrayal of the healer-patient partnership stands as a testament to what many people feel since their lives were changed forever—the structures fell, the relationships grew. If you knew Chris, and his family, you'd understand why. He was raised to know the importance of reaching out with a loving heart. Marie Felix kept each phase of this project moving and made it look easy, all the while carefully proofing—without complaint—each version.

My Dad is no longer alive to see this. Monsignor Joseph W. James was father in his stead—always encouraging, helpful, frequently directing, and occasionally demanding. Although he never put pen to paper, he was my writing partner. Mom read the drafts. Of course, she thought they were wonderful—even the versions that weren't. Thanks, Mom. I love you, too.

Most important though, I bow to the greatest Healer of all, the Divine Source, recognized by all cultures throughout history as the origin of these healing arts and known by many as the supreme grantor and keeper of covenants. May this work and those who read it reside within the embracing spirit that flows from such an abundant and generous fountain of love and caring. And may the world—and health care—be healed.

Part 1

FOUNDATIONS OF HEALING

From the earliest days of human social life, the healers of the community were recognized to be in contact with the most powerful and uncontrollable forces known—those of the divine. The evidence that this was the case is compelling. We know this was true of those ancient groups that left us written records. We know this is true in tribal life today from anthropologists' studies. We intuit this to be true among the ancients who left only their artifacts from the way those items were preserved and arrayed. Healers lived and practiced the healing arts—which were viewed as gifts from the divine—within the context of relationships that were held to high standards of conduct. The material and social rewards for a healer were great. The responsibilities were also immense.

To embrace those relationships and promise the community that the healing practices would be only for the good of the patients, healers followed the example of others in the community who made sacred commitments to one another. These commitments were called covenants. Like the divinely blessed relationships between husbands and wives, fathers and sons, kings and subjects, they adopted a covenant with those they served in their healing roles. Within this covenant, healers called upon their gods to witness their engagement in important, life-supporting arts for the good of each patient, their intent to practice within high standards of technical and ethical care, and their wish to be held accountable for their performance. They even invoked a curse upon themselves if they broke this oath to their patients and communities. Covenants—as sacred matters—were serious matters.

In those days, the high technology, extraordinary science, and complex interplay of today's health care had not yet developed. In those days, the community was small and much more isolated than today's six billion global "neighbors." In these days, we approach challenges our forebears could not have imagined as biomedical science, health care technology, patient demands, global travel, and world trade confront us. In these days we have the benefit of the "grounding" that the first healers established for us with the model covenants they created. These healers sought to care for patients and communities alike and took their responsibilities seriously as indications of the sacredness with which they protected these relationships. Many of today's healers practice within the covenants established long ago and call their patients and communities into the covenant with them. More healers should. Covenant is the foundation of all healing practices and the world today depends on it.

Chapter 1

Healing as Divine Gift

*The government of the United States, under Lyndon Johnson,
proposes to concern itself over the quality of American life. And
this is something very new in the political theory of free nations.
The quality of life has heretofore depended on the quality of the
human beings who gave tone to that life, and they were its priests
and its poets, not its bureaucrats.*[1]

William F. Buckley, Jr.

Stepping Into Healing Streams

Angels might have feared to tread into the world of government-guaranteed health care. President Lyndon B. Johnson did not. In 1965, he conceived an extension of President Franklin Roosevelt's New Deal and called it "The Great Society." It was a social safety net woven by a government acting as a leveler for the economic inequities of the day. The Great Society birthed Medicare and its sibling, Medicaid. These programs formalized an emerging social contract between people and their government. It also brought our national and state governments deeper into the patient-physician relationship in a new way. It used health care to heal the national disparities in income and the ills of poverty in the elderly and the disadvantaged. It infused health care systems with new resources for providing care and, in return, it targeted health care as a tool for redistributing the incomes of the American people.

The Great Society institutionalized access to health care. It assured that elderly or poor people (and many elderly at that time were also poor) would receive health care services and would not suffer from their diseases simply because they were old or economically vulnerable. It was not the first time that this or any other government had delved into healing. The U.S. government had cared for its military in times of peace and war and had provided pre-paid health care for the merchant marine at a time when marine trading routes were essential to national commercial growth. It had also conducted research and practiced public health.

Other governments and rulers, as recorded in documents as old as the Code of Hammurabi in 1800 B.C.E., had established hospitals, regulated the healing arts, set its fees, and developed medicines. But with Medicare, it was the first time that the U.S. government became a party to the one-on-one healing encounters of its general, civilian population. It was also the first time that American healers were asked, as a group, to balance a national policy objective with the covenant to care for patients. The American Medical Association objected at the time. The result was a political compromise in which the government agreed to subsidize, rather than fully cover, physician fees.

In the end, however, whether paying for all or part of the bills, the government, intentionally or not, stepped into intimate healing encounters. It also stepped into a stream of expectations, relationships, social values, and traditions that had been flowing for thousands of years. This stream had swift currents of standard practices, oaths, and mores of the profession. It had undertows of theology and ethics that could trap the unwary and uninformed. Healers, whether in the earliest days of Hippocrates or during the legislative era of Medicare and Medicaid, were engaging powerful, magical, and sometimes mystical forces. American public policy—and public policymakers and interest groups—joined them.

Today, public policy enjoins healers all the more. Federal and state health care programs have grown as populations have aged, as research funds have increasingly flowed from tax-supported sources, and as governments themselves, acting as employers and providers, have purchased health care goods and services. The Clinton Administration's proposals for health care reform and universal coverage were spurred by the desires of Americans for more care and their needs for a funding source that would insulate them from the costs of that care. Failed as these proposals were in their government-driven approaches, they were neither the first, nor the last, government incursions into care. Notably, however, from the outset, the American government engaged healers in its public policy agenda without embracing the healer's covenants. The time has come to do so. The time has come to engage others as well—not just government, but patients, communities, and corporate providers of health care in today's healing enterprises.

Historical Connections to the Sacred

Scholars suggest in their interpretation of the earliest historical evidence that ancient societies believed they received two gifts from their deity, or from the deities in the case of polytheistic cultures—the law and the healing arts.[2] Whether granted by Isis, Ishtar, Dhanvantari, Asklepios, Apollo, YHWH, or a Heavenly Father, both were gifts. Each of these gifts was fundamental to the orderly course and nature of human life. Each structured the nature of community relationships and personal behavior, and each offered a certain security in the face of the harsh unknowns of life. There is ample evidence that this was the case in the origins of the three major monotheistic religions of the more modern eras—Judaism, Christianity, and Islam. It is also the case in the major cultures of Asia. It can be inferred for primitive societies by observing the few remaining native, indigenous, and aboriginal societies, as well as from the artifacts that some prehistoric societies left behind.

The law provided the vehicle for managing the seemingly uncontrollable behaviors of people in society. Suffer an injury at the hands of your neighbor and there was recourse to a judge to set matters right between you and your neighbor. The healing arts, in contrast, helped manage forces that were more mysterious and uncontrollable than your neighbor. Suffer from an invasion of some unknown spirit or ill humor causing an illness and there was recourse to a healer to set matters straight between you and your god. This was particularly true if it was your god who sent the malady or if your benevolent god was viewed as more powerful than the offending evil cause. Both—the law and the healing arts—were central to the destiny of the individual and the community. Both contributed to the orderliness of society and day-to-day personal, family, and community life.

Powerful legal forces and healing forces emerged in those communities. Rulers and healers were among the most valuable members of society. The sacredness of the social pacts between them and their communities tempered the power they had been given. They were, after all, not only responsible to their people, but to the gods from whom their skills flowed. These pacts were modeled after the covenant experiences of the day. There must have been abuses of legal and ruling power, but the many good kings and judges remain respected in history and lore. Effective healers were legend as well. Sometimes, a single individual like Emperor Vespasian was given both gifts of ruler and healer. He was said to cure blindness, in one case by anointing the cheeks and eyes of a man with his saliva and in another by allowing a woman to kiss his knee. King Pyrrhus of Epirus was another. He could allegedly heal with his big toe. When his body was cremated after death and the toe did not burn, it was placed in the temple as a holy relic and used for subsequent healing.

Mysteries of Health and Disease
More often, the healers were not the rulers, but the priests, priestesses, or shamans of the society. In coping with mor-

tality and the more unpredictable and sometimes terrifying forces of health and illness, people sought comfort in the folds of religion. Lacking the most basic knowledge about the mechanics of the body and unable to even theorize about the nature of genetics, infectious disease and sanitation, their conditions were often shrouded in mystery about cause and effect. As they sought safety from annihilation at the hands of their fellow men under the protection of laws, people likewise sought understanding of the mysteries of life, harmony with their gods, protection from disease and relief from physical pain and death from healers. If a patient died, healers were often called upon to ease the transition to the other world through ritual burial as well. In some societies, as in the case of some Greek traditions, healing was a power not gifted by the gods but stolen from them by man. This made the human healer an even more revered figure. Monetary or some other compensation for healing was granted, but in many societies it was secondary. The real benefit of the healing art was the honor bestowed upon the healer in keeping with the power of delving deep into mysterious forces, confronting them and doing battle with them on behalf of the needy patient.

The intertwining of medicine with mystery and sacred texts is as undeniable as was the rationale. Disease in most societies was associated either with the will of the divine or the work of the devil. It also might be the result of an interplay between both. An entire book common to the Judeo-Christian tradition scripture recounts such a tale. It describes the life of sixth-century B.C.E. Job, detailing all manner of physical, psychological, and social suffering. This suffering was the result of two mysterious forces beyond the control of this acknowledged upright, seemingly invincible man. One of those forces was demonic, the other divine.

Other texts describe similar forces at play and, unlike Job, recount effective actions to keep the evil forces at bay. In Egypt, it was Sethapop who was the great spirit of evil that caused illness. In Babylon and Assyria, the demon Alu attacked the chest, Labasu caused epilepsy, and Nergal was the god of pestilence. In India, Tokman was the cause of fevers. In Persia, six archfiends and thousands of minor demons supported Ahriman, the god of evil. Among the Greeks and Romans, Febris was the god of fever. To this day, our description of illness involving fevers is described as "febrile." In ancient China, families burned bonfires at the edges of property to keep evil spirits and their sicknesses away. In medieval Europe, Pope Clement VI did the same. He sealed himself in his private rooms and surrounded himself with burning fires, seeing no one, in an attempt to protect himself from the unknown causes of the plague that ravaged the continent in the fourteenth century. More than half of the clergy of that period died. The pope survived.

Justice, Retribution, Mischief, and Malevolence

If not the work of evil spirits, disease might also be seen as the whim of the gods, the result of offended spirits, the malevolence of witches with powers of sorcery and magic. Disease could also be the result of violating God's laws and, therefore, the wages of an individual's sin. King Antiochus, as he lay dying in 164 B.C.E., attributed his death to his past evil deeds of plundering and pillaging Israelite territory (Maccabees 6:1–13). In modern times, we refer to his belief as "immanent justice reasoning," a view that has been a prevalent throughout history. Even Job's friends thought he must have done something wrong to deserve the disasters that befell him.

This view of immanent justice was so strong in the Middle Ages that entertainment was rejected as a form of healing. A group of healers drew upon the recommendations of ancient Greeks to use comedy as a therapy for illness. The approach was much like that of Norman Cousins using Marx Brothers' movies in his own cancer treatment and Dr. Patch Adams using humor in his hospital. Religious groups of the day protested that any entertainment must, of necessity, be the devil's work, as it was proper for man to suffer. Try as they might, promoters of humor and laughter were unable to convince religious healers that a bit of entertainment might help body and soul. Comedy, they reasoned unsuccessfully, might even allow men to return to the rigors of life with a strengthened capacity to defeat evil, sin, and the bodily pleasures that destroyed their souls. The religious healers of the Middle Ages ignored the documentation in Proverbs 17:22: "A joyful heart is the health of the body, but a depressed spirit dries up the bones."

Culturally, the church of the Middle Ages, with its practice of canonizing martyrs and saints, sanctified pain and suffering. Illness held a powerful sense of meaning, as is captured in the prayer of seventeenth-century philosopher Blaise Pascal:

Prayer to Ask God for the Good Use of Sickness

Make me fully understand that the ills of the body are nothing else than the punishment and the encompassing symbol for the ills of the soul. O Lord, let them be the remedy, by making me aware, through the pain that I feel, of the pain that I did not feel in my soul, deeply sick though it was and covered with sores. Because, Lord, the greatest sickness is insensibility ... Let me feel this pain sharply, so that I can make whatever is left of my life a continual penance to wash away the offenses I have committed.[3]

The view of immanent justice was so strong throughout history that it was extended to the sinful condition of mankind generally. Biblical evidence of the suffering required in childbirth, cited in Genesis 3:16, Galatians 4:27, Isaiah 66:7, Isaiah 13:8, Isaiah 21:3–4, Revelation 12:1–2, and Hosea 13:13, indicates that birth was intended to be a painful process as a reminder to women of the "curse of Eve." This view was so predominant that it was used to deny women anesthetic and amnesic drugs, even during difficult deliveries. In fact, it was not until the endorsement of the Lamaze Method of natural childbirth by Pope Pius XII, 100 years after chloroform was first administered to women in labor, that any method to address the pain of childbirth was condoned by the church.

The view of immanent justice was so strong in 1980s America that the HIV/AIDS infection became a major controversy between some religious groups and government efforts to find cures. It is a prevalent view among patients today with chronic pain, and it remains a view held by the educated and elite in the modern era. When asked if contracting a mysterious, serious, and deadly illness could be related to the etiology of the disease, nearly 30% of college students in a recent study agreed that it could.[4] Obviously, the relationship between sin and pain or illness is unrelated to the condition, the era, or the education of the believer.

To protect oneself or to reconcile with the gods, the individual required the assistance of higher, more powerful forces. These forces could be engaged with the help of the healer. This was the case in some societies, because the gods had granted the healing skill. In other societies, the healers had demonstrated that they could control the divine forces or conquer the evil forces personally. This belief was most pronounced in the shaman tradition, in which the healer traversed the underworld of illness and death and returned to the world of the living. To assure the cure and protect from evil, healers would incant, cajole, pray, and employ relics and holy objects. The healer would prescribe prayers in conjunction with herbs, medicines, and other therapies and personal, sometimes penitential, rituals. If none of these techniques succeeded in calling forth the gods or in subduing the evil, the priest-healer would invoke the greatest force and mystery of all—the will of the divine.

Wisdom of Divine Law
In Western traditions, formal health care prescriptions and

the sacred meet most clearly in Mosaic Law. The ancient Hebrews were no strangers to the power of pestilence and disease. In 1250 B.C.E. they had been saved by God from the diseases inflicted on the Egyptians who held them in captivity, but they were threatened with a similar fate if they disobeyed the commandments delivered by God during their wanderings in the desert following the Exodus. These commands were given directly to Moses, written down, and contained in the biblical book of Leviticus. It stands as a remarkable public-health text, with explicit dietary, sanitation, infectious disease, and public health instructions.

Following those instructions was a part of the law that engaged the community's covenant with God, but it was also a prescription for health, disease prevention, and longevity. Life was dichotomized into "clean" and "unclean" foods, persons, houses, clothes, and utensils. The "clean" could be touched, the "unclean" could not. The "unclean" was segregated from the community, and anyone coming into contact with it required "purification" before they could rejoin society. In characterizing some food as "unclean," requiring ritual cleanliness, and limiting food sources, the Hebrews reduced the potential transmitters of disease. Trichinosis was avoided in the prohibition of pork, schistomiasis avoided in the prohibition of seafood. Refraining from touching dead animals, eating dead meat, or consuming blood all prevented disease contamination of the human community. Inspecting, draining, cleaning, and salting meat kept a major protein source safe. Isolating mothers and their newborns following delivery protected both from the harsh realities of ancient life at the time when their mortality risks were the greatest. It assured the growth of the population despite harsh living conditions in hostile climates and during warring times. Hand washing and avoiding persons with infectious diseases were common practices with the obvious benefits we preach, but rarely practice today. Disinfecting property and clothes to the point of burning dangerous items and vacating homes was also good for the individual's and the public's health.

It was many centuries before public health science would confirm the wisdom of these practices and modern communities would resurrect and promote the simple, clear regulations of this ancient society. Unfortunately, that understanding did not come in time to save a community of European Jews. Because these practices were so effective, there were devastating consequences during the time of the great plagues of Europe. Dr. Balavignus, a Jewish physician who was cognizant of Old Testament law, the Talmud, and the writings of the famous twelfth-century Rabbi and healer Maimonides, recommended to the leadership of the Strasbourg Jewish ghetto that it institute practices similar to those prescribed by Moses. In particular, he advised the cleaning and burning of refuse, and the protection of the water supply from contamination. This reduced the size of the rat population transmitting the plague and reduced mortality in the ghetto to five percent of that of the main Christian city. The survival rate differential was so noticeable, even in the absence of formal public health studies and epidemiology, that the Jews were blamed for the plague and thousands were massacred in retaliation.

Other Ancient Texts and Practices

Even older than Hebrew traditions, Sumerian texts from more than six thousand years ago contain similar references to medicinal gifts from the divine to priests for their use as healers. Buddhist texts of that same period show the relationship between healing and the sacred as unmistakably clear. In those, Brahma, the First Teacher of the Universe, provided healing information within the Ayurveda, or the Science of Life. This text consisted of 100,000 hymns and all knowledge concerning medicines and healing. The legends describe the gods conquering demonic forces of illness through ritual; through more than 1,000 herbs derived from heaven, earth, and water; and through medicines, rituals, and chants. Disease was seen as the result of sin and, therefore, confession was required. Therapies were effective only when they were combined with prayer and ritual. Buddhist monks and sages passed down the wisdom through an oral tradition, and its current written form, which is still quite extensive and enjoying a renaissance, is considered to be more limited than the original instructions.

In ancient China, oracle bones were used for divination of the recovery of the patient and then pounded into medicines. Around 2000 B.C.E., the Second Celestial Emperor developed the national pharmacopoeia by personally testing over 1,000 herbs and 70 poisons—one of which finally killed him. Healing by acupuncture was the gift of the goddesses Scarlet and White to the Yellow Emperor, around 500 B.C.E. An alchemist Taoist priest, Ko Hung (300 B.C.E.), taught that his elixirs could provide protection from an interesting array of clinical conditions—including ghosts and digestive disorders—and that they could raise the dead and confer immortality.

By 900 B.C.E. the Greeks had institutionalized the gift of medicine from the gods to the point of creating temple hospitals. Apollo was the most powerful god-physician, using epidemics for punishment and healing wounds as rewards. Angry gods caused physical and mental diseases. Appeased gods provided medicines for the favored, especially soldiers. When necessary, the Greek physicians used incantations to secure a healing. Chiron, a centaur, had two famous pupils: Achilles and Asclepius, the son of Apollo. Achilles did not become known as a healer. In one 490 B.C.E. depiction he was shown as inept in applying a tourniquet and causing the patient great pain. Nearly invincible himself, he perhaps had no great incentive to be a compassionate healer. Asclepius, in contrast, learned the secrets of medicines to relieve pain. A heavy price was exacted from Asclepius when he ignored the limits to the healing arts imposed on his practice and the risks involved in challenging the gods with too much success. Having committed the unpardonable sin of raising a dead man to life, Asclepius was slain by Apollo with a thunderbolt. Because the serpent and the cock were sacred to Asclepius, they were frequently portrayed with him. One serpent, entwined in Asclepius' walking stick, remains the predominate symbol of this healer. In prehistoric times the snake was associated with regeneration, owing to its ability to shed its skin. That practice of using snakes in healing rituals continued for centuries, and the image of snakes remains dominant in medical symbols today. Hippocrates, who was born and lived on the Greek island of Cos around 460 to 361 B.C.E., is said to have stolen the prescriptions of Asclepius before destroying the god's temple, claiming the medicine and snakes as his very own.

Hippocratic Mystery and Medicine

The Hippocratic tradition is rooted in early observational medicine and nearly worshiped today as the beginning of a new, rational era of thought applied to the study of disease. Modern mythology holds that Hippocrates launched the practice of medicine into its current technical and more scientifically based state. In reality, the Hippocratic practice was actually similar to other spirit-related medical traditions of ancient societies and was by no means free of mystery and magic. Anyone who doubts this connection between Hippocratic medicine and religion need only attend the medical "oath-taking" reenacted for visiting medical VIPs on the island of Cos today. It is an unmistakably religious ceremony, shrouded in ritual and symbol common to religious traditions of the West today.

At the hands of Hippocrates and his students, the cult of Asclepius, complete with snake, spread throughout Greece and to Rome. The god was accompanied by his daughters Hygeia (hygiene), Panacea (cure all) and Telesphorus (convalescence), and his priests built temples of healing where diseases were cured and preventive measures were taught. It was said, in that day, that everyone who entered the sanctuary of the temples was cured. By 239 B.C.E., when a pestilence descended on Rome, the locals consulted with the Asclepians at their temple. As they did, a snake emerged from the temple and boarded the Roman ship that had transported the delegation. Believing this to be an omen, the cult became entrenched in Rome, giving way only gradually with the emergence of Christianity many hundred years later. We still pay an homage, of sorts, to the grand old patriarch of medicine—Asclepius—not with temples but with wallets. To this day, his dominance of healing the sick overshadows the call of his daughters to prevent disease or support caregivers through the convalescence of the patient.

The Greek cults and systems of medicine spread not only to Rome, but also throughout the Arabic world, gradually coming to coexist with Islam. Unlike the emerging Christian traditions in Europe in the same era that addressed mainly the spiritual health of the patient, the Qur'an spoke to the physical as well. Although the believer was subject to divine aspects of health and illness, there were physical and natural causes of illness also. A believer was thus advised to bear sufferings for the merits that the trials would bring, but to seek secular healing when the disease became intolerable. The Prophet Muhammad instituted measures much like the public health directives of Moses, and compassionate caring for the sick was a practice of the Prophet himself.

Christian Mystery and Medicine

By all accounts, healing was a significant part of the ministry of Jesus of Nazareth, on whose life the Christian tradition is built. He healed physical and mental conditions. He did not theorize about them, he simply cured them. He denied that illness had anything to do with the sin of the sick person or that of his parents (John 9:1–12). Occasionally he viewed illness as the result of evil spirits, as in a man possessed (Mark 1:23–28, Luke 11:14–20). He

---

believed that there was an evil force loose in the world. This evil was part of a larger picture, and illness was only one manifestation of the death it caused. Sickness and death of both the physical and emotional body were part of the realm of the ministry of Jesus and were not intended to end when he departed the earth. Instead, he assigned the closest of his followers with the commission to go forward and, as stated by the Apostle Luke, himself a physician, "cure the sick" (Luke 10:9).

Unfortunately, medieval Christianity did not take a step forward in either the science or the art of medicine. Medicine was subordinate to the study of theology. By this time, theology had shifted away from an imitation of the healing practices of Jesus, and now focused on an imitation of his life. Suffering acquired new meaning. The practice of medicine as a secular art, which had emerged in 200 C.E. with the work of Galen and other scientists, was considered to be inferior to the state of priesthood. Illness was judged to be either the result of sin or a test of faith. Suffering the trials of pain or disease to gain rewards in heaven was, therefore, the patient's most appropriate response. The love of the healthy body and intellectual curiosity about its functions, which were "givens" within the Greek systems of health care, were not appropriate avenues for salvation of the soul, the more important purpose of life on earth. The dissection of cadavers was forbidden, and the mechanics of the body's inner workings remained mysteries. Healing the patient or curing the disease was not necessarily good, except when that happened by the hand of God or His representatives—especially saints and their relics. In fact, healing could actually interfere with God's plans for the individual.

Nonetheless, cults of saints grew up among the people and flourished during this time as their intercession for healing was sought. As practitioners of the healing arts, saints were largely specialists. The image of St. Sebastian, martyred by being shot with arrows, merged with that of

Apollo, the archer-healer of the ancient Greeks. The saint was credited with saving Rome from the plague in 680 C.E., when a church was built in his honor near the city. From that point forward, he became the recourse for the plagues that would all too often and all too suddenly curse the European continent. The word "plague," whose Latin root means "blow, stripe, or stroke" of punishment, was, in that case, a fitting term for the meaning attributed to the sudden and widespread illnesses over which the people had little control. The devastation of a plague must certainly have felt like punishment. The hand of St. Theresa of Avila was said to cure jealousy and indigestion. Diluted blood from Thomas of Canterbury cured blindness, insanity, leprosy, and deafness. The saints Cosmas and Damian appeared to a physician in a dream to teach him mastectomy procedures. Apollonia—a saint whose teeth were knocked out during her martyrdom—became the patron saint of toothaches. St. Anthony was invoked against erysipelas, or St. Anthony's Fire, as it came to be known in the eleventh century, and numerous cures were ascribed to him. Having a relic in the home, the church, and the nation was an indispensable tenet of health care. Saintly body parts were cut up to be dispensed as relics, becoming talismans against misfortune for the rich and powerful.

Secular Healing Traditions

Although many of the Christian rituals that emerged were quite similar to those of the Asclepians, there was a major difference. Christians established a tradition of taking in all patients. Even when non-Christian healers were aligned with a strong sacred healing tradition, they frequently avoided caring for patients they knew would not recover. They discriminated against the truly ill. A Christian healer ideal emerged out of this practice, and the priest-physician was institutionalized in Europe within the religious communities that cared for the sick. In the Christian community, all the sick were welcome. St. Benedict was one of the early founders within this tradition. He established monasteries that, in addition to other monastic endeavors, cared for the sick. They also grew and studied the various herbs and other prescriptions for treating disease.

During the Middle Ages secular-healing practitioners grew in number, coexisting with religious healing for many years, sometimes at odds and at other times in harmony. There is ample evidence that the powerful religious leaders of the day—popes and priests—sought secular remedies. Conversely, secular healers reciprocated. In Europe they adopted the formal study of herbal healing as it emerged from the Christian monasteries. Nonetheless, frequently, and especially when the secular healers were women, they were fined, excommunicated, exiled, and persecuted as witches who used the black arts and invoked Satan in their work.

Secular healers invited retribution from the religious powers because of the patients they treated. This might seem like a conundrum, but it is not. Unlike many other healers throughout recorded history, and even beyond the ethics of the Christians, secular healers were the "healers of last resort" and were the least likely to screen out the most critically ill and dying patients. Even the Christian healers who cared for all patients, including the dying, eventually abandoned the care of terminal patients to the providence of God. This was particularly true if patients suffered with pain. The etymology of the term "pain," after all, is derived from the Latin "peona," or punishment. Suffering was sanctified by saints, and it was sanctifying of souls. As a result, the overriding theological preference for many was to suffer. The writings of St. Catherine of Sienna, for instance, who today is regarded as one of the major teachers within the Catholic tradition, describe her choice to suffer on earth rather than in eternity. Death was the last opportunity to assure eternal life, and meddling with the eternity of the soul was theologically incorrect.

It was at this point that patients sought secular village

healers for the "alternatives" they offered. These healers took on the cases that others had abandoned as terminal or incurable. Some historians believe that these so-called witch-healers even created their own myths and instilled fear about their potions to frighten away the uninformed, who might otherwise experiment with their powerful herbs—some of which, like digitalis, are still used today. They created this fear by giving common but powerful herbs names that would frighten away the uninitiated and limit experimentation by the uninformed. *Digitalis purpurea*, a biannual plant with a stem of bell-shaped flowers known as Foxglove in our gardens today, was called "Dead Man's Bells" in the Middle Ages. Other herbals were named "Snake Milk," "Graveyard Dust," and "Beggar's Tick." Only the most foolhardy would dare venture into the "witches'" garden. This blend of fear and respect protected the unwary patient, but endangered the secular healer.

If patients judged incurable were treated by one of these secular healers and lived, the healer must certainly have touched a power that challenged God's own. In the early centuries of healing, such a power was expected of healers. In the European Christian era, it was heresy. As a result, the healer became vulnerable to the political retaliation of the most powerful social institution of the day: the Church, with its ordained healers and its eye on salvation. Once a secular healer emerged in the community, became known, and acquired a reputation for success, the healer— and this was usually, but not always, a woman—lived in a dangerous political predicament. Success in healing could bring charges of conspiring with Satan. Deaths in healing, on the other hand, could bring charges of incompetence and murder. Were her "Dead Man's Bells" a tool of the devil to prevent the afflictions sent by God? Or were they used to kill the patient, without benefit of clergy at bedside? Either way, the secular healer was at risk if she had run afoul of the local church authorities.

Throughout the ages, healers, with physicians carrying

the heaviest burdens, had been held accountable for their failures. This is the primary reason why some healers took great care in selecting patients. But practicing without benefit of "license" granted through religious vows carried the most serious consequences of all—regardless of whether the patient lived or died. Hildegard von Bingen, an eleventh-century German abbess whose work in herbals and healing is enjoying a renaissance today, most certainly learned from and taught secular healers of her era. As much as their secular practices were similar to hers, as a vowed religious leader, her practices were ordained as safer and more likely to be in tune with the divine.

Happily, the conflicts were eventually resolved. The Protestant Reformation, particularly Calvin's insistence that salvation come through grace alone rather than through the works (including suffering) of man, separated the body from the grip of the church. Within the church, peace came when all healing, regardless of its nature and regardless of the nature of the healer, was declared to be a "miracle" from God. Furthermore, the church recognized the limitations and frailties of its own religious healers. The powers and prestige of healing and law were abused by some practitioners, and ecclesiastical circles acted in the twelfth century to curb abusive practices by the religious healers. To clip the avaricious wings of its healing angels, several church councils ruled that monks and "canons regular" were no longer allowed to study jurisprudence and medicine for the sake of temporal gain. The practice of healing and law were permitted, but financial compensation was banned.

This was the Middle Ages, several millennia after the first mentions in ancient texts of the sacred gifts of law and medicine. The two essentials of civilized society provided by God remained squarely and unmistakably in the hands of the priestly class. And, for the first time, healers were decreed, by the highest authorities, to provide uncompensated care in their practice of the healing arts.

Shamanic Mystery and Medicine

Anthropological studies of native cultures and their reemergence in modern days confirm the historical interpretations of the sacred aspects of healing in those cultures that left no written records—especially with regard to the shamanic tradition. The shaman was a particular type of sacred healer. He or she, by virtue of heredity or "election," was "called" upon by the community to serve not only in the more secular, herbal healing roles, but in spiritual healing roles as well. The shaman was healer, priest, and, when necessary, undertaker. He engaged in healing arts, reconciled the soul to the gods, and accompanied the soul to the afterlife. It was for this reason that the "calling" was so important. The shaman was the keeper of the collective soul of the community and the healer of the specific souls who sought his care. Initiated into the shaman role through dreams and personal crises of sickness, hardship, and brutal rituals, the shaman experienced the death, dismemberment, and resurrection of his own consciousness. Having come to grips with his own spirits—good and evil—and now in control of them, the shaman was a technician of sacred ways and was able to employ them for the benefit of others. The term "shaman" means literally "he who knows," and it was clear to the community that shamans knew the many mysteries of the forces of power.

The perceived causes of disease and the prescriptions to treat them are similar in the shamanic traditions of those groups that we know better through written records. In the Australian aboriginal tribes, the shaman healers use both spiritual and herbal techniques, and they are evaluated to ensure they can produce miracles. Aztec shamans traced the cause of some diseases and herbal remedies to the rain god Tlaloc. Water-related deaths, such as edema and drowning, were signs that the individual had been chosen to live with Tlaloc in the afterlife. To thwart the god's intentions to have the patient join him, the healers employed diuretic herbs to cleanse the body and relieve swellings.

Native North American tribes held similar views and placed the shaman within the priestly class of the culture. Diseases were seen as the result of evil spirits and soul wanderings. Healing occurred through god-given herbs and rituals. Even when, as in some tribes, the rituals were thought by the medicine men themselves to be tricks and "sleight-of-hand," much like our modern-day placebos, they were used ethically and considered effective because the gods sanctioned such tricks for the purpose of restoring health. Like saints in the Middle Ages, native shamans tended to specialize, both in the types of diseases and conditions they would treat, as well as in the types of treatment techniques they would employ.

When European medicine met tribal medicine during the American colonial period, the shamans did not fare well. Both traditions were highly superstitious, and neither was far removed from invoking the mysteries of the gods. Nonetheless, early European observers of Native American healing characterized it as uninformed and ineffective. Descriptions by traders, missionaries, and captives denigrated both the native practitioners and the patients for practices that were virtually identical to secular and sacred traditions in Europe. Although Europeans believed that "possession" by the devil was a cause of illness, with healing achieved by "casting out" the offending spirit, similar practices among the Native American tribes were discounted as savage. Europeans recognized devils by name and exorcised them. Cherokees, as well, named several dozen spirits, each with a specific ritual for "casting out," but they were viewed as primitive. French Jesuit priests decried the use of charms and totems among the Native American Indians, but mixed water with dust from the tomb of an Iroquois girl, Kateri Tekakwitha, to perform miracles. She was later declared a saint, in part because of those miracles. Native healers remained respected and powerful within their culture despite these attacks, however. In fact, because of their power, they were viewed as a threat to the possibility of assimilation of native groups into white civilization. As a result, early government strategies to transition Native Americans into the mainstream civilization included undermining the respect for the native healer.

Many native healers went underground to survive, to maintain the traditions of the tribal society, and to protect the healing covenants they had established with their communities. For example, Christian names gradually replaced the Aztec native names of herbs to protect the healer from being denounced during periods of inquisition. *Peyotl* became "Mary's rose," and *yauhtli*, one of the two principal remedies of Aztec medicine, became "Saint Mary's herb." Traditional, non-Christian, sacred-origin practices could then continue in safety. Even today, modern Mexican shamans, called *graniceros* or "hail people," make yearly pilgrimages to caves that are swept with "Saint Mary's herb" to assure that evil spirits do not deprive the healers of their powers. Once inside, a blue cross, the symbol of the rain god Tlaloc, is worshiped in a combination of ancient and Christian ceremonies. Just to the north of that region, the U.S. Public Health Service accommodates traditional healing practices in its medical-care system for Native American tribes. Its hospitals include special rooms for important native healing rituals. Medical personnel and native healers practicing among the tribes have reciprocal referral relationships in their practices on reservations. Community Health Centers treating immigrant and native populations with strong tribal-healer traditions incorporate those healing methods and personnel into their base of care and networks of referrals.

Modern Mystery and Medicine

The shamanic tradition is reemerging globally, and so are other sacred-method healing approaches. In the 1980s, New Agers adopted shamanic practices in such numbers that Native Americans protested that the proliferation of sweat lodges, ritual dances, and spirit healing was a theft

---

of their cultural and religious traditions. While some of those practices might be extreme for most people, the trend to incorporate the sacred into the secular practice of healing is growing, and the effectiveness of these approaches is being demonstrated. Even within the most traditional practices of medicine, there is a resurgence of interest in the connection between the sacred and healing arts. In fact, sacred healing approaches are being tested in clinical trials and have been demonstrated to be helpful adjuncts to modern secular techniques.

A number of clinicians and scientists are advocates of the connections between the spiritual and healing within the current practices in health care. Some, like Bernie Siegel, M.D., are physicians who have suffered severe illnesses and in the course of their care recognized the relationship of the mysterious and sacred forces to their healing. Others, like Harvard-trained Andrew Weil, M.D., saw the limits of contemporary allopathic medicine in the course of caring for others, particularly when the task was to promote wellness and not just to cure disease.

Some of the connections between the spiritual and modern medicine maintain the mystery of the sacred. Physician and former hospital Chief of Staff Larry Dossey incorporates prayer in traditional clinical practice and is comfortable with "not knowing" exactly how it works. Some of the connections attempt to demystify the sacred, as in Herbert Benson's prescriptions for simple exercises in *Relaxation Response*, or with scientific measures in Doc Childre and Howard Martin's book, *HeartMath Solution*. Regardless of whether the mystery is penetrated, however, the unknowns and the sacred connections to healing are unmistakably present once again as we care for patients and research disease. Nutrition and wellness expert Dr. Dean Ornish also promotes the value of intimacy. Medical intuitive Carolyn Myss describes the relationship between biography, biology, and chakra spiritual centers. Meditation, imagery, art, and music—those sources of nourishment typically considered food for the soul—have become medicines for the body as well. Not only have the mind and the body connected in these times, both have welcomed the soul to the party. Prayer of all sorts is once again present—this time in the healing encounters and enterprises of modern American health care.

A new magazine, *Spirituality and Health*, is on the newsstands. Amazon.com lists over six thousand book titles dealing with healing, and a substantial number draw on religion and spirituality as the prescription for the path to health. Weekend healing seminars and tent-meeting opportunities flourish. Faith-based communities offer spiritual and physical healing alternatives, expanding their roles into prevention and primary care, hiring parish nurses, and offering immunizations after Sunday services. They also continue to provide institutional care and maintain their missions in the wake of Medicare cut-backs and managed-care competition. Jews, Baptists, Lutherans, Adventists, and Catholics merge their spiritual missions with their medical acumen and manage major health care operations. The largest of these is a $40 billion Catholic enterprise comprising 10% of the country's hospitals.

Prayer is not necessarily a subject that lends itself to traditional clinical instruction. Nevertheless, in just the past five years, nearly one-third of the medical schools in the United States have added courses on prayer and healing to their curricula. Prayer is not the common subject of health care administration seminars. But managed-care executives are holding conferences on the subject of prayer in medicine and taking it seriously enough to look ahead to its financial aspects. "Coverage," they state for the record, will depend on "proof that it works." Over 850 studies have examined the relationship between involvement in spiritual activities and mental health status and three-quarters of those studies have found positive relationships in adaptation to stress. In examining the impact on physical health, a majority of 350 studies found a positive correlation.[5] The effect of a spiritual life on health was, in fact, substantial. One study indicates it might have the survival impact of abstaining from smoking[6], or adding between 7 and 14 years to one's lifespan.[7]

Proving that it works will take some research, and prayer is not the usual subject of our studies in health care. Yet, researchers are now examining the proper analytic methodologies for investigating its effectiveness. Physicists are hypothesizing the energetic mechanisms responsible for healing through prayer. Ethicists are debating whether prayer should be researched at all.

Ronald Kydd, in *Healing Through the Centuries, Models for Understanding*, describes six models of miracle-focused healing in which the success rates are within the range of the placebo effects of standard clinical interventions in medicine today:

- In the "confrontational" model, healing is done within the model of Jesus, as a direct confrontation with evil and intervention in the lives of men.

- In the "intercessory" model, those who led exemplary lives on earth and are now saints are called upon to request the assistance of God on behalf of the patient.

- In the "reliquarial" model, the remains, possessions, or burial places of holy people are the means for healing.

- In the "incubational" model, patients enter into healing sanctuaries in which they are prayed for over time to achieve the healing.

- In the "revelational" model, God reveals information to the healer to assist in the healing.

- In the "soteriological" model, best exemplified today in the healing ministry of Oral Roberts and most active in the Pentecostal church, God routinely "breaks in" on the lives of men for the purpose of healing and salvation.

None of these models are mutually exclusive, and they are frequently employed in combination. Common to each of these models (with the exception of the incubational) is that the healing will occur instantly.

What is useful in Kydd's work is the construction of a language for different healing models that will enable the closer examination of miraculous healing in the modern world. The bulk of miraculous healing is based on self-reports from patients without verification of clinical diagnostics—but then, a portion of our current traditional medicine is based on measures of patient satisfaction that are not dissimilar.

The Sacred and the Secular: A New Partnership?

Whether or not one is religious, honors the sacred, or prays, it is undeniable that disease is still frightening and the ordinary terrors of life are still as uncontrollable for us as they were for our ancestors. Healing today may well be even more mysterious. The biogenetics revolution creates even more fear, because it reveals that the causes of disease are not just the external evils of demons or the result of our own weaknesses; rather, the uncontrollable ticking bombs of ancestral programming await detonation within us. In the best of these scientific and clinical times, we may also face the most trying of times in integrating the sacred with the secular in pursuing the public policies for our modern care systems. In the worst of these post-September 11 times, we turn to law enforcement to protect us from the offenses of our global neighbors. We also turn to our healers to help us with the new stresses caused by bombings and the new risks created by weapons of a biological nature.

On the jacket cover of physician Larry Dossey's latest book, *Prayer is Good Medicine: How to Reap the Healing Benefits of Prayer*, Ayurvedic physician-guru Deepak Chopra, M.D., says, "With the elegance of simplicity and the precision of science, Dossey shows us how we can create a lasting partnership between faith and medicine." In *The Scalpel and the Silver Bear*, the first female Navaho surgeon weaves her fascinating story of transformation from a mechanistic technician trained at one of the elite medical schools to a healer integrating the native with the new. At a recent meeting of the American Psychiatric Association, Dr. Robert Palmer, a psychiatrist of Ojibway Anishinabe descent, discussed his use of traditional healing methods. Despite the fact that only a small percentage of his patients were of Native American ancestry, he employs a medicine wheel, a Mishomis (or grandfather stone), and ceremonies in his healing.[8] The sacred basis of healing appears to have come full circle and has arrived in modern health care. It will feel at home in the twenty-first century. It will be needed in this post-terror era, as suddenly, the mysteries and our fears loom larger than ever.

Does it feel at home in this, and other, countries? How strong are these traditions within the minds of patients and healers? How important is this history to the process of healing in a contemporary society? Do governments feel prepared to abide within the traditions that are at the source of healing and health care and may influence the process of care? Are policymakers prepared to recognize that those who function within the healing enterprise do so within a complex multicultural, ethical, spiritual foundation? Will public policies accommodate the attitudes and perspectives of these traditions that are harbored so fundamentally within patients? Can governments that step into healing streams now swim in its waters easily, not only for the elderly and the poor it set out to help, but also for the rest of the world whose health it increasingly influences?

A Short History of Medicine

I have an earache.

2000 B.C.E. Here, eat this root.
1000 C.E. That root is heathen, say this prayer.
1850 C.E. That prayer is superstition, drink this potion.
1940 C.E. That potion is snake oil, swallow this pill.
1985 C.E. That pill is ineffective, consider an implant.
2000 C.E. That implant is artificial. Here, eat this genetically engineered root.
2050 C.E. That genetically engineered root has harmed other life forms. Here, say this prayer.

Chapter 2

Healing Within the Covenant Tradition

*The Medicine Trail is a manner of approach, an attitude, like a
color of dawn, something that reaches out to touch things any
way it can, unformed, created only by the desire to connect.*[1]

Stan Rushworth, on Cherokee Healing

Covenants . . . sacredness . . . healing. These are emo-
tionally charged terms. I imagine them echoing
through empty hallways in health care enterprises across
the country. The halls are empty because everyone has
retreated into the recesses of their private offices lining the
corridors. I can almost hear them saying, "God forbid that
I would be drawn into anything new. I don't have time.
Things are tough enough. I have patients to satisfy, budgets to balance, and financial losses and premium increases to explain. If it's not the latest accreditation group, quality group, or Government Accounting Office (GAO) study
group coming to visit, then it's the Inspector General
knocking at my door. I've got a business to run—no, a
business to save. I've got reporters and trial lawyers looking for trouble. I don't have time for covenants and sacredness in healing." Take this message to other countries and
too many of them will have serious objections as well. After
all, within, on average, forty nations each year, they are not
fighting inspectors or the competition, they are fighting
wars.

As a health care system under stress, it is natural to
reject new ideas that sound like impossible new demands.
As Americans, we separate church and state, and these
words feel church-like in a state-focused, if not state-con-

trolled, health care economy. As clinicians, policymakers, and payers, we separate soul and science, and words such as "sacred" and "covenant" sound too much like soul in an era that demands scientific application to everything pertaining to health care, including the art of medicine. Besides, for many of us in health care, even our own souls have taken a beating in the course of the caring for people. Is this what we signed on for years ago when our education began? How can we initiate a dialogue like this? How can we possibly engage in a dialogue like this? How can we give even more of ourselves to patients, communities, or the world when all we get in return is hostility? How can we heal others when we are suffering ourselves?

Nonetheless, it is undeniable that these "sacred" concepts are rooted in every culture. They are embedded in our language and, like it or not, they frame our debates. Scan the reactions to the AMA announcement that it would support unions for physicians who work as employees: covenant was an implied foundation of these comments. Articles and editorials across the country were outraged that physicians would consider violating their oath and subliminally reminded physicians that they cannot dare to do so. No reporter or editorial writer explicitly connects the oath with its traditions and origins in the sacred or in covenant. No writer needs to do that. The concepts of covenant, oath, sacred, and healing are so embedded in our traditions that we take them for granted. They are like the ground on which we walk.

Health, healing, holy, priesthood, and sanctuary are inextricably linked in our language. "Heal," "holy," and "sanctuary" arise from the same ancient root word, "hal." The term and its usage grew from life experiences and became entwined in our deepest linguistic origins. These concepts reside within the Judeo-Christian influences that dominate our mainstream culture, and they resonate as well with the Islamic, Buddhist, and Hindu views that are increasingly a part of our national consciousness—and certainly a part of our world view. These ideas, as different as they may appear in the nature and expression of their theology, come together in their recognition of the sacred within the healing encounter.

Covenants: Origins and Meaning

It was not only the language of healing but also the structure and relationships within which healing occurs that grew from the sacred. That structure was provided within covenants. It is unclear in the literature whether covenants, as well as healing and law, were viewed as being endowed originally by the divine. What is clear, however, is that "covenants" were employed by God on notable occasions and used for divine purpose—including health and healing. The most notable of these is found in the covenant between God and Moses at Sinai. As a result, the practices of healing developed in communities alongside the emergence and practice of the covenants that structured the patient-healer and community relationships to support the health of people. The elements of covenantal relationships and covenantal thought were embedded in the original medical oaths and remain today in oaths and principles of ethical practice.

Both biblical and ancient secular texts are crowded with examples of what covenants were and how societies and covenants developed. Some covenants were between a king and his people, while others were between communities, between fathers and sons, between teachers and apprentices, and between husbands and wives. Early Akkadian and Hittite covenants, among the earliest known, established a "covenant formula." Within the formula, covenants contained essential elements. The obligations for a king's vassals, the blessings for obedience, and the curses for disobedience were clear. Earlier Hittite covenants not only came from the king and carried the force of his law but were also witnessed by the gods of the society, who were incorporated, by reference, into the agreement. Later, biblical covenants would follow that established rule. These covenants—both ancient and modern—structured the nature of the relationships between the parties in a particular way. We use the term covenant today, but, frankly, we use it carelessly when compared to usage in ancient times from which our current medical ethics grow.

In the context of today's usage, a covenant is:

> An agreement or promise to do or not to do a particular thing; to enter into a formal agreement; to bind oneself in contract; to make a stipulation; a promise incidental to a deed or contract, which is either express or implied; an agreement, convention, or promise of two or more parties, by deed in writing signed, and delivered by whichever of the parties pledges himself to the order that something is either done or shall be done or stipulates for the truth of certain facts.[2] [270 P. 2d 276, 278]

Our current usage of the term covenant comes from our current codification of our own laws and distinguishes between several different types of covenants. "Dependent covenants" are those in which the obligation for performance depends upon the actions of another to perform some prior action or meet some condition. "Concurrent covenants" are those in which one party is required to perform his obligation when the other party is ready to perform his. "Independent, or mutual, covenants" are those in which performance must be done, without reference to the performance of the other party. Other specifics in the definitions of covenant relate mainly to issues of land, title to land, transfers of land, and matters relating to estates. These are not the concepts intended in the use of similar terms in the biblical and ancient texts.

In ancient texts, covenants, by their very nature, involve more fundamental elements of relationships. They are mutual, binding, and alter the life and the life-course of any party who enters into them in significant ways. Covenants are typically created between greater and lesser partners—

as in a grant of property between a father and son. They reflect the dependency of the weaker party on the stronger party and the superiority of the stronger party over the weaker one. They may or may not bind both parties equally and mutually to a set of expectations, but they are binding and cannot be reversed. Unlike our modern versions in legal definitions, the performance of one is not dependent on the other; nor is it necessarily concurrent with the other or done in isolation from the other. A covenant, once established, determines the actions of both parties from that point forward, no matter what. And there is more.

In contrast to contracts, covenants are forever. As a result, they transform the identity of the parties. Covenants are not highly detailed. They do not anticipate each of the possible aspects of the relationship over time; to do so within a covenant would not be possible. Because covenants act within relationships and between ever-evolving parties, the nature of the covenants themselves is a moving target. As the parties to the covenant grow and change, the obligations evolve. In covenants, the giving and receiving is endless and goes deeper over time. The parties to a covenant are continually mutually responsive and alive within the covenant. Medical ethicist William May said it well:

> A contract has a limited duration, but a religious covenant imposes change on all moments. A mechanic can act under a contract, and then, when not fixing a piston, act without regard to the contract: but a covenantal people act under covenant while eating, sleeping, working, praying, cheating, healing, or blundering... Initiation into a profession means, in effect, that the physician is a healer when healing and when sleeping, when practicing and when malpracticing.[3]

Covenants of Grant and Obligation

Religious covenants are of two types: "covenants of grant" and "covenants of obligation." These distinctions are important in health care today because of the way in which

---

medical oaths were structured. Understanding medical oaths in the context of these types of covenant points the way to possible solutions to a number of dilemmas we face in health care today.

Covenants of grant describe a unidirectional relationship, in which one party establishes a relationship of giving—a promise, for example, with no requirement that the other party return the favor. This was the type of covenant between the Hebrew God of the Old Testament and Noah. In this covenant of grant, God promises that He will never again destroy the earth by flood. Noah and his family do not promise and are not expected to perform anything in return. Although they are invited to "Be fertile and multiply and fill the earth" (Genesis 9:1), they do not promise to do so, nor are obligations imposed on them to do so. The only promises are made by God. These promises are numerous, and they are significant. And yet, for all the consequences of the promises, Noah is not expected to reciprocate:

> God said to Noah and his sons with him: "See, I am now establishing my covenant with you and your descendants after you and with every living creature that was with you: all the birds, and the various tame and wild animals that were with you and came out of the ark. I will establish my covenant with you, that never again shall all bodily creatures be destroyed by the waters of a flood; there shall not be another flood to devastate the earth." God added: "This is the sign that I am giving for all ages to come, of the covenant between me and you and every living creature with you: I set my bow in the clouds to serve as a sign of the covenant between me and the earth. When I bring clouds over the earth, and the bow appears in the clouds, I will recall the covenant I have made between me and you and all living beings, so that the waters shall never again become as a flood to destroy all mortal beings. As the bow appears in the clouds, I will see it and recall the everlasting covenant that I have established between God and all living beings—all mortal creatures

that are on the earth." (Genesis 9:8–17)

This type of covenant of grant is not unlike the one that currently exists between patients and HMO-contracted physicians. Stronger parties—the employer, Medicare, and Medicaid, working with the HMO—arrange for physician care for the weaker party, the patient, at the time of an illness. The physician provides a prescription to relieve the symptoms or treat the disease. The weaker party—the patient—is under no obligation whatsoever. He may choose whether or not to arrive at the appointed time for the visit, whether or not to give the physician complete clinical information, to consent to diagnostic tests, to take the prescription, or to abide by the advice given. Like Noah and his family, the patient does not need to promise anything in return.

The second type of covenant is a covenant of obligation. The best-known covenant of obligation in the Western religious world is the one described between God and the chosen people of Israel. It was to become the central organizing principle of the relationship between God and man, first in the Israelite tradition and, later, in Christianity. This covenant was engaged at Sinai:

> Moses went up to the mountain of God. Then the Lord called to him and said, "Thus shall you say to the house of Jacob; tell the Israelites: You have seen for yourself how I treated the Egyptians and how I bore you up on eagle wings and brought you here to myself. Therefore, if you harken to my voice and keep my covenant, you shall be my special possession, dearer to me than all other people, though all the earth is mine." (Exodus 19:3–5)

The God of Moses grants the covenant, binds the human partners to obligations—to God and to each other—and describes His retributions for their failure to perform. In the chapters of Exodus that follow and throughout the book of Leviticus, mutual obligations are detailed.

The Israelites are instructed on virtually every aspect of their individual, family, and community lives. Faithful adherence to those requirements brought territory, prosperity, fertility, and special favors. Failure to perform would bring punishments, such as the extended stay in the desert that befell the community. Unlike a covenant of grant, a covenant of obligation established reciprocal duties and requirements for each of the parties to the covenant. There was no escaping the covenant. There were no exit clauses. No party could "buy out" the rights, obligations, or prerogatives of the other. Thus, care from God was linked to loyalty to God. This relationship with God also spilled over to frame the relationship between men. It was in specifying this covenant that the melding of the sacredness of the healing gifts from the divine become united with the sacredness of the expectations of the covenant between God and man and between men. It was a critical framing of the oath and ethical perspectives of healing and medicine today.

In this biblical example, as well as in other covenants, the formation of the covenant is preceded by the receipt of a gift. According to Professor May,

> "... gifts precede the promise—just as the gifts of courtship precede a marriage vow, and in the Scripture of Israel, the exodus precedes Mt. Sinai. The Jews bind themselves to God at Mt. Sinai as those who have already received an astonishing gift, the deliverance from Egypt. A covenantal ethic positions human givers in the context of a primordial act of receiving a gift not wholly deserved, which they can only assume gratefully. God tells the Israelites: When you harvest your crops, leave some for the sojourner. For you were once sojourners in Egypt. Givers themselves receive. Benefactors ultimately benefit."[4]

Professor May, in his work on this type of covenant—the covenant of obligation—and its relation to the medical profession, notes that a gift is also present here. Physicians receive an education, which is a gift from predecessors who came before and learned the skills to impart, and from the communities who supported the educational institutions within which the learning occurred. Gifts come to patients as well: they receive the care and healing. The two—physicians and patients—step inside the covenant.

Covenants of Hippocrates and Maimonides

Notions of covenant were reflected in the two best-known ancient medical oaths. The most widely known and used is the Oath of Hippocrates, which is an artful combination of both types of covenants. In this oath, healers—in this case, physicians—enter into a covenant of obligation with fellow members of the profession. They do this by promising to share their knowledge and goods with each other, and to care for each other and their families as if they were one family. They also enter into a separate covenant of grant with patients. In this other type of covenant, they swear to do only good for the patient, protect privacy and confidentiality and practice by ethical principles. The gods witness the covenant agreement, the terms of which are specified, and the rewards and punishment for failure to perform according to the covenant are invoked:

> I swear by Apollo the physician, by Aesculapius, Hygeia, and Panacea, and I take to witness all the gods, all the goddesses, to keep according to my ability and my judgement the following Oath:

> To consider dear to me as my parents him who taught me this art; to live in common with him and if necessary to share my goods with him; to look upon his children as my own brothers, to teach them this art if they so desire without fee or written promise; to impart to my sons and the sons of the master who taught me the disciples who have enrolled themselves and have agreed to the rules of the profession, but to these alone, the precepts and the instruction. I will prescribe regimen for the good of my

patients according to my ability and my judgment and never do harm to anyone. To please no one will I prescribe a deadly drug, nor give advice which may cause his death. Nor will I give a woman a pessary to procure abortion. But I will preserve the purity of my art and my life. I will not cut for stone, leave this operation to be performed by practitioners (specialists in this art). In every house where I come I will enter only for the good of my patients, keeping myself far from all intentional ill-doing and all seduction, and especially from the pleasure of love with women or with men, be they free or slaves. All that may come to my knowledge in the exercise of my profession or outside of my profession or in daily commerce with men, which ought not spread abroad, I will keep secret and will never reveal. If I keep this oath faithfully, may I enjoy my life and practice my art, respected by all men and in all times; but if I swerve from it or violate it, may the reverse be my lot.[5]

Lesser known is the oath crafted by Maimonides in the twelfth century, which he presented in the form of a prayer. Jewish communities viewed medicine as a divine calling. Doctors were given a special protecting angel, and religious authorities directed that a doctor should always be called in time of illness. Unlike others in the community, physicians were allowed to work on the Sabbath, because saving a life was an important task for the community and blessed by the divine. Maimonides was explicit in his view of how physical and spiritual health was linked. This is a mission statement to which to aspire, even today (some might say, especially today):

The purpose of the practice of medicine is to teach humanity the causes of ill health, the correct hygiene, the methods of making the body capable of useful labor, how to prolong life, and how to avoid disease. It thus directly elevates the human being to a higher moral plane, where the pursuit of Truth is possible and where the happiness of soul is attainable.[6]

The alignment of natural and spiritual concepts is evident in this physician's daily prayer. This is also the first appearance of a covenant of obligation between the physician and patient. Maimonides' prayer calls the patient into a covenant of obligation by requesting that patients have confidence in the physician and his healing art, that they comply with the directions and prescriptions he offers and that they not take advice from potentially harmful quacks and uninformed family members. Maimonides speaks to reciprocity in the physician-patient relationship that is ignored by Hippocrates. He steps out beyond the Hippocratic Oath, and its description of the more limited covenant of grant between patients and physicians. Maimonides prays:

> All-bountiful! Thou hast formed the human body in Thy complete wisdom. Thou hast united it in ten thousand times ten thousand parts that function continuously to preserve the harmony of the beautiful entity, the mortal integument of the immortals. Ever they are active in complete order, harmony, and unity. The moment, however, that frailty of matter or passions disturb this order and disrupt the unity, the forces engage in conflict and the body is reduced to its dust. It is then that Thou sendst to man beneficent messengers, the diseases, who announce to him the danger and urge him to avoid it.
>
> Thy Earth, Thy rivers, and Thy mountains are blessed by Thee with healing substances: they can heal. They assuage the suffering of Thy creatures and heal their wounds. Thou hast granted man the wisdom to unravel the secrets of his body, to recognize order and disorder; to draw the substances from their sources, to seek out their forces and to prepare and apply them according to their respective diseases. And Thy eternal foresight has chosen me to watch over the life and health of Thy creatures, and I now go forth to follow my calling. Stand by me All-bountiful, in this great undertaking so that I may succeed, for without Thy aid, man has no success even in

the most trivial things.

Inspire me with love for my art and Thy creatures. Do not permit that thirst of grain and greed for fame interfere with my calling, for these are enemies of truth and philanthropy, and they might also lead me astray in the mighty enterprise to further the weal of Thy creatures. Preserve the strength of my body and soul, so that they may be indefatigable at all times to help and to stand by the rich as well as the poor, the good and the bad, the enemy as well as the friend. In the sufferer always let me behold only the human being.

Enlighten my understanding so that I may grasp what is present and correctly surmise what is absent or hidden. Allow it not to sink, so that my judgment may not fail to recognize what is evident but also that it may not overestimate itself and see what cannot be seen. For fine and imperceptible are the boundaries of the great art, and of watching over the life and health of Thy creatures! Let not my intelligence be abstracted. At the bedside, let no extraneous matters rob my spirit of its watchfulness. Let them not disturb in its quiet labors. For great and holy is the search for the preservation of life and health of Thy creatures.

Grant my patients confidence in me and my art, and imbue them with obedience to follow my precepts and directions. Ban from their bedside all quacks and the army of advice-giving relatives and too-wise nurses, for they are a terrible band, who, through their vanity, harm the best intentions of the healing art and frequently cause the death of Thy creatures.

If wiser artists seek to improve and instruct me, let my spirit be thankful and obedient; for great is the field of the art. When, however, conceited fools berate me, then let the love of the art steel my spirit and insist on truth, regardless of age, fame, or standing, for to retract in such a case would mean death and disease of Thy creatures.

Grant to my spirit, gentleness and calm, when colleagues, vain of their years, repulse, scorn, or sneering try to correct me. Let this also be to my advantage for they know some things that are foreign to me and their self-conceit shall not offend me; they are old and old age is not the master of passions. For I too hope to be old before Thee, All-bountiful!

Grant me contentment in all things, save in the great art. Permit not the thought to awaken in me: You know enough; but grant me strength, leisure and the urge always to enlarge my accomplishments and to add to others. True art is long, but man's mind penetrates even farther. All-bountiful, Thou in Thy mercy hast chosen me to watch over the life and death of Thy creatures. I now go forth in the pursuit of my calling. Stand by me in this large undertaking, so it may be successful, for sans Thy help man is not successful, be it in the most trifling matter.[7]

The Prayer of Maimonides is not commonly part of the oath taken by modern physicians, and more modern forms of the Hippocratic Oath have emerged. One such standard revision is:

I do solemnly swear, by whatever I hold most sacred, that I will be loyal to the profession of medicine and just and generous to its members. That I will lead my life and practice my art in uprightness and honor. That into whatsoever home I shall enter, it shall be for the good of the sick and the well to the utmost of my power and that I will hold myself aloof from wrong and from corruption and from the tempting of others to vice. That I will exercise my art solely for the cure of my patients and the prevention of disease and will give no drug nor perform any operation for a criminal purpose, and far less suggest such thing. That whatsoever I shall see or hear of the lives of men and women which is not fitting to be spoken abroad, I shall keep inviolably secret. These things I do promise and in proportion as I am faithful to this oath, may happiness and good repute be ever mine, the opposite if I shall be foresworn.[8]

The Islamic Code of Medical Ethics provides a physician's oath that is similar:

I swear by God the Great; To regard God in carrying out my profession; To protect human life in all stages and under all circumstances, doing my utmost to rescue it from death, malady, pain, and anxiety; To keep people's dignity, cover their privacies, and lock up their secrets; To be, all the way, an instrument of God's mercy extending my medical care to near and far, virtuous and sinner, and friend and enemy; To strive in the pursuit of knowledge and harnessing it for the benefit but not the harm of mankind; To revere my teacher, teach my junior, and be brother to members of the medical profession joined in piety and charity; To live my Faith in private and in public, avoiding whatever blemishes me in the eyes of God, His apostle, and my fellow Faithful; And may God be witness to this Oath.[9]

Regardless of the particular form—old or new—the oaths in use in medicine today abide by the elements of covenants established many millennia before. Whether ancient or new, the oaths are witnessed by the gods and specify the duties of the greater partner (the physician) to the lesser partner (the patient). They create loyalty to their more knowledgeable partners (teachers), describe standards of conduct, and invoke rewards and (though less so in modern times) penalties for the quality of the performance.

Did the oaths influence the practice of medicine in those days? It is hard to know. Do oaths influence the practice of medicine today? The Foundation for Medical Excellence, with funding from The Robert Wood Johnson Foundation, studied how oaths and ethical norms governed medical practice in 1997. In results presented at the Institute of Medicine (IOM) in 1998, the investigators noted that there was widespread familiarity with medical oaths, that physicians referred to the oaths frequently, that the oaths influenced their practices (particularly when the physicians were women), and that ethical beliefs and integrity in practice were a critical concern.[10]

Another recent phenomenon is also instructive. In 135 of the 145 U.S. medical schools, first year medical students are now "cloaked" in "white coat ceremonies" in which they swear to an oath. Some schools use the traditional Oath of Hippocrates, others update it or use other versions, such as the one by Maimonides. Columbia Professor Arnold P. Gold, whose leadership resulted in the first of these ceremonies, has noted that taking the oath at the start of medical training is a return to the ancient apprenticeship days of medical education and that it is embraced enthusiastically by students.[11] The ceremony has been promoted as a return to the humanity of medicine at a time when the profession feels its professional values are being assaulted from all sides. It is also an unmistakable return to covenant. This movement has expressed itself in greater involvement of students in the development of oaths. The Student American Medical Association and the Association of Academic Health Centers have weighed in with encouragement for oath-taking and for developing student versions of oaths.[12] In one particularly innovative style, the oath is structured as a dialogue between the swearing class and the patients they serve. It contains the essential elements: the class swears by all they hold sacred, recognizes the gift of medical education, and enumerates the duties they will perform and the ethics they will hold dear. This style of covenant also includes some implied obligations on the part of the public, most notably to be "partners in care."[13]

Physicians: In the light of all we hold sacred, we make this covenant with the persons we will serve.

Public: As representatives of humankind, we acknowledge and accept your covenant with us.

Physicians: We are enriched and humbled by centuries of research and experience in the healing arts.

Public: *May the inheritance enable you to enable nature's healing power.*

Physicians: We are indebted to you for our education: the resources, the institutions, the support, the freedom, and your willingness for us to practice our fledgling skills upon you.

Public: *And we are indebted to you for your long hard years of study, your anxious years of stress, your risks and sacrifices, your dedication.*

Physicians: We feel called to our healing profession by divine direction or the cry of human need.

Public: *We are grateful for your high calling. Recognize that we, too, are individuals who have callings, goals and ideals; that we, too, serve humankind with our talents.*

Physicians: We respect and cherish life and the lives of individuals.

Unison: We are all individuals who live and love, who dream and sorrow, who laugh and cry, who think and feel, who cherish life and other humans.

Physicians: We will strive always to be sensitive to your feelings, needs, and thoughts.

Public: *And we, to yours.*

Physicians: We earnestly seek to alleviate pain and suffering and to sustain human life.

Public: *But to do so only so long as both are compatible and appropriate.*

Physicians: We know there are times when maintaining life seems not worth the suffering.

Public: *We each differ when that time comes. Argue with us, but honor our decisions.*

Physicians: We will. But we will never desert you.

Public: Cure if you can, alleviate if you can't, but listen and comfort always.

Physicians: We will, and we will never desert you. We will act in your best interests.

Public: But discuss with us our "best interests." Consult us in weighing risks and planning outcomes.

Physicians: Yours are the governing goals, and ours are the medical means.

Public: We are partners in our care.

Physician: There can be no deceit between us.

Public: Make known to us all matters concerning our health, whether good or bad, certain or suspected.

Physicians: And you make known to us all matters concerning your health, whether good or bad, certain or suspected.

Public: Protect our confidences as best you can and tell us wherein you cannot.

Physicians: Pressures come from all quarters: government, families, agencies, and organizations.

Public: But we are your patients. It is our will you need to know, not government's, not family's.

Physicians: We will be your advocate.

Public: Guided by our will.

Physicians: And by the laws and regulations of the land.

Public: So long as they are just and democratically determined.

Physicians: When forming public policy, we will do justice.

Public: Be rational and impartial.

Physicians: As human life is infinitely precious, so it is infinitely complex. It far surpasses human knowledge.

Public: Moreover, we are each unique in our complexity.

Physicians: Certainty eludes us, mistakes will happen: we are not gods; we work, explore, and serve. Our craft is art and science.

Public: We understand the stress of uncertainty and applaud your willingness to work within it.

Physicians: We will be the best we can and do the best we know.

Public: We cannot ask for more.

Unison: As physicians and patients in the sight of each other and in light of all we hold sacred, we make this covenant with each other. So be it.

These oaths were historically structured as covenants and remain so today, even in these recent, very modern interpretations. The dominant oath taken today remains the Oath of Hippocrates. It is a covenant of obligation, but only among the members of the profession of medicine who take the oath as well. Unfortunately, in most oaths, patients are not yet a party to any covenant of obligation with their physicians. Furthermore, communities are not called into the covenant in the way that the ancient Hebrews were called to act as a group to ensure healthy and viable people. Rarely are the specific duties or obligations of patients mentioned, nor are patients held accountable for their behavior. Patients are not asked or required to take a vow. They are not called to act in any particular way. They will not suffer the consequences of any failure to comply with a physician's orders. The Hippocratic Oath, if it describes a covenant between physicians and patients—and I believe it does—describes a covenant of grant. Is this distinction important? I believe it is.

The Emergence of Contracts Within the Medical Covenant

Physicians face a daunting task in the United States to provide clinical care under a Hippocratic-style oath. They practice within both types of covenant simultaneously. The covenant of obligation among members of the profession promotes progress in the healing arts and sciences. It facilitates the development of new knowledge. It also creates a fraternity and provides the support to sustain a difficult life of practice.

But by virtue of the Hippocratic oath, healers also practice within a more limited—and for them, more demanding—covenant of grant with patients. Physicians provide, but patients are not expected to reciprocate. There are clearly some returns for physicians that derive from patients—primarily income and respect—but the patient is not, by covenant, engaged in joining the healing venture. Healing is treated as if it were the domain and responsibility of the physician alone, acting within the scope of his knowledge and skill and with the help of the divine. Without the reciprocal obligation of the patient to likewise participate in the healing, it is little wonder that the physician would need to rely on the assistance of the divine. Unlike the values suggested by Maimonides, patients are not enjoined to follow the prescriptions of the physician or to avoid the bad advice of family and friends. Unlike the modern covenant-dialogue between physicians and the public, there is no recognition that health is a partnership. If patients were engaged in a covenant of obligation rather than the more limited covenant of grant, they would be more likely to follow directives and assume more personal responsibility for their care. As it is, the physician-patient relationship does not call upon them to do so. To complicate matters for the physician today, the covenant is established with patients, but the process of providing care and the payment for care is established by contract with other parties acting on behalf of the patients' and others' interests. Physicians, acting within covenant, cannot abandon patients. Individual clinicians cannot abandon individual patients, and the profession as a whole cannot turn back several millennia of calendar pages to abandon society.

The emergence of contracts has complicated the demands of healing for any of the healing professions that take, and feel bound by, the covenants as they are intended to function. A contract is defined as:

> A promise, or a set of promises, for breach of which the law gives remedy, of the performance of which the law in some way recognizes as a duty. [1 Williston, Contracts §1.] The essentials of a valid contract are "parties competent to contract, a proper subject matter, consideration, mutuality of agreement and mutuality of obligation." [286 N.W. 884, 886]; "a transaction involving two or more individuals whereby each becomes obligated to the other, with reciprocal rights to demand performance of what is promised by each respectively." [282 P. 2d 1984, 1088].[14]

The law specifies several types of contracts. Bilateral contracts are between two parties, cost-plus contracts allow for costs plus a percentage profit, oral contracts require no written documents, and output contracts require delivery and receipt of all the products of the work. In contracts, the exact duties and responsibilities of each party are clearly specified and carefully reviewed by attorneys or representatives of the parties. Contracts contain exit clauses and time limits. They limit the rights of the parties in explicitly described ways. Contracts assume at the outset that each of the parties acts solely from self-interest. In that case, it is in the "interest" of one party to guard against the "self-interest" of the other by building in carefully described requirements. Contracts require payment for the expected performance. In contracts, non-performance is anticipated and, therefore, legal enforcement provisions and penalties are built in. Contracts can be enforced in courts.

As a party to a contract with health plans and payers, the physician becomes a contractor. A contractor is defined as "one who is a party to a contract; also one who contracts to do the work for another."[15] A physician is considered to be an independent contractor, or "one who makes an agreement with another to do a piece of work, retaining in himself control of the means, method, and manner of producing the result to be accomplished, neither party having the right to terminate the contract at will."[16]

Acting within a covenant, as May has said, requires that a physician live within a "24/7" lifestyle. Being "on covenant" is much more difficult than being "on call" in a physician's practice or "on contract" with a payer. There is no time off from the covenant. There is no time outside the covenant. There is no canceling a covenant. For each of the twenty-four hours of the day and each of the seven days of the week, physicians are bound by the covenant in Hippocratic Oath, with obligations to fellow healers. They are also bound by the covenant in the Hippocratic oath to "grant healing" to their patients. They receive support from fellow healers, but there is no such reciprocity on the part of patients. Regardless of the time of day or particular activity, a healer is a healer—whether in relationship to fellow healers or to patients. Regardless of what the office schedule or managed care contract reads, physicians are always "on call," if you will, in the context of the covenant.

In addition to the parameters of covenants of obligation and grant, today's physicians also practice within the context of a contract. Contracts specify, in greater or lesser detail, how the physician will carry out the covenant. Increasingly, those contracts are specific about how the physician will be expected to practice. Few contracts recognize the comprehensiveness of the binding covenant relationships within which physicians practice, nor could they. As a result, the compensation for performance under the contract is inadequate for the level of responsibility that we expect from these healers as they practice their art. And then it gets worse. The accelerated introduction of new medicines and technologies places additional demands on physicians who must work under capitation contracts and live within the covenant. How? Physicians, obligated under covenants to provide care, must adopt the new technologies they feel are viable for healing patients. Yet no contract recognizes the increased costs associated with those innovations. As a result, the physician is left in the untenable position of failing to treat for lack of resources, yet living and working constantly within the covenant. The "market" today does not recognize or value that the modern healer/physician lives a demanding, unrelenting, obligation to patients. Is this a realistic or fair and reasonable expectation in today's world? Is it any wonder that physicians, in particular—though they have not been the only healers to feel the tensions of managed care—have bristled under the demands of managed care? Regardless of the circumstances of the contractual relationships, they were still obliged by their covenantal ones. Is the nature of covenant antiquated? Is it outdated in today's pursuit of health and healing? I think not.

Engaging Covenants in Health Care Today

Although they have ancient roots, notions of covenant and sacred origins of the healing arts are not outdated. They continue to be central to healing enterprises today. This is a critical time to be more explicit about these foundations of healing and return to them in whatever ways possible to address the health care needs of the nation. Doing so will help us come to grips with the challenges and maximize the opportunities in health care today. Failing to do so will stretch our healers to the breaking point and will fail to recognize that patients and communities, who heretofore have been passive recipients of healing largesse, must become more engaged in assuring their health. Covenants should be central to each of the practices within health care and must be among the fundamental considerations of everyone in healing endeavors. "Everyone" means every individual patient, scientist, clinician, health care executive, government bureaucrat, legislator, employer and community.

This notion is not new. It was proposed by Dr. Donald Berwick, president of the Institute for Health Care Improvement, and others in a *British Medical Journal* editorial, "An Ethical Code for Everybody in Health Care," published in 1997. In it, Dr. Berwick notes the dilemmas created because important leaders and stakeholders have not adopted ethical codes. This is worse than it might seem, as ethical codes translate into standards and norms of practice. In an informal survey of attitudes, for example, he found that 83% of the health care executives who responded indicated that a surgeon who develops a new technique to reduce hospital length-of-stay and control post-operative pain is ethically obligated to share his discovery. Only 56% believe that an HMO with similar insights is likewise obligated. Do we really want the corporate healers to abide by different ethical standards?[17]

Everyone should be invited into a covenant—a covenant of obligation, that is. For some, particularly physicians, this will mean re-engaging, re-invigorating, and re-inventing the covenants they have held for so long. For others, particularly for patients and communities, this will entail crafting a covenant where no explicit covenant has existed in the past. For still others—those who support clinical care in the health care infrastructure of research, education, management, advertising, legislation and payment bureaucracies—this will require a radical recognition that they, too, work within the same healing enterprise as clinicians, have the same responsibilities to patients, and, therefore, should be brought into covenants with each other and with patients. At the heart of the crises in health care today is an opportunity to design symmetry and synergy in the relationships between healers and patients, among healers, and within communities.

Seeking covenant alone will not resolve all of the issues

we must address to achieve the promises of the healing arts and sciences today, but it will help tremendously. Failure to do so will surely contribute to the further decline of the healing enterprise; hence embracing covenant in the fullness of its potential should be considered as an important step in advancing the health arts and sciences. Failure to do so will ignore the fact that we can no longer afford business-as-usual tweaks to financing formulas, more burdensome regulations of providers, and hand-wringing over patient noncompliance. There are too many diseases to treat. An aging population is destined to have more of them than ever before, and this shrinking globe is bound to bring more of them to our shores.

The concept of covenant, itself, is not radical. It is really quite conservative. To recreate and enliven covenants in health care would be restorative and potentially healing for individuals, for the system, and for society as well. It is precisely the notion of covenant that would enrich health care relationships and allow us to craft the public policy debate on more fruitful ground.

Without such a restorative attempt, we will continue to drift in a direction that strays from its sound origins and is likely to collapse under the weight of its own conflict and confusion. This conflict should be resolved by returning to the foundations of our relationships as healers and patients. This confusion should be addressed by engaging each other in dialogue about what we value within health care and how we will pursue it jointly as patients, healers, and communities.

Each of us, at one time or another, participates as a patient in health care today. Even healers become patients, since—as in ancient times—today's healers turn to other healers when they are in need of care. We have the incentive, then, to take an especially close look at the role of patients in the process of healing, including the most important health care measures of all—those practiced by patients between clinical visits, when the critical prevention and treatment regimens are managed at home. Further, we are all, patients and healers alike, members of communities whose decisions about safe water and food, traffic safety enforcement, unemployment, poverty, warfare, and tax-supported health care will impact on our ability to be healthy.

There is no room in this discussion for old professional jealousies, territoriality, secret incantations of science, and mystical methods of clinical discernment. There is no room for segmenting health and healing from other aspects of our lives, social systems, and economics. This is a time for entering the heart of the conflicts that drive us apart to find the values that bring us together as individual patients, healers, and communities—not only in this country, but throughout the world. This should be done by addressing health care covenants at the three levels at which they are broken, weak, or unformed: first, among those who are healers; second, between individual healers and patients; and third, among those in communities at the local, state, national, and even international levels.

The New Covenant Among Healers

The model covenants were created for physicians in the Hippocratic Oath and prayer of Maimonides, and it is the physician oaths that are best known. But others in the healing professions take oaths as well.

Pharmacists swear:

> At this time, I vow to devote my professional life to the service of all humankind through the profession of pharmacy. I will consider the welfare of humanity and relief of suffering my primary concerns. I will apply my knowledge, experience, and skills to the best of my ability to assure optimal drug therapy outcomes of the patients I serve. I will keep abreast of developments and maintain professional competence in my profession of pharmacy. I will maintain the highest principles of moral, ethical and legal conduct. I will embrace and advocate change in the

profession of pharmacy that improves patient care. I take these vows voluntarily with the full realization of the responsibility with which I am entrusted by the public.

Nurses take the Nightingale Pledge:

I solemnly pledge myself before God and in the presence of this assembly: To pass my life in purity and to practice my profession faithfully; I will abstain from whatever is deleterious and mischievous and will not take or know- ingly administer any harmful drug; I will do all in my power to maintain and elevate the standard of my pro- fession and will hold in confidence all personal matters committed to my keeping and all family affairs coming to my knowledge in the practice of my calling; With loyalty will I endeavor to aid the physician in his work, and devote myself to the welfare of those committed to my care.

Members of the American College of Healthcare Executives pledge to:

Abide by its Code of Ethics; Contribute to the advance- ment of our profession by exemplifying competence and leadership in healthcare management; Commit to life- long learning by maintaining a personal program of continuing education; Contribute to the improvement of my community's health status; Enhance our profession through leadership in a wide range of community and professional activities; Uphold and further the mission of the American College of Healthcare Executives to advance healthcare leadership and management excel- lence.

To engage new covenants with patients and communi- ties, healers today should re-engage their own covenants first. This should be done in several ways. To begin, those healers in medicine, nursing, and pharmacy with existing oaths should revise and expand their oaths. It is unlikely

---

that, under examination, they will choose to abandon the covenant of obligation that they feel now toward each other. It is likely, however, that they will need to reconsider how those obligations flow to those who are in other related healing professions. For example, it is unlikely that physicians, nurses, or pharmacists will decide that they will no longer impart their skills to the younger generation of students, interns, and residents learning in the ranks behind them. Even those healers who are uninvolved in formal medical education have the opportunities, and use them, to impart their knowledge to the young.

It is likely, however, that they may consider broadening their view of peer relations to other professional groups who have recently emerged as having particular specialty skills or who have demonstrated the ability to enhance patient healing. Pharmacists come to mind. Recent advanced education, coupled with computer information systems and a plethora of new medicines, have made pharmacists a more important addition to the clinical care team. No longer relegated to counting pills, pharmacists increasingly use their clinical acumen to counsel physicians and patients on appropriate prescribing, dosing, and compliance with medicines. As a result, they are no longer subordinate to the prescribing clinician; they are capable clinicians in their own right on whom physicians and patients are heavily dependent. Pharmacists are the only healer today capable of monitoring the increasingly common and potentially deadly practice of patient self-medication with combinations of prescriptions, over-the-counter, and herbal remedies. It would be a missed opportunity for all involved to neglect to marry the professional covenants together in such a way that the obligations do not flow freely between the two.

Critical to all the covenants of the healing professions, the elements contained therein should provide the structure for a true covenant of obligation with the patients they serve. It is the stronger party, after all, who creates the relationship and its requirements and invites the other to join. By virtue of the knowledge of the professional and the vulnerability of the patient, it is the professional who must take this first step. This step will involve determining how responsibilities of the patient should be engaged to optimize the healing encounter and support the health of the patient throughout life—on those days when patients are healthy and on those days when they are not.

Having accomplished this task, healers with reinvigorated covenants should lead the dialogue with others in health care who support clinical care and healing. Where necessary, this may mean engaging the others in an oath similar to the one offered to health profession graduates generally. At graduation, some schools offer a more general oath for those entering the healing professions, including those in health administration, public health, and management:

> I will devote my professional life to the service of humankind through my chosen profession. I will consider the welfare of humanity and relief of human suffering as my primary concern. I will apply my knowledge, experience, and skills to the best of my ability to assure optimal therapeutic outcomes for the patients I serve. I will keep abreast of developments and maintain professional competency in my profession. I will maintain the highest principles of moral, ethical, and legal conduct. I will embrace and advocate change in my profession that improves patient care. I take these vows voluntarily with the full realization of the responsibility with which I am entrusted by the public.

Or, if necessary, this may entail developing an oath more specific to the needs of the particular responsibilities of the profession within health care. It is less important whether the oaths in health care are general or specific. It is critical that there are oaths, and that they are pledged and lived by those engaged in healing enterprises today. By everyone, I do mean everyone. On this list, I include without hesitation everyone providing health care products and services for the benefit of people's health. I also include those who facilitate the delivery of healing products and services. This directs every individual engaged in healing—physician, nurse, technician, scientist, administrator, manager, marketer, insurer, legislator, regulator, or government bureaucrat—to become a party to a healer's covenant. This also includes pharmaceutical and medical device companies, e-commerce health care ventures, architects designing health care and living facilities, wholesalers managing the supply chain of goods, and telecommunication and financial service companies providing information and financing products. Everyone who participates in or supports healing enterprises is acting as healers did in the past. They are simply doing it in more sophisticated ways and to larger numbers of patients. Our societies are more complex and sophisticated today and so, too, are our healers.

Those who now seek to enter the healing arena in the family caregiver, alternative, or complimentary arenas of practice should be a party to the healing covenant. My mother is healthy and active today, but what happens when she needs more care than her twice-yearly checkups and daily prescriptions, and my brothers and I have to turn to an eldercare consultant, a nursing home, a home-care agency, a physical or speech therapist, a surgeon, a hospital, a hospice, and each other for her care? Whose patient will she be? She'll be our Mom, for sure, but she may also become our patient, along with other medical entities and individuals who help us care for her. Her physician will see her less often and will have less impact on the quality of her life and her health than the rest of us. All of us who care for her, whether we are her children or her home health aides, would become parties to the covenant that will care for her. All of us should be willing to embrace the ethics and the values that healers have through the ages, for that is what we will become.

Nobel Peace Prize winner Joseph Rotblat believes that scientists should take an oath similar to that of Hippocrates and vow to do no harm. Even if it is merely symbolic, he believes that it would lead scientists to consider the ethical and social issues involved in their ventures. I agree. I would add that everyone involved in such a critical arena as health care owes patients that same consideration regarding the wider issues.

This covenant of care would extend to those who do not currently see themselves as part of the healing enterprise. Take, for example, those who watch and report on health care and medical issues, or who manage health-related Internet sites. The *Boston Globe* recently announced that in the interest of public health they would no longer run tobacco advertising. They join a small, but growing group of newspaper publishers, including the *New York Times*, *The Christian Science Monitor*, the *Seattle Times* and the *San Jose Mercury News,* who have made similar pledges. Additional steps might now be taken in their reporting and advisory editorial content. A Canadian medical journal study found recently that advice in 50% of medical columns directed at the general public was inappropriate and 28% was dangerous to the point of being potentially life-threatening.[18] Similar studies should be undertaken to assess the accuracy of health advice on television network news and talk shows, and the media should be responsible for its health content. Our weather is provided to us by meteorologists accredited by the American Meteorological Society. Why not some similar assurance for our health information? Beyond the dangerous is the inflated or the incomplete, as well as the unbalanced view. According to a recent study conducted by the National Council on Aging, nearly one in four news stories about research and older women omits critical information. Internet health care providers add to the mix and add greatly to the confusion. Modern patients risk receiving the wrong information, becoming overwhelmed with variously accurate and inaccurate information and being underserved by it. There is a positive side and evidence that the media can act as healers. For example, 240 affiliates of the ABC Radio Network will soon launch a partnership with the Department of Health and Human Services. This effort will reach over 90% of African Americans in the U.S. with information about local care providers, public health issues, and ways to improve health. The project will be supported by an Internet website and will attempt to "Close the Health Gap" and reduce the disparities in care that so many African Americans face.

Leaders in health care can make great strides in reclaiming the positions they have lost over the past fifty years by initiating a dialogue to shift the paradigm back from contracts to covenants, and from covenants of grant with patients to covenants of obligation. These shifts must go beyond the mere mission and vision statements created in corporate climates of medicine. They must reach back to the foundations of care laid down in early civilization and project ahead to the needs of healing today and in the foreseeable future. Those forebears of modern healers may have lacked the scientific basis for their practices and cannot guide us today in the technical aspects of care, but they had a clearer perspective on the importance of the climate within which care should be delivered. Whatever they lacked in science, they possessed in soul. Whatever we have gained in data, information, and knowledge in the past several centuries, we seem to have lost in wisdom. Has science placed such a mountain of information in our path that everything we know is becoming a barrier to treating and healing in ways that are more fundamental, perhaps lower priced, certainly more satisfying, and perhaps more effective?

In the early 1980s, former President Jimmy Carter posed just such a question to a group of public health experts. He posited that we did not solely need more research to improve the health of most Americans. He believed that there was already substantial knowledge that we were not using in the best ways for the benefit of the nation. He wanted to know what could be done with existing knowledge to improve health and how he could best help in any such venture. The deliberations on his question were not easy, because the targets of opportunity were so numerous. In fact, he was right. We already know what we need to know to prevent and treat a vast majority of the diseases in this country, and certainly to prevent and treat diseases that are most costly. To answer President Carter's question, public health experts assessed disease and risk-factor categories for him. He was advised on conditions such as obesity, smoking, alcoholism, and accidents to determine how to change behavior. Should he have looked at the nature of the relationships instead? That is, at covenants? If the physicians who know the road to good health and the patients who are asked to walk it day-by-day had better relationships, would behaviors change? Would risks be reduced? Would the results have been more productive if his advisors had approached the underlying nature of the care-giving paradigm? Where would we be today if covenants had been considered in the early 1980s?

Crafting Covenants Between Healers and Patients

The model covenants created among healers should then be used to construct a covenant between individual healers and patients. These covenants should be developed initially by groups of healers and patients working together and then modified for the particular practices in health care where they need to be applied. The nature of the relationship and responsibilities of healers and patients within primary care, for example, may be specified somewhat differently than the nature of the relationships in critical care. The ease of access that patients expect for a preventive care visit is different than the access expected for a suspected heart attack or stroke. The parties to the healing of a child will be different than for an adult engaged in self-care. The case of an asthmatic child, for example, involves more than just the patient, parent, and physician. The school is involved as well, and in today's climate of "zero-tolerance" drug policies, asthmatic children who cannot carry inhalers are likely to be less compliant with drug dosing regimens and suffer more attacks. Likewise, the healer's expectations of the patient differ. Healers anticipate that patients can follow the directions for the tablet medicines they prescribe with relative ease, but caring for a home-infusion drug delivery system is altogether different. Physicians and pharmacists anticipate that patients and families providing for high levels of care will need additional training to assure compliance and proper use. Responsibilities, as well as rights, of each of the parties may vary by the type of care and need to be explicitly recognized.

With examples and models of healer-patient covenants in hand, each individual clinical healer should invite each patient into the covenant in a new way, building on the longstanding covenant of grant with patients, and encouraging and even requiring them to participate in a matured covenant of obligation. This covenant would establish the basis for reciprocity and mutual obligation that is so desperately needed now. This reciprocity should go beyond bill paying and social courtesy. Most physicians I know would gladly forego a good restaurant table for a more satisfying practice of the medical arts. It should promote the active participation of patients in the remedies that will promote and restore their health. It would involve those elements of lifestyle and personal responsibility of the patient and their families that would support the continued health of the patient, whether through prevention, treatment, recovery, or maintenance activities. Maimonides, for instance, included patients in his covenant, seeking their compliance with his remedies. He also included their families, hoping to protect patients from the bad advice of meddlesome relatives, and warning that their intervention could result in the patient's death. That was a beginning. On that foundation, a paradigm can be built to include patients within a modern covenant of obligation. From the paradigm will come the practices that will, over time, create new insights into the care of individuals and communities.

This dialogue is needed, particularly in an era in which patients' rights and the allegations of health care failure are so prominent in national policy dialogue. The reciprocity of rights and responsibilities of both parties—healer and patient—must be taken into account. Without defining the relationship—the covenant—in terms that call for patients (as well as healers) to take responsibilities as they secure rights, the goal of achieving health or relieving disease will not occur. This, by the way, is not easy for healers to do. Steeped within the covenant of grant that has framed their relationships with patients, the natural inclination of healers is to accept all the responsibility for the health outcomes of their patients.[19] Nonetheless, healers should shake themselves from that habit and initiate this debate. It is increasingly in their interest to do so. In the absence of such a covenant, healers will continue to bear the burdens of patients' failures to engage in responsible acts. To the degree that the healers and their enterprises are capitated, it is the healer, not the patient, who bears the most immediate and identifiable impact. It is true that patients who do not take their medicines eventually suffer the consequences, but healers paid under capitated contracts suffer as well. This is particularly true if their practice patterns, financial performance and public relations are monitored by quality groups, Wall Street, the press, and, in the late 1990s, tobacco-settlement-era trial attorneys. Failure to take medications will lead to longer spells of illness and sometimes hospitalizations. Failure to be immunized will do likewise. Failure to eat well, lose weight, and exercise will increase the costs of preventive care for hypertension. Inappropriate uses of over-the-counter medicines cause overdoses, accidental poisonings, and adverse-event inter-actions with prescriptions. Self-treatment without learned guidance can cause crises.

Respected health policy observer, Eli Ginzberg, reflect-ed on his own experiences when he asked,

> What is the most important lesson I derived . . . over a span of 70 years? Americans think of illness and disabil-ity as a condition that can be fixed by an expert, in this case a physician. Accordingly, they want more medicine, more research, and more physicians—all with a lower cost and equitable distribution. This was the case in 1930 and it is still the case today at century's end. However, the fact that each individual is ultimately responsible for the maintenance of his or her own health is a lesson that most Americans still need to learn.[20]

Reaching Out Toward a Covenant with Communities
The notions of covenant in healing should extend beyond the person-to-person encounters among physicians and between physicians and patients. Communities themselves are parties to health and should be invited to establish covenant relationships as well. What is a community? A community is any group that assembles itself into a recog-nizable unit. A community is a group of employees who work for the same employer; it is a town, a county, a state, and a nation. In a shrinking world, with the prevalence of the Internet and the ability of people and diseases to travel the globe within a matter of hours, community extends beyond our borders to include the entire planet. A commu-nity is fluid as our affiliations change, and we are all mem-bers of multiple communities. Are all communities of con-sequence to health? Potentially. Even the Internet, as we now know, is an important community. It does not just pro-vide information to the 60 million Americans who went on-line to search for health information last year[21], it is a "set-ting" in which disease can be transmitted. As research has demonstrated, people who search the Internet for sex are a high-risk community with higher rates of sexually transmit-

ted diseases than those who do not.[22]

What about the covenants among the members of the community? The most stunning advances in health have been made because of community-level action over the past 100 years. Increasing life span and improvements in the day-to-day quality of life were achieved not by medical care, but by the nearly invisible work and unsung heroes of public health. Modern science traces its understanding of public health back several hundred years. Ancient texts trace public health at least as far back as the divine edicts of God to Moses. Our living together, sharing common water, shelter, storage, and sewage enables our sharing of common plagues and bad habits. Our support of the public health infrastructure is, therefore, critical. Unfortunately, our funding of public health is appalling, and our recognition of its importance occurs only when the infrastructure breaks down and diseases break through. Experiences with E. coli contamination of food at state fairs and fast food restaurants, rabies exposure of children at petting farms, and West Nile Virus Encephalitis should be enough to raise our awareness about the importance of maintaining the public health infrastructure, even in a highly developed nation such as ours. Experiences with tuberculosis, HIV/AIDS, and bioterrorism should be enough to raise our awareness about the importance of creating global networks of disease prevention and management.

Public health today means more than just the safety and security of the community's infrastructure. It also includes our personal risk-taking behaviors. We increasingly impinge on the quality of each other's lives. We smoke, abuse alcohol and drugs, carry guns, drive fast, forget seatbelts, neglect immunizations, shun pre-natal care, and spread sexually transmitted diseases. When these risky behaviors result in high-cost illnesses and disabilities, we burden the tax-based and employer-paid systems that reimburse healers and health care enterprises for our care. Just as the ancient Israelites learned the interdependencies of personal and public health, so must we today. We must extend our understanding to include the reality that all of the health care we receive—especially when it is paid for in whole or in part through third-party mechanisms—is rarely an individual matter. It is all, now, a community matter.

The Fordham Institute for Innovation in Social Policy has reviewed the data of the past quarter century and concluded that the nation's Social Health Index is declining. The American Dream may be easier to realize, but as a nation we "feel worse." Why? The Institute measures sixteen aspects of social health: infant mortality, child abuse, children in poverty, teen suicide, teen drug abuse, high-school completion, average earnings, health insurance coverage, unemployment, poverty among the elderly, highway deaths due to alcohol, the homicide rate, affordable housing, food-stamp coverage, and the gap between the rich and poor. Ever since the mid-1970s, as the GDP has increased, the social well-being index has been falling, and the gap between the GDP and the Social Health Index is widening yearly. We must expect that these factors, which are so integrally related to the conditions within communities, do have an impact on health status and on health care. Particularly for those measures that relate to the health and well being of children and families, the measures have been declining most markedly in recent years.[23] Unless communities address these and other factors, the pressures on health, health care, and health costs will continue to grow. For too many nations beyond our borders, the challenges of poverty-related disease are even more staggering.

Communities must create the reciprocal relationships that will support the health of all their members, and they must work in partnership with other communities as well. An employer community can hardly expect a healthy workforce if the local municipal community does not support a clean, safe environment. Dealing with the health of communities is perhaps one of the most pressing needs in health care today. Not only do we have individual, private, and confidential matters concerning our own personal and separate health care needs, we also have needs in common with others. The community is the setting in which our needs and those of others are placed in conflict and can be brought into harmony. Increasingly, our communities have neglected this aspect of collective life. Some of our most contentious public policy issues arise from the collective relationships of community, and some of the greatest potential for resolution lies there as well. Some of the most important ways to improve health and reduce health care costs are born within communities. Smoking, food safety, gun control, traffic safety, immunizations, clean air and water, hazardous waste, rabies in urban animals, and pest infestation are community, not just personal health, concerns. Yet resolving each will require larger budgets and less liberty—tough issues for any community. Addressing these tensions will be one of the essential challenges of the next generation. Resolving them will require that the other covenants are acknowledged, in place, and practiced if we are to address the critical challenges that an aging population, advances in medical technology, and patient demand place upon us. Fortunately, a number of communities are leading the way in models that define health in terms that satisfy their needs and that address the social, economic, behavioral, public health, and clinical care imperatives of meeting those needs.

The Interdependence of Covenants

These new, modern covenants of obligation extend the reciprocity in the relationships in a number of ways. They extend the covenant of obligation among physicians to include obligations among all healers, between individual healers and patients, and among members of a community. They establish obligations of patients for the first time. They reach out to communities in a new way and call on them to be accountable. They create the foundation on which a new dialogue can be engaged in between healers and patients within a community, a state, a nation, and around the world. The healing enterprise today, now more than ever, depends on the actions of interdependent parties, acting in reciprocity in the context of a covenant of obligation.

As they currently stand, the relationships between healers and patients rest on the patient's dependency on the physician. This is a role patients have been encouraged to assume. Employers and health care financing systems have facilitated that dependency. In recent years, that dependency has shifted from a clinical dependency on physicians (with financial support from third parties) to clinical and financial dependency on the managed care organizations that contract with those physicians. Dependency, however, evokes a parent-child paradigm that is wholly unsatisfactory for the fulfillment of health goals and the development of mature health systems today.[24] Remaining child-like in the approach to our own health and healing deprives us of the opportunity to grow toward a greater potential that accepting responsibility entails.

This growth process may be painful. Change and growth frequently are. Without a deliberate covenant dialogue, however, we risk taking steps toward change that will be unproductive. We all remember adolescence and the developmental imperative to assert independence. Today's relationships in health care are taking on the appearance of the familiar rebellions of that stage of life. In many ways, patients are becoming independent. We are not taking our prescription medicines, we are ignoring the advice of physicians, and we are turning to alternatives on our own initiative. It is projected that nearly half the population is now using alternative and complementary therapies and that visits for alternative therapies exceed visits for primary care. Counting visits and the costs of products, Americans spent over $30 billion in 1997, paying for it mostly out-of-pocket. We are combining the prescription and over-the-counter medicines in ways that may be harmful. We are venturing into the land of herbals and unregulated, unproven products as if the "natural" is always better than today's health care offerings. We're not reading labels and may be mishandling many of the medicines we take. We trust the anonymous sources on the Internet more than the trained and licensed practitioner in the neighborhood. This type of rebellion may, in fact, be a necessary phase of development in human growth. It would be an unfortunate place for health care systems to get stuck, however. The same foundations of science and education that support traditional, clinical care should support self-care and alternative and complementary medicine as well. If managed care today required patients to use these alternatives without the benefit of the Food and Drug Administration (FDA) or other regulatory agencies' assurances of their safety and efficacy, we, as patients, would object.

Neither dependence nor independence is an attractive or satisfying state for adults. Childhood and adolescence are both necessary stages of human development, but each would be a horrible place to get stuck. Baby boomers are poised to use their political power to demand more from health care, and they should. But they should make those demands with the awareness of their responsibilities. The parents of the baby boomers were given entitlement reassurances through Medicare and employer-based reassurances through health insurance. Both created dependencies on modern health systems that are not capable of meeting the demands of the growing elderly population, which will become increasingly vocal and powerful as baby boomers age. With luck and some hard work, especially on the part of the health care community, we may be able to weather the storms of rebellion of this adolescent period in our national patient-driven maturation. With policy and political restraint on the part of the legislatures, we might succeed in reaching adulthood without institutionalizing the dependence and independence that are most common today.

The aim for individuals, as well as for society, should be to progress toward "interdependence." If healers, particularly physicians, wish to resume the effective and powerful roles that are deeply embedded in our tradition and culture, they must make the first moves toward creating and offering new covenants. They have both the historical and the legal prerogatives to do so. They remain, by law and tradition, the more responsible of the partners—both among healers and with patients. They should initiate the dialogue with each of the other parties involved in the healing enterprise. They must provide leadership.

When physicians have succeeded in creating a broader group of healers who have adopted and developed practices within covenants, they can then approach the tasks of dealing with patients as individuals and in community. In much the same way that good parents help their children to grow up, the healers of our society should take the initiative to confront the dependencies that they and their forebears have created in the patients they treat. This applies not only to those healers who are directly engaged in patient care, but also to those who are supporting and peripheral in medical care—including those in public health, health care company management, research, or public policy. The inclination of all these healers today has been to take too much responsibility from the shoulders of patients and place it on their own.

As a result of assuming all the responsibility and shielding patients and communities from difficult choices, the health care enterprise today finds itself in constant turmoil. It bears the internal conflicts over the allocation of power and professional practice. It struggles with how best to allocate the scarce resources given to it by the community. Its own identity is in crisis as it is being reformed by forces from the outside. It faces controversy with patients and the broader community on every front. Its costs are too high, its quality too low. More and more of its patients—estimated at upwards of 47 million at last count—have no health insurance. It has become responsible for limiting access and is being sued for succeeding in that responsibility. Its new products and services are perceived as too expensive. Its most valuable practices are second-guessed and under-paid. It is a target of fraud investigations by the Inspector General, the Justice Department, and the FBI. Neither its patients nor its healers are satisfied.

These are crises, but they are also opportunities. It is the opportunities that are the most exciting. We know that much of disease is lifestyle-caused and that a change in lifestyle can improve health. We know we can relieve sub-stantial illness, injury, cost, and suffering through the appli-cation of new treatment and care paradigms that create behavior change. We know that we can affect the clinical course of certain diseases by changing patient and family dynamics. We know that working with patients within the healing context can save lives. We are learning that the sta-tus and involvement of the patient in the healing process will differentially determine the effectiveness of the drugs we prescribe to heal him. We know that communities that support the health of their citizens can enjoy better quality of personal and collective life. Whether we are pushed by threats or pulled by opportunities into covenants, it is the next worthy step to take.

Part 2

AMERICAN CHALLENGES
AND OPPORTUNITIES

Each day arrives bearing gifts. Some are readily recognizable. They are the gifts of freedom, relative safety, good health, longevity, and prosperity far beyond what is enjoyed by the rest of the world. Even in trying times, Americans are among the most privileged. Even challenges and crises can be gifts. They provide us with the opportunity to examine how we live our lives, value our freedoms, express our compassion, resolve our conflicts, accept our responsibilities, care for our dying, and allocate our resources. These challenges and opportunities require that we address the immediate concerns for health and healing while we accommodate the different cultural, ethical, social, and political perspectives of heterogeneous communities in the United States.

How we care for the youngest, oldest, and weakest among us will be a reflection of our character. In the future, whether or not we decide to invest in biomedical research, patient-centered care, new communications, and the Internet, infrastructure development and public health will show how visionary our instincts are compared with those who came before us. How we reach out to the rest of the world with our health care technologies, or whether we reach out at all, will evidence our degree of health isolationism and our interest in the global community. How we study our genes, meet the demands of an aging society, and balance our rights and responsibilities will demonstrate the degree of maturity we attribute to patients and healers. How we monitor and manage the work of healers will indicate how much we continue to trust the covenants to which they ascribe are active influences in the practice of medicine and the healing arts.

These challenges and crises are gifts, because they will push the limits of defining ourselves as human beings, as members of communities and as participants in healing. They are not unique to this nation, our health care system, or cultural realities, but because we are the richest nation in the world we have a luxury to use these issues to explore our values about ourselves and our systems of healing. These challenges and opportunities will force us to examine each other and ourselves at the depths of who we are and what we view as important. Each can prompt a rich dialogue and can lead us to new, creative solutions to seemingly impossible dilemmas—especially, I believe, if these challenges and crises are examined in the context of the gifts of healing and in the presence of covenants of care.

Chapter 3

Interdependence

Covenant in Patients' Rights

*Historically, governments that provide rich legal rights to their
citizens have been endangered, not when the community
demanded that those who have rights also live up to their
social responsibilities, but when this was not done.[1]*

Amitai Etzioni

Early Roots of Rights and Responsibilities

Even in the earliest days of recorded civilization, the
relationship between healers and patients was structured and provided patients with rights. The Code of
Hammurabi is the oldest known example, and it is not
unlike today's quality-controlled, cost-managed, and
patient-rights environment. It established the relationship
between the healers and the patients of the day. It held
physicians accountable for bad clinical outcomes. It regulated access to care. It also set compensation.[2]

It is believed to be based on even older—3000 B.C.E.—
practices. If that is true, managing the relationships—
including the business relationships—between healers and
patients has been a long-standing practice in human history. American insurance systems and health policy didn't
invent it through employee benefits, union negotiations,
rules, regulations, or appropriations. It seems, though, that
even after 5,000 years of practice, we still can't seem to get
it right. Perhaps that will bring some comfort to those in
healing systems and managed care today. Perhaps it will
be both humbling and enlightening to those of us in health
policy circles. Apparently, we have not been as creative as
we believed about structuring health care. It is not as easy

as we might have hoped. Our thoughtful health care management plans and proposals are nothing more than the clinical and business relationship patterns established millennia ago, and we are still working to achieve the most palatable refinements. Our health care enterprise today is much more complex, but it does not operate much differently when it comes to the fundamentals.

The Healer's Accountability for Quality

Like their earlier counterparts, healers today are accountable. Physicians, nurses, and pharmacists are monitored and measured and have been since the earliest days of regulation in this country. They take exams, disclose personal information, and are subject to state licensing board reviews and Inspector General investigations. They have also been tracked in a National Provider Data Bank (NPDB) and monitored for criminal and malpractice experience. Hospitals and other institutions are assessed as well. The Joint Commission for the Accreditation of Health Care Organizations (JCAHO) assesses the quality of the care they deliver, and the stakes are high—slip in the ratings, and the care will not be reimbursed by third parties. In ancient times, governments sometimes took over production of herbals to assure their purity. Today, the quality of pharmaceutical and medical device products is monitored by government agencies.

These methods to measure healer performance and hold them accountable have improved over the years. We have become better at defining what we want in quality care and better at making the measures of it. The number of organizations doing the measuring has grown as well. The National Committee for Quality Assurance (NCQA) drives quality improvement for employers paying for care using its Health Plan Employer Data and Information Set (HEDIS). The Leapfrog Group has likewise created new standards and issued calls for improvements on behalf of leading employers. The Foundation for Accountability

---

(FACCT) is developing more "outcome-based" quality measures to track patients' experiences across an entire episode of care. The Agency for Health Care Research and Quality (AHRQ) is the federal government agency that is taking the lead in quality assurance. It has developed a comprehensive consumer satisfaction survey (known as "CAHPS") that complements HEDIS and other clinical assessment tools and enables consumers to compare the performance of health plans and providers. Peer Review Organizations (PROs) are physician-owned quality review organizations that assess quality, and each hospital and health insurance plan has its own method to track healers as well. Public and private sector purchaser coalitions measure quality to incorporate it into contracting and buying decisions. Esteemed private groups such as the Institute of Medicine[3] and respected individuals like George Lundberg[4] of the *Journal of the American Medical Association* examined medical error, quality, and trust problems and articulated them for the public and professionals alike to review. Unlike those days of old, we don't remove a surgeon's hand when an operation is unsuccessful, but we do remove operating privileges when we judge that too many surgeries result in bad outcomes. Physicians, other clinicians, and institutions are vilified in the press, held accountable in the courts and by Congress, and lose their licenses to practice as healers. Unlike those days of old, we don't make a physician pay for the life of a slave who dies under his care, but we do sue physicians for lost wages and damages if patients die and the healer is judged to be at fault.

The Healer's Accountability for Access and Cost

Historically, healers also played a role in assuring access. In ancient societies care was sometimes subsidized by the ruler, or by employers (as in the case of slaves), but healers were required to cooperate to assure access by yielding to a fee schedule. This fee schedule was not only based on the nature of the healer—surgeons were paid more than physicians and pharmacists—but also on the nature of the procedure and on a sliding scale to fit the status of the patient. Yesterday's gentlemen of rank paid more for the same services than did tradesmen or slaves. Tradesmen paid fees equivalent to half of what a gentleman would pay; owners of slaves paid half again as much for care of their slaves. Physicians were expected to treat patients without regard to payment status and, in fact, to provide charity care as required.

Similar fee arrangements are true today. Today's "gentlemen" and "persons of rank" are the insured or the wealthy that can afford care. This coverage is provided largely because the "gentleman" receives a health care benefit from an employer. In addition, as an employed person, some of these "persons of rank" can afford to pay out-of-pocket for care because of their individual wealth. These payment systems allowed a certain amount of cost shifting within the healing enterprises that developed in this country, and, with some subsidies from governments for the care of the very poor or the elderly, health care systems were able to sustain the infrastructures needed to survive and grow. This did not absolve healers of the responsibility to provide free care, however.

Recent years have brought changes to this delicate balance. Increasingly, new payment relationships are common. In some cases these are out-of-pocket arrangements. Some people seek complimentary and alternative treatments or care from alternative healers whose services are not reimbursed by third parties. In other cases, however, traditional healers have opted out of health payment systems and are offering—and individuals are accepting—arrangements in which traditional health care services are paid for directly by the patients themselves. Some physicians, for example, are opting out of third-party systems altogether and structuring practices based on exclusive, cash-only arrangements with limited numbers of people.

This situation changes the "balance of payments" that has been the foundation of the cost-shifting methods of financing care. "Persons of rank" and charity care from healers have subsidized care for others. This was so common and so embedded in our tradition of healing that we came to expect that the poor and the uninsured would receive care and that the health care safety net would be woven by our healers. We have come to expect that some care will be delivered at low- or no-fee because some patients are not economically privileged. Since the earliest days of practice—and in particular, since church councils ruled that healers, at least those associated with the religious healing traditions, should not practice medicine for profit—we have come to expect that some care would naturally be uncompensated.

There is no evidence from early times that society as a whole neglected to pay for its care. Even the religious healers of the Middle-Ages Christian tradition were paid. They were restricted only from profiting from their healing over and above the other tributes that were paid them by the local flock in their care. How unlike health care in contemporary America, where there is increasing resistance to paying for the cost of medical care. Furthermore, there does not appear to have been any collective effort on the part of buyers, even when the buyer was as powerful as the emperor, to leverage buying power, or to unite to purchase jointly at better rates. Not so, today. Concern for the cost of care has led governments and employers to take steps to reduce the financial liabilities associated with health care commitments. In turn, healers have counteracted these moves by changing age-old commitments to provide care to all, even at no charge.

Increasingly, powerful buyers and buying consortia are forming to get such low rates that the health care infrastructure is weakening. It is harder to get appointments with doctors and dentists. Hospitals are no longer staffed adequately for the intensity of care required by patients.

Institutions are strapped for cash and unable to make improvements in the data and information systems that would support more effective care. Added costs of patient care, training, and research in teaching facilities are not covered adequately. Training programs for medical residents, long supported by private and public sector payers, are underfunded. Pediatrics, in particular, has been hard hit. The best and the brightest centers of academic excellence are suffering and in danger of closing. Costs that shifted from one payment center to another years ago and that were covered by wealthier and more willing payers are in jeopardy because buyers today are prudent to the point of being stingy purchasers. Costs cannot be distributed across patients and payers refusing to pay for anything other than what they, alone, receive. As a result, research, teaching, and indigent care are falling by the wayside. Investor capital is drifting away from health care, envisioning a future where returns do not justify the risks of investment. Purchasers are getting the best bargain today, but scant assurance about the infrastructure for tomorrow. Healers of old had few tools for addressing disease problems, but apparently could be well paid for it. Today's healers have the tools, but greater difficulty in applying them in such adverse payment climates.

Lack of Reciprocity in the Covenant Relationship
Today's health care climate is adverse not only in terms of payment but in terms of responsibility as well. This, too, originates in the relationships of old. The Code of Hammurabi is consistent with other covenants of grant. Like the Oath of Hippocrates, it does not mention the responsibility of individuals, patients, and family members to care for themselves and each other, nor does it include directions to the community to do likewise in providing for healthy environments. There are no directions or requirements for healthy living. Hippocrates may have felt no reason to mention it because prevention, wellness, self-care,

---

and love of the body were already embodied in ancient Greek lifestyle. At any rate, the ancient codes which are the foundation of our practices today not only insulated patients from bad outcomes at the hands of physicians, they insulated people from the bad outcomes of their own unhealthy behavior and poor lifestyle choices. The codes also ignored the responsibilities of communities. Responsibility was shifted from the person (or patient) and community to the healer. Individuals and communities reaped all the benefits and bore none of the risks.

In a society in which prevention was the norm, the healer was respected, and his nostrums taken as directed, this imbalance between benefits and risks might not be so problematic. In today's climate of inadequately practiced prevention and eroded confidence in the practice of healing, this imbalance creates immense challenges. It traps today's insurance-financed, HMO-managed healers in a maddening descent into hell, defined by customer and community expectations, but not balanced by reciprocal obligations of any sort. There is plenty of evidence to detail what the public believes is wrong and how it now holds healers, and managed care in particular, responsible for the problems. Polling, focus group, marketing study, editorial, litigation, and talk show data abound. Complaints— and there are plenty of them—produce the easiest insights. Americans today are quick to comment on the length of office-visit waits, the cost of prescriptions, the conditions in nursing homes, and the surliness of hospital staff. We are ready with wish lists for quick fixes, cures, and easy answers to tough disease problems. Oh, and another thing: we'd rather not pay for it. Someone else should—either employers or the government—and, barring that, the providers themselves should be capable of footing the bill, especially for new developments in technology. At the same time, though, we neglect good personal health practices that could reduce the cost of care. As individuals, we eat too much, smoke too much, exercise too little, and take risks too often. We carry guns in the streets and in our schools. Then, as our behaviors make us sick, we want the providers of the care to patch the traumas and cure the sickness, at little or no extra cost. Or, so it seems.

But if patients are discontented, healers are even more so. Patients deal with the frustrations of today's health care episodically. The fact is most of us are healthy for the vast majority of our days. It is a minority of us who are ill at any given time, or have chronic or terminal illnesses that require constant care. We confront waits in outer offices on rare occasions. Healers, on the other hand, deal with their frustrations continually, so it is no surprise that healers want changes in health care as well. Many are as angry as their patients. Their work is no longer satisfying. They wonder if their clinical education has been wasted on filling out reimbursement forms, attending committee meetings, and dealing with bureaucratic dictates. Managed care pioneers who believed they were on the verge of finding the solutions to health care dilemmas have been excoriated in the press, blistered in Congress, and bankrupted out of business.

Communities are also concerned. Health care costs, unemployment, teen pregnancy, violence, and guns have taken a toll on community life and drained resources from the coffers that would otherwise support education, the arts, and business development. Not only are some people unhealthy, some communities are unhealthy as well. At a time when the armamentarium for clinical care and public health is at its best and is positioned to add value to life and years, it isn't clear who should make the first move to create the necessary changes that will re-inspire confidence and rebuild relationships.

Limitations of the Current Covenants of Grant

We're stuck in these doldrums because our health care system today has not progressed beyond ancient times in an important way—our health care system is still a covenant of grant in which patients and communities receive from, but do not reciprocate with, their healers. It is a covenant of grant in which health care payment systems further insulate patients and communities from the financial consequences of unhealthy behaviors. It is a covenant of grant that reinforces a dependency on healers that is frightening in its implications as the population ages. Making changes will be difficult because the covenant of grant has been further entrenched within the contracts of managed care.

Today's patients and communities are dependent on healers not only for health care services, but also, with the dawn of managed care and capitation, for the financing mechanisms to cover cost of the care. The patients of Hammurabi's era would have considered the economic costs of a clinical visit. Today's patients with third-party coverage—especially in managed care—have few such worries. What we as patients have gained in access, we have lost in incentive for personal responsibility. It is not just ancient societies that were guided by myths; ours is as well. A new mythology has arisen in our modern culture that is dangerous for healers, patients, and communities alike. We have come to believe that it is more in the interest of payers, including employers and managed care—or the newly merged healer-payer of managed care—to care for patients, than it is in the patient's interest to care for themselves. This mythology ignores that individual people, themselves, reap benefits that merit some contribution of their own in time, effort, or financing. It ignores the fact that some of the best health care a person can get is not the clinical care in the healer's office or hospital, but the preventive measures and lifestyle choices made in their own homes, workplaces, and communities. Whatever our healers do for us in choosing diagnostic measures and available therapies, the most important choices people make are those between visits to healers. It is not the clinical decisions healers make that create the best value in health, but the lifestyle choices patients make and communities support day to day.

The benefits of prevention are too often stated in ways that promote this mythology, holding the managed care healer-payer responsible for assuring that patients take even the most clear and simple preventive measures. For example, one HEDIS measure assesses quality according to the number of patients who receive influenza vaccines. Why should managed care be responsible for assuring that its patients are protected from flu? How far do those responsibilities reach? With information? With patient tracking and recall systems? With free vaccine? How could any adult today not know that flu is seasonal, that a vaccine can prevent or ease the disease, and that it is cost-effective for the individual—not just for the managed care healer-payer or the nation—to receive it? What additional information and shot clinics should managed care possibly provide? What should it need to provide when a multibillion dollar cough and cold products industry advertises extensively each year about the symptoms of flu, and visiting nurses, WalMart, and neighborhood pharmacies offer easy and inexpensive access to the vaccine, at a cost equivalent to a few soft drinks? Local news broadcasts track the arrival of the offending viruses. Families suffer as parents and children alike lose work and school days to the illness. Yet, how often have patients resisted and avoided even painless, low-cost, affordable items like the influenza vaccine? It is an indication of our covenant of grant in health care today that administration of flu vaccine is a measure of managed care healer quality and not patient responsibility.

Like other preventive measures, vaccines are too often viewed as benefiting the employer or the payer more than the patient. As people, in our dependency on our healers we too frequently say, "The payer (government, HMO, or employer) should pay for my vaccine, my check-ups, my health club, my obesity medications, because it will save them money in the long run." Legislatures too frequently agree. An entire industry has developed to make cost-effectiveness calculations, and it has flourished on the notion that health care benefits accrue to employer payers and managed care of a population's health care costs. This notion can reach extremes. One state legislative proposal is aimed at requiring HMOs to cover weight loss surgery for Medicaid patients at about $15,000 per patient, with the rationale that it will save money in the future by avoiding the costs of the ancillary diseases associated with obesity, such as diabetes and hypertension. Surely there are other less costly strategies for reducing obesity short of radical surgery. Is it that patients will not comply with lifestyle changes? Why should it be so much in the payers' best interests that even extreme solutions and doubtful procedures are mandated? Why aren't changes in behavior and lifestyle demanded of patients? These are important questions for this new era.

The dependency of patients and communities on their healers, which was established in the Oath of Hippocrates, reinforced in tradition, embedded in the culture of medicine, and facilitated by today's health financing systems, has exacerbated the current health care financing problems. This dependency has transferred too much of the responsibility in health care from the patient and the community to the healer. Healers are too often assigned responsibility for all aspects of care, cure, and cost. For the capitated health care provider today—and for the managed care systems that contract with employers and governments to provide care—attempting to provide care within a paradigm that expresses patient rights but not patient responsibilities is "mission impossible." By covenant and by contract, the healer is bound to care for the patient. The patient, on the other hand, is in no way obligated to reciprocate by practicing healthy behaviors or following orders.

Hypertension provides another example. In the care of the patient with high blood pressure, healers are obliged to use epidemiology and population studies to identify individuals who may be at risk of the disease, screen them for hypertension to diagnose the condition, counsel them about diet, smoking cessation, and exercise, prescribe anti-hypertensive medicines, and subsidize the cost of the drug. They are also expected to monitor compliance, remind patients to take the medicine along the way, and assess the outcome of the therapy, making changes as needed. The patient, on the other hand, need do nothing. The patient, living within the current covenant of grant with the healer and under financing plans with his employer (or government), is not required to show up for appointments, follow the dietary or exercise advice, stop smoking, or take the medicines. If the patient continues to come for care, the healer will be expected to repeat all the care-giving steps. If he does not come for care, the healer will be expected to find out why and encourage him to show up. If the patient has a heart attack or stroke—both likely outcomes of unmanaged hypertension—the healer will be expected to provide the access and quality of care for the emergency services, intensive care, surgery, and rehabilitation required to ensure survival and good quality of life afterwards. And the healer, particularly within the current managed care paradigm, will be expected to provide all of this within the negotiated, preferred, capitated rate.

What is the patient's responsibility? Few oaths address the reciprocity in the relationship between healers and patients. No oath addresses how to deal with the conflict in health care today over the increasing cost of care and any responsibility of the individual to help control those costs. Yet those opportunities to control costs are myriad, and the implications of not embracing these opportunities are frightening for providers of care. In today's capitated world of health care, it is the healer who bears the fiscal consequences of the failure of people and communities to practice good health behaviors. It is also the healers who have the best insights into how to reduce those costs through responsible behavior. As such, it will fall to the healers to address this issue in the individual contacts they have with patients, in the contracts they sign with managed care or health payers, and in the public policy settings within communities. There are a number of targets ripe for discussion—compliance, self-care, health behaviors, and public health.

In 1998, HBO aired a documentary entitled "Six Months to Live," which portrayed a patient's heroic efforts to comply with a healer's prescription. This documentary traced the experience of people facing terminal illness and seeking alternative paths to healing in addition to the traditional medical approaches of their clinicians. The story of one woman was compelling. In addition to dietary, attitudinal, and other therapeutic approaches, she visited a Native American healer. His prescription for her, in part, was that she spend a night, underground, naked, and alone, with Mother Earth. Her family spent that night praying for her above ground as she, wrapped in a quilt, descended into an underground, dugout space much like a small sweat lodge. The intention of the healer was that she contemplate her mortality and eventual return to the earth. It was, no doubt, an attempt to require her to deal with the fears about her eventual death, if not from this terminal condition, then from some other in the future.

The nature of the prescription is clearly unusual in the context of today's healing practices in mainstream American medicine, and so is the response of the patient. She did it. She really did it! She spent the night, naked and alone, underground. How different from many patients in this country today, who will fail to take even one antibiotic tablet per day for ten days. Studies have shown that between 20% and 30% of patients do not fill their prescriptions, and of those who do, many take incorrect doses, take medicines at the wrong time, forget to take doses, and stop medicines too soon. Logic would say that this is because the cost is too great. But surveys indicate otherwise. It is more often because they doubt the effectiveness of the medicine, fear side-effects, and decide they do not need it.[5] They do this independently, by the way, without consultation and benefit of their healer's guidance.

Self-care and the practice of prevention are other ways to reduce costs. We have the ability to control the most common contributors to death and health care costs: immunizations, tobacco, diet and exercise, and alcohol use. These behaviors drive infectious diseases, heart disease, cancer, accidents, chronic obstructive pulmonary disease, diabetes mellitus, and chronic liver disease.[6,7] They make their marks quickly on health care costs. In as short a time as 18 months, those who fail to practice prevention and engage in high-risk behaviors will use more health care resources.[8] Frequently, these factors combine, so it is difficult to sort out the individual contributions of each risky behavior to the cost of care. It is clear, however, that the costs to society are high.

Because we, as individuals, have failed to manage our own health practices, our behaviors are driving up costs. Although we suffer some of the consequences in life lost or quality of life reduced, we have not suffered financially as much as we should perhaps, because we have been largely insulated from the health care costs and the community consequences, including those in the workplace. In some ways, our healers have failed us in this respect—they have not been vocal enough about the cost implications of these lifestyle choices. In some ways, our payers have also failed us—they have paid for lifestyle-induced disease, further removing the responsibility we have to practice prevention and encouraging our dependencies on them to take care of us in any case. In some cases, our communities and employers have also fallen prey to accepting the parental role of providing coverage and care, without consequences.

Smoking-related medical expenses for the 48 million Americans who smoke, for example, hit an estimated $50 billion in 1993, or about $2.04 for every pack of cigarettes sold. These estimates are believed to be twice as high when they include workdays lost due to smoking-related illnesses. Smoking is linked to heart disease, respiratory infections, chronic bronchitis, stroke, emphysema, miscarriages, low-birthweight infants, and ulcers. Secondhand smoke is related to asthma and respiratory problems and to deaths from lung cancer and heart disease. Smoking by women has caused the lung cancer death rate among women to rise more than 400% from 1960 to 1990, making it the number one cause of cancer deaths among women, surpassing breast cancer. Overall, more than 400,000 people die each year due to tobacco-related diseases. Sixteen percent of high school students are frequent smokers, and that number has been on the rise.[9]

Add to that the costs from sedentary lifestyles and poor nutrition. In 1999, the total health costs of treating adult obesity in the United States was $238 billion—or roughly 25% of total health care costs.[10] People who are overweight are at increased risk for heart disease, stroke, cancer, diabetes, and osteoporosis. Obesity is considered the cause of more than 300,000 deaths per year. Estimates indicate that from 15% to 20% of children and 20% to 50% of adult Americans are overweight[11], and the matter is of such great importance that the Journal of the American Medical Association devoted an entire issue to obesity in October 1999.[12] Pharmaceutical companies believe that obesity drugs are possibly the world's biggest market. Analysts predict that sales of obesity drugs could exceed $26 billion in the United States alone. Treating only 25% of the patients at a cost of $3 per day would generate sales at that level.[13]

Limitations of Covenants of Grant with Communities
This same covenant of grant has been extended to communities, and with similar outcomes. Communities that fail to maintain a strong public health infrastructure and address social problems are insulated from the direct and immediate health care costs associated with those decisions. Over time they suffer from lost productivity and economic growth, but the immediate consequences are large-

ly hidden. A Harris Poll conducted in September 1999 indicated widespread support for public health measures, such as infectious disease control, immunization, safe water, air and waste disposal, and education for healthy lifestyles, particularly among the best educated and most politically influential.[14] Yet even those in favor of public health programs admitted that public health measures lacked the excitement of modern medical miracles, leaving political support for funding weak. Since it's modern miracles they expect, it's modern miracles they get; and, like patients, communities pass the bill on to "others." Too frequently, communities expect that local employers who pay for care and managed care organizations that provide it will continue to do so, absorbing the costs of innovations as they spill from research pipelines.

New medicines, devices, and surgery compete for other financial resources; in particular, the public health programs that care for communities. If adequate public health resources are unavailable, problems will become greater in the coming years and disease outbreaks will result. Food-related diseases, for example, have become increasingly common, with 76 million illnesses, 325,000 hospitalizations, and 5,000 deaths each year. The odds are one in four people will become ill from a food-borne illness each year.[15] One in 25 children is at risk of lead poisoning in the wake of inadequately funded screening programs.[16] A number of Healthy People 2000 goals were unmet, and some measures actually got worse. West Nile Virus (WNV) Encephalitis affected the Northeast in 1999. Once the crisis of new cases subsided, regional health commissioners worried aloud about how they would pay for local mosquito control programs to prevent outbreaks in future years.[17] Rabies is once again a problem. Three thousand children were exposed to a rabid goat at a travelling fair and required treatment at $1,500 each. Rabid raccoons released by hunters at a club in West Virginia have transmitted the disease to wild and domestic animals through the east, causing public health officials to advise that any contact with an unknown animal on the eastern seaboard must be viewed as a potential rabies contact and, tragically, causing severe injuries to at least one baby, who was attacked at his home in suburban Washington, D.C.[18] Air pollution continues to cause an estimated 50,000 to 120,000 premature deaths and $40–50 million in health costs annually from exposure to outdoor pollutants.[19] An outbreak of avian H5N1 influenza in Hong Kong recently alarmed the world medical community and demonstrated our vulnerability to a major outbreak. For influenza experts, this drove home the need to prepare for an expected pandemic. Since they are fully aware that there will not be adequate supplies of vaccine, some communities, particularly in areas of poverty, will be disproportionately adversely affected. The implications for physician and hospital costs are clear.

Besides shoring up the public health infrastructure, there are other notable social health targets. As a result of the failure to address the social issues of teenage sexuality, the U.S. has the highest teen pregnancy rate among developed countries. About one million teens become pregnant each year. Ninety-five percent of these pregnancies are unintentional, and one-third end in abortion. The cost of teenage pregnancy was $120 billion from 1985 to 1990. Forty-eight billion dollars could have been saved if the mother had waited until she was 20 to bear a child.[20] Other infants—more than 2,000 each year—are born with fetal alcohol syndrome (FAS), which causes growth retardation, facial abnormalities, and central nervous system dysfunction. Children often suffer lifelong consequences from *in utero* alcohol exposure as a result of their mother's drinking, which rose four-fold between 1991 and 1995. In 1992, the National Institutes of Health (NIH) estimated the annual cost of FAS from mental retardation to be $1.9 billion.[21]

Despite public health programs and a new endeavor to

apply epidemiology to the problems of injuries, they are one of the most frequent causes of death and among the most costly to the economy. Including homicide and suicide, injuries are the leading cause of years of potential life lost before age 75. The cost of injuries from automobile accidents, firearms, falls, fires, poisonings, and drownings is $260 billion. Of that amount, $69 billion (in 1993 dollars) was spent on health care costs for injury victims. That is 12% of all medical spending.[22] Injuries account for 46% of all emergency department costs, 10% of all hospital costs, and 16% of all outpatient costs.[23] Traffic crashes continue to be a leading public health problem and are still the leading cause of death for people aged 6 to 27, with total economic costs of $150 billion a year.[24] Despite widespread education and the availability of free car seats, 40% of children ages 1 to 4 years are still unrestrained and nearly 80% of safety seats are improperly secured.[25] The rate of death from firearms in the United States is more than eight times that of other economically developed nations, and the costs are also high. In 1990, firearm injuries cost over $20.4 billion in direct and indirect costs of health care, long-term disability, and premature death. At least 80% of those costs are paid by taxpayers.[26] Finally, in 1991, the costs associated with head injury or death from head injury due to bicycle accidents was $3 billion. It is believed that 75% of bicycle-related fatalities among children could be prevented if all children wore helmets. Every helmet worn saves this country $395 in direct health care costs and other costs to society. If 85% of children wore helmets for one year, the medical savings are estimated to be between $109 million and $142 million. One person who survives a head injury may cost $4 million in health care services over a lifetime.[27]

As individuals and communities, when we fail to address these drivers of health costs, the burden is shifted to employers, payers—including taxpayers—and healers. Payers are increasingly resistant to covering these costs and require that the healers bear the fiscal consequences of our illnesses and injuries. Too many of us prefer not to care for elderly parents and turn to healers to do it for us. We choose to allow guns on the street, keep guns at home and at school, repeal or fail to enforce helmet and traffic laws, and turn to healers to provide us with emergency care to tend our critical injuries. When we survive the accidents our risky behaviors have caused, we turn to healers at rehabilitation centers to restore lost function to damaged limbs and brains. When we fail to address the social issues driving teen pregnancy, we want healers to provide the neonatal intensive care that will keep our low birth-weight grandbabies alive—and they will. Healers are fast running out of strategies that control costs by tinkering with their own systems, however. In the future, patients and communities will need to take responsibilities for health approaches that will yield the desired cost-management results. Accepting personal responsibility, understanding risk in the population, developing targeted group interventions, case management, and multidisciplinary teams that will deal with social, juvenile justice, and education problems will be required. These programs will be invasive in the life of the individual and the community, but they will be necessary if we are to address the real needs of health and health care in the future.

Unfortunately, nowhere in the discussion of the modern miracles of medicine have healers confronted their individual patients, communities, or the nation as a whole with the true cost of the behaviors contributing to health care inflation. Likewise, nowhere do we systematically address the questions of conflicts the public must resolve as we confront the difficult issues of changing personal health and social behaviors. Even worse, nowhere have we systematically confronted the fact that some of the changes—like gun control—will challenge values and liberties.

Rationale for Covenants of Obligation with Patients and Communities

Much of today's disease is preventable, yet all indications are that we cannot assume that even the most advantaged of the citizens in this nation will practice good preventive health or adhere to a healer's advice. Our rates of medication compliance are low, we gain weight and lead sedentary lives, shun immunizations, drive fast on the highways and drive up costs that employers, taxpayers, and health care providers are expected to absorb. Over the decades of modern medical progress, healers have provided and people have come to expect medical solutions to all manner of physical, emotional, and social disease. Live a lifestyle that results in obesity, and healers have solutions for us. If they can't make us slim again, they can at least medicate or surgically correct the arthritis, diabetes, and heart disease that will result. If we choose to delay childbearing, healers will help us conceive with fertility medicines and *in vitro* fertilization.

This perspective is frightening, as too often the patterns of disease associated with the aging population have been taken as uncontrollable givens. In fact, they are not. Patterns of disease can change as patients and communities modify behaviors and improve public health systems. Patterns of disease had better change if we are going to retain employer-based systems of financing and solvency in federal programs like Medicare. As long as the nation avoids confronting the responsibilities of the individual and the community, health care today will be on the verge of a crisis that cannot be resolved with mere tinkering of per-member-per-month financing formulas, tighter Diagnosis-Related Group (DRG) payment rates, patient rights legislation, or HMO litigation.

How is this a matter of covenant? In much the same way that the divine edicts to Moses in Leviticus defined interrelationships in the life of the tribes of Israel, these questions present similar issues to us today. Our living together, sharing common water, shelter, storage, and sewage enables our sharing of common plagues and bad habits. Those who choose to practice bad public health habits place the health of their neighbors at risk. Unvaccinated individuals transmit preventable diseases to others, which is a consequence for the community, not just for the unvaccinated individual. Food service workers with lax hygiene transmit Hepatitis A to their customers. Areas with contaminated ground water transmit E. coli O57H:17 to children at state fairs. Towns without animal control operations leave their babies vulnerable to attacks by rabid raccoons. Polluted air keeps asthmatic children and adults from work and school. Drunk drivers and gun-toting teens kill others in their path.

In addition, we not only live together, we pay our health care bills together. Payers, and in particular managed care, might feel the first pinch, but ultimately, the buck stops with every worker and every taxpayer. As a result, we are jointly financially responsible for the costs of each other's healthy or unhealthy behaviors. Whether we pay taxes, buy insurance, or pay for care out of our pockets, the costs of irresponsible personal and health behaviors that increase the costs of care are borne by everyone. Risk in health care financing is never "assumed," it is "spread." As a result, few patients pay the true cost of their health insurance or their own care. Those who do pay—whether through insurance payments, lower wage rates, out-of-pocket payments, or taxes—bear the costs, to some degree, for all the care that is delivered—for other taxpayers and insured persons, but disproportionately for those whose high-risk behaviors result in high-cost care. The young person, insured or not, who rides a motorcycle without a helmet and suffers an accident most likely incurs high costs for the health care he will require for the rest of his life—up to $4 million is the likely expense. Even if the costs initially are borne by insurance, it is unlikely that insurance payments will be sufficient to cover them all. If, as is the case in so many high-risk/high-cost behaviors, this young person requires extensive care over some long term, he would most certainly require tax-supported Medicaid or other indigent charity patient support. Costs, when they exceed the billings, must be passed somewhere. There may be "free care" for an individual in a particular health care encounter, but there is no "free care" for an individual over a lifetime, for a community or for the nation.

Our personal and high-risk behaviors increasingly impinge on the quality of other people's lives. Likewise, our collective decision to fund or not fund community health programs increasingly impinges on us. The most stunning advances in health have been made at the community level in the past 100 years. Increasing life span and improvements in the day-to-day quality of life were supported not by medical care, but by community public health programs and personal lifestyles. Communities must create relationships that lead to reciprocity among their members to ensure health and conquer disease. This is perhaps one of the most pressing needs in health care today.

The community covenant of healing creates reciprocal relationships between healers, patients, and communities. It recognizes a reality of health care today: Not only do we relate to one another as individual patients and healers, but we do so within a context created for us with communities. What we do to protect and maintain our own good health benefits not just ourselves, but others as well. Conversely, steps taken by communities to protect the health of the public at large also have an impact on each of us as individuals. That impact might be directly related to the quality of life and health we enjoy, or it may be related to the overall cost of care that we all support. We have needs and depend on others to meet them. Others have needs and depend on us. This is precisely the reciprocity of relationship of a covenant of obligation.

Some of our most contentious public policy issues are embedded in community covenants. Resolving them will require that the nature of the other covenants be acknowledged, in place, and practiced. There is no other way to address the critical challenges that the advances in medical technology and patient demand place upon us. Some of these public policy issues are simmering on Main Street. Others are boiling in the halls of Congress. Still others have spilled over to Wall Street. They are most ready for change on matters regarding patients' rights.

The Patients' Bill of Rights

We are not facing these issues as much as we are backing into them. The health care world of the future is one in which costs will increase because of technology, demand, and demographics. It is one in which patients and communities are likely to remain dependent on healers. It is one in which, along with the mythologies of health care financing, we will add the fallacy that much of the new demand for services will be absorbed into previously negotiated capitation rates. Health policy "wonks," managed care executives, and some employers know we're at the breaking point. Consumers and communities, however, believe that an endless supply of health services and resources will be available—with little demand on their wallets and even less constraint on their lifestyles.

It is into this covenant-bound and contract-driven world of health care that patient expectation, frustration, and fear associated with managed care cost controls and large medical bureaucracies has finally spilled over into legislative debates. The most contentious of those are about the rights patients should have as they deal with today's healers, particularly those in managed care. Specific state and federal legislation has been debated for the past several years, proposing one sort of protection or another as patients and, occasionally, clinicians feared they were increasingly vulnerable to the large forces of corporate medicine.

Federal patient rights debates address two principal

---

concerns: access to care and slippage in quality, as corporate forces govern the healer-patient relationship. The list of patient rights is extensive and goes well beyond the contracts negotiated for patients by the employers and governments that arranged to pay for the care. Patients want guaranteed access to care in times of emergencies, access to specialists, and access to healers from outside the plan's negotiated network. They also want access to all pharmaceuticals and clinical trials for experimental treatments. They want continuity of care when switching plans. Patients want assurances that disadvantaged groups are not discriminated against, that medical records are kept confidential, that they can get help in a confusing medical marketplace, and that health plans will produce comparable information so that consumers can make better choices. They want quality. They want quality improvement processes within managed care, data collected to measure and monitor quality, and utilization review programs that are rational and based on good criteria. When there are disputes about care, patients want a timely review process to settle the dispute, if necessary, by outside, disinterested parties. They want the relationship with their own physician to be protected from business intrusions. They want doctors shielded from "gag orders" that prevent candid discussions of treatments and from medical necessity guidelines that are imposed by the HMO instead of accepted by the profession. When all else fails, they want to be able to sue the administrators of the plan providing the care. These demands reached the floor of Congress because there were problems in the halls of medicine.

States have also been an active ground for clarifying patient rights, and one in which protections have not only been debated, but enacted. In early 1994 the American Medical Association developed a model law, The Patient Protection Act, which was used the following year as a guide for states' legislation. It provided the template through 1996 and was later expanded to address

Managed Care Consumer Bill of Rights initiatives, which were more consumer-oriented. More than half the states have adopted some type of "Patient Bill of Rights." Included in the new state laws are provisions that address continuity of care, emergency care, direct access, freedom of choice, mandated benefits, consumer grievance procedures, bans on gag clauses, bans on financial incentives, provider protections, and provider profiling. Freedom of choice was a legislative proposal in 22 states, and mandated benefits were enacted in 26 states, requiring coverage of particular treatments and prescriptions. Financial incentives to compensate providers for ordering minimal care for patients are now banned in 25 states. Continuity of care legislation in 22 states addresses the problem of continuity when the individual's provider is terminated or disenrolls, or if the enrollee changes HMOs. In 42 states, emergency care legislation ensures that managed care organizations provide some type of reimbursement for the cost of emergency care services. In 37 states an individual may select an OB/GYN as their primary care provider, in three states individuals are permitted to use their chiropractor as their primary care provider, and in two states dermatologists can be considered as a primary care provider.

Harnessing the Voices of Patient Rights

The most articulate voices for patient rights are among the most advantaged in our society. Although these voices represent the poor, they more often represent the interests of the employed, who, unlike the growing number of Americans without health insurance, have some form of assistance to pay for most of their care. These vocal patients don't rely on charity care or government-funded programs. Unlike the poorest and unemployed Americans, they have the income to pay for those services that are not covered at all or require copayments. In today's economy, they are in stable relationships with employers, and their employers are providing a non-cash benefit that, for some with personal or family illnesses, will exceed the value of their salary earnings. For those who will not experience catastrophic events, the benefit brings a certain peace of mind from knowing that the protection against potentially devastating health care costs will not bankrupt family finances.

These vocal patients are precisely the people we would anticipate might be able to accept responsibility for the condition of their health. If they are currently healthy, we would anticipate that they would stay healthy. They would use fitness facilities, watch their diets, get flu shots, and take over-the-counter remedies well and in compliance with the label. If they are not in good health, we would anticipate they might be most able to make the behavior changes required to improve it. If they need medicines, we would anticipate that they would be most capable of following the prescription regimens or guiding their own self-care with advice from the local pharmacist. If they need more services than their insurance plan subsidizes, we would anticipate that they would be willing and able to spend some of their discretionary income on care for themselves. If they feel compassion for those less fortunate, we would anticipate that they would contribute to financing for others who cannot otherwise afford it.

We would expect those who are vocal to be the leaders in their communities. They would most probably be politically active. They would be among those we call the "elites," as we poll for public opinions. They are the people we would expect to have the best knowledge and understanding of the health care financing systems that are so stressed today. They would be capable of engaging in a dialogue to retrace how these dependencies were created and how relationships can be better structured to preserve the benefits that twenty-first century miracles can bring us.

Amidst their dissatisfaction is an opportunity to engage them, and other Americans—patients, healers, and their communities—in a discussion of how to better achieve what is most desired by everyone in promoting and assuring good health and access to health care. There is an opportunity to grow past the dependencies that are so widespread in our system today and move into the interdependencies on which everyone can thrive and realize their potential. Creating covenants that address both the rights and the responsibilities of the parties involved is one way to do that.

Creating Covenants of Obligation

Even after years of debate, no federal or state patient rights proposal encourages a covenant of obligation in healing among healers, patients, and communities. National patients' rights debates took a backseat to national security issues and provided health care players with a "cooling off" period for crafting new relationships in the post-terrorism era. Would it be possible to do so? I believe the answer is "yes."

The evidence is compelling. Increasingly, employers and health plans are responding with programs that assure many of the rights that patients have sought. More now have direct access to specialists and obstetric-gynecologic care, experience fewer referral barriers, and obtain quick external reviews when there are disputes with plans.

Would it be possible now to gain the reciprocal involvement of patients within the covenant? I believe this answer is "yes," too. Individuals can come to recognize that good health is its own reward and a worthwhile investment. They can come to understand that they themselves benefit much more from good health than their employers, payers, HMOs, and governments ever will. They can continue to struggle for more patient rights, care, and financing, but they can also recognize that with those rights must come the reciprocity of responsibility.

And what of communities? Can they be engaged? Again, I believe "yes." Communities, likewise, can continue to demand more miracles in medicine, but they can also recognize the value of public health systems and fund

---

them. Communities can work to improve public safety, prevent disease, and not shift the burden of illness to the healers in clinical practice. The nation can continue to expect efficiency and effectiveness from its healers, but it should balance any demands with expectations that people will accept their responsibilities as well. This will be possible if individuals, communities, and the nation will reconsider their covenants in health care, moving from the current covenant of grant and into covenants of obligation in healing.

Immunization for influenza provides one example of how a covenant of obligation among the three parties might work. Healers have a number of responsibilities. Public health officials are the healers who monitor the nature of the influenza strains, predict their occurrence in the country, define the vaccine cocktail, and encourage widespread immunization. Vaccine company healers are the ones who produce the vaccines, seek regulatory approval to market them, and ship them to immunization sites. Clinicians and other healers (including employers in some cases) provide immunizations to those who need them. Individuals have a number of responsibilities as well. They should seek the vaccines and, I believe, pay for them if they are employed. The vaccine is reasonably priced, and even with administration fees is rarely more costly than a few soft drinks. It is a worthwhile investment in personal and family health, and it is one way to prevent not only suffering from the disease, but transmission to others—including those we encounter in our work lives. Preventing disease in the workplace is a personal responsibility that translates into health expenditure savings for the employer, and this benefits all employees and shareholders of the company. The community should be responsible for making the vaccine available through public health clinics for those too poor to afford to pay through public health funding.

Those who fail to uphold their responsibilities should be accountable, and in recent years, it has been the individual who has been least subject to that criticism. Too many people have chosen not to receive influenza immunizations. One employer in Kentucky has developed a method for encouraging immunization. The company provides influenza vaccine at no charge to employees. Those who receive the vaccine and become ill with influenza during that year's season are given paid sick leave. Those who refuse immunizations are not given paid sick leave if they become ill. A managed care organization might consider something similar—offering reimbursement for antiviral products for influenza disease only for those enrollees who have been immunized.

Covenants of obligation should build on the existing covenants of grant and call for change in a number of areas. As in the case of any covenant, only the parties to it can adequately define its terms; only healers, patients, and their communities will be able to specify what they expect from each other and how they will agree to abide within the covenant relationships they will establish. It would be presumptuous to offer more than a directional paradigm here, but some items are clear and are called for implicitly within the dissatisfactions expressed by patients, healers, and communities today.

A covenant of obligation, with its rights and responsibilities, would address each of the players—the healer, the individual patient, and the community—and their mutual, interlocking relationships. A covenant would recognize that the health of the individual is dependent on the behavior of the individual patient, the healer, and the community. Likewise, the success of a healer's practice depends on the individual patient, the healer, and the community. The health of the community depends on behaviors of the individual patient, the healer, and the community. For example, a person will remain healthy to the degree that he practices prevention, has access to quality care, takes the advice of the healer, and lives in a community that provides safe water and streets. A healer's practice will yield successful results to the degree that the healer maintains a level of skill, has patients who follow medical advice, and practices within a community that provides financing for patient care—whether through employers or with public funds for those who cannot otherwise afford to pay. A community's health will be assured to the degree that patients follow good health practices, healers use peer review to monitor the quality of the care rendered, and the community invests in prevention and public health measures.

Other aspects of these interdependent relationships will lead to the health that the patient, the healers, and the community strive for, but those can only be determined if all the parties work collaboratively to make the choices about their mutual responsibilities to the others.

- Patient responsibilities. Each individual might assess their personal health practices and determine where they can make changes to improve the quality of their own health and life. Each of us, no doubt, can list any number of dietary, exercise, and risk-reducing practices that would prevent disease, reduce health care costs, and add years of enjoyment to our lives. Increasingly, there are health care, employer, Internet, and community resources available to help us make those changes. Patients can take personal steps to get the information they need—it is widely available today—and they can take the steps to change their behavior. In addition, each individual should assess the personal, family, and social problems they face in today's world. They cannot unilaterally resolve the problems that may contribute to their diseases and drive their need for health care resources, but each individual and family can make inroads toward improving the quality of their lives and their health. They can become politically active in creating community change to address the social problems that threaten their health and safety and drive health care costs. Patients can reconsider how to balance their expectations of healers with their own responsibilities for health. Patients might thoughtfully examine whether they expect the skill of their healers to compensate for the lifestyle risks that cause disease and disability. Patients might actively seek healers who will encourage interdependence in the healing encounter.

- Healer responsibilities. For their part, healers might now draw on the vast public health literature, with its information on how to prevent illness and improve health, and engage patients, employers, and community policymakers in a discussion of how to better address the patients' responsibilities. Healers might challenge why, wittingly or not, national policy has played into the current dependency dynamics, creating cost-quality access tensions that are impossible to resolve. Healers might question why patient rights bills are silent on the matter of patient responsibilities. Healers negotiating contracts with health payers might assure that the plans are written to make patients more responsible for the lifestyle that creates illness and drives medical expenditures.

- Community responsibilities. Communities must reconsider the nature of the public health and social infrastructure that supports the health of individual citizens and the community at large. There is some evidence that many communities are beginning to do just that. More should. Communities might find the way to support public health programs, educate legislators and public administrators and improve funding, even in the absence of "crises." Communities might assure that public health programs are not defunded when they are successful. Communities might resolve the social issues that drive health care costs, exploring the role of schools, families, businesses, law enforcement, and churches in working to reduce the factors that drive healing costs.

- Policymaker responsibilities. Policymakers and legislators might consider the dynamics of addressing
  issues this complex in political settings. The national
  and state governments that shepherd decisions on
  questions like these—if they are posed at all, and
  they rarely are—are geared to giving constituent voters the most for the least tax dollars. As a result,
  when the questions are posed, the answers yield not
  a balance among tradeoffs, but new benefits.
  Policymakers might search for other settings, off the
  "Hill" of politics that can more successfully resolve
  the tensions in health care today. If there are none,
  if politics is too intractable a venue, they might
  explore how politicians can avoid further entrenching
  the dysfunctional policies that promote today's
  dependencies and remove responsibility from
  patients and communities. Legislators might call a
  moratorium on mandated benefits until those mandates are coupled with patient and community
  responsibilities. Legislators might balance the
  responsibilities of managed care with rights for those
  organizations. They might, for example, allow managed care organizations to hold communities
  responsible for a portion of costs incurred for care
  when a public health failure results in widespread
  disease.

Can we bring a set of rights and responsibilities back
into balance? Can we shift our expectations from one of
total dependency on our healers to interdependency with
them to assure the best in access, quality, and cost for
everyone? The answer to these questions is yes, but only if
we succeed in creating something new in society's healing
enterprise—a true covenant of obligation in which the relationships offer rights, but require responsibilities. This will
require a level of reciprocity among patients, healers, and
communities. For patients this will mean embracing a new

way of living and accepting responsibility for their health. For healers, it will mean shedding the parental role, and some of the power and prestige that goes with it. For communities it will mean entering into new ventures of health and healing. For everyone it will mean creating, for the first time in American health care, a truly new covenant in healing.

Chapter 4

Curing Disease

Covenant in the Animal Research Conflict

> *I am writing a report on animal abuse. Please send me materials about what you do.*
>
> *Dear Researcher,*
> *I admire your dedication. Your ability to help people is really amazing. I hope one day to be someone like you. You have saved many lives. Thank you.*[1]

Letters from children to an association for biomedical research

Recognizing Needs and Filling Gaps

There are healers that patients rarely see. They are the researchers that explore the unknowns of the human body and push the limits of science in search of cures. Some work at the bedside, others work at the bench. Regardless of whether they ever treat patients successfully, their search for the answers to the challenges of health and the mystery of disease makes them valuable assets in the world of medicine today. Many of them are physicians and ascribe to a physician's oath, but even those who have not formally taken an oath operate within a covenant of sharing knowledge with their peers for the benefit of the patients they seek to help.

Their work is based on thousands of years of explorations about the nature of illness. Whether exploring evil forces, ill humors, or errant enzymes, they have worked tirelessly, sometimes outside the law—as in the Middle Ages, when dissection of cadavers was illegal—to systematically explore the workings and failings of the body. Despite the millennia of effort, the largesse of researchers, and the cures that they have provided us in modern American medicine, there are still quite a few diseases that can be neither prevented nor cured. The healers who treat us and the researchers who have developed the treatments have tremendous expertise. But even so, some of the therapies they have developed to prevent, treat, or cure our ills are expensive, painful, distasteful, and difficult for us as patients to comply with.

Whether scientists make advances to discover new, less expensive, more palatable solutions for our suffering will depend on a number of factors. Key among them will be our support of researchers' work and innovation. We support innovation through investments in biomedical research, adequate reimbursement for new and better alternatives, and a good supply of well-trained researchers working in well-equipped laboratories. After that, we rely on the hard work of those healers among us who have chosen the path of discovery, the advancement of knowledge, and the serendipity of science.

We have debated and lobbied each of these various ways to support innovation since government entered the biomedical research world in mid-century. The government contributed to research in a number of ways: providing research funding to agencies, training researchers, and hiring them. The government also granted rewards to the private sector for engaging in discovery. As the government gradually assumed the funding role of wealthy individuals and philanthropic foundations, the matter of biomedical research became a public domain. Research was conducted principally through the National Institutes of Health, though it was also conducted by other agencies, including the Centers for Disease Control and Prevention and the Departments of Agriculture, Labor, and Defense. Public funding allowed all eyes to focus on the nature of research in public institutions, its funding and its management. It allowed us to peer into the organizations, politics, and personalities that guided research for the nation. As discovery in the private sector was recognized as important, investors decided to risk their capital in hopes of finding discoveries and public policies changed to support innovation. Through the tax code, patent laws, purchasing decisions, and trade policy, rewards could be granted to those in the private sector using private capital to create the discoveries that would benefit the public. It was in the nation's interest to ensure that the research ideas and resources flowed freely into the search for cures and the improvement of health. The implications and the dollars at stake were substantial.

As a result, through its public, private, and not-for-profit institutions, the nation invested a small portion of its total health care spending—but still a hefty amount of funds—into its research enterprise. Total biomedical research funding in 1997 from both public and private sources was estimated to be $42 billion.[2] No total funding estimates are available since then, but from two sources alone—the National Institutes of Health (NIH) and the American pharmaceutical companies—the research investment exceeds $50 billion annually. Investments from the private pharmaceutical sector have doubled every five years since 1980.[3] These investments have yielded substantial progress. The span of our lives is longer and the quality of our lives better. Infectious disease no longer claim the lives of so many of our children; surgical techniques have improved outcomes and led to the wonder of human organ transplants. Research spending to develop therapies and prevent disease created benefits for the economy. For example, diabetes research spending of $181 million resulted in savings of $1.2 billion in annual Social Security Disability payments and returned income tax dollars to the Treasury as diabetics were more able to continue working at their jobs.[4] Kidney research spending of $9.8 million resulted in drugs that save $93 million annually in other health care costs.[5]

The examples could fill this book. Research stocked our shelves with over 5,000 prescription medicines, 300,000 over-the-counter products, and countless medical devices and surgical techniques to manage our health. Research also fueled an abundant and promising pipeline for the future. At this time, research costing over $24 billion is testing 500 new medicines for a dozen uncured diseases that currently cost us over $600 billion annually to manage, and without preventative or curative answers to just these dozen diseases, medical costs will rise even higher as the nation ages.[6] More solutions are on the way, for these and other conditions. Computer technologies will create "smart" medical devices; home- and self-care demands will create new products; and molecular medicine, minimally invasive procedures, and organ replacement options will become common. Research and discovery have never been more promising or worthy of support.

Debating Research

It might seem as if research ventures, as productive as they are, would constitute one of the more placid arenas of public policy. They do not. Lobbying and debates about research programs have had their contentious moments. HIV/AIDS activists fought for increases in research support in the 1980s, convinced that "low" levels of funding were the result of the bias against the groups who had contracted the disease. In the wake of their success in obtaining funding increases, a variety of other groups countered that women's health, children's health, cardiovascular health, and other disease conditions were actually more widespread and more deserving of funding than HIV/AIDS. Debates such as these could be protracted and were always political, but they had rarely become truly incendiary, except in one special area: research that uses animals as subjects. Whether and when to use animals in the course of making discoveries for the benefit of humans is an issue of longstanding controversy.

Controversy, per se, is not new or unusual in research. There are disagreements in virtually every aspect of research. Some of these disagreements are about the priority of the project, the level of funding for particular areas of investigation, or the qualifications of a designated researcher. Others are about the inclusion or exclusion of certain age, gender, or racial groups in the studies, the acceptable degree of patient risk, and the nature of patient consent. The peer-reviewed nature of research helps to surface such disagreements, and by addressing the differences of opinion of the various parties to the research, those projects actually improve.

Scientists do not shy away from controversy because it is often productive discourse. Disagreements are eventually resolved, largely through compromise. For the most part, these discussions yield better results of greater utility. Over time, research methods have been refined and have become more efficient, women have been included in clinical trials, drugs have been developed for children, rare diseases have been studied, consent procedures have improved, and human subjects have been better protected through external monitoring of research projects.

One type of research is notable because the conflict seems intractable and relationships among those who might resolve it are deteriorating. In the dispute concerning the use of animals in research, we seem unable to resolve our differences. We cannot even agree to disagree. Instead we have come to blows and bombs. It is only in the area of animal research that scientists must face the reality that their life's work, even when it creates a cure, will certainly create escalating, violent opposition.

Coming to Terms with Animals as Research Subjects

On April 5, 1999, an estimated $2 to $5 million worth of damage and lost research was sustained by two biomedical research facilities at the University of Minnesota.[7] Vandals damaged lab equipment, spray-painted walls, smashed computers, and released over 100 animals. Some of the animals were later recovered, dead or hungry, along roadsides. Press reports noted that the Animal Liberation Front claimed responsibility, and a student animal rights group held a vigil in support of the break-in several days later.

The break-in was a violation of the Animal Enterprises Protection Act, and the U.S. Senate had just passed a bill to strengthen the penalties under the Act. Would stiffer penalties be effective? Ingrid Newkirk, co-founder of People for the Ethical Treatment of Animals (PETA), thinks not. She told the journal *Nature* that the Senate action was nothing more than a "knee-jerk piece of legislation," adding: "Nobody in any social movement has ever been deterred from breaking and entering or arson because the penalties have been elevated."[8]

Incidents and attitudes such as these are typical of those who oppose animal research and create disruptions in many parts of society today. Children in elementary and high school science classes refuse to perform the types of animal dissections that were once rites of passage for their parents. Medical company executives are targeted for bombings and are followed as they drive home at night. Researchers, their families, and neighbors are attacked and harassed at home and at work. Protesters march outside government and university research facilities, sometimes breaking in, releasing animals, and destroying research records. It's enough to make some researchers want to quit—and some have.

In news reports, school children and Hollywood personalities are visible, but it is biomedical researchers who are the most highly vulnerable and who bear the day-to-day consequences for our society's disagreements over animal research. They bear the burden of the nation's failure to address these disputes immediately and tangibly. Sick people suffer, too, though not always visibly and rarely immediately. Anyone today who lacks an inexpensive, palatable, readily accessible prevention, treatment, or cure for which an animal model is key to the discovery or development of the therapy suffers as a result of these disputes.

Even people who are healthy today are affected, as everyone can anticipate that someday they are likely to need cures that will flow from research using animals. Any employer or health care payer that funds care for unrelieved disabilities or pays for palliative care where there are no cures also suffers. Although it is not widely recognized, most people and health care payers are affected by our unresolved conflicts over the use of animals in research.

Addressing the Tensions and Conflicts

Can we engage in a reasoned and rational debate about the use of animals in the biomedical research endeavors that advance medical discoveries? Should we be willing to use animals for research, including the dogs and cats that so many of us see as near-human companions, in experiments that are painful or in ways that restrain them in laboratories? How long will we tolerate animal experimentation while we search for alternatives to animals? Will we stop research in most disease areas because the nature of some animal research is repugnant to some of us? Will patients with today's incurable diseases be allowed to have a voice in these decisions about animal research? Can we resolve this issue peacefully, or will violence continue to hound the biomedical research community? These are the questions we must address together as we move into this century.

Yet as a society, we have failed to address these tensions. As a result, those healers who have dedicated their careers to research are under fire. Skirmishes and wars surround them and there is no demilitarized zone to assure their safety. There is no truce on the horizon, much less the promise of peace. There are neither cease-fires to anticipate, nor sanctuaries wherein to live and safely conduct research until a treaty is negotiated or animal replacements found. Worse, in the failure of our society to confront this issue, we have turned a blind eye to those who will ultimately bear the brunt of our inability to resolve this conflict:

the patients.

How did this happen? Will groups opposing animal research succeed in one of their goals—to end animal research by the year 2020–2030? What will happen to patients who rely on the discoveries that animal research enables? What is the impact of demonizing those on whom scientific progress depends? What perspectives of each side in this debate would enlighten the other? What motivates animal rights groups that might enliven our covenants with each other? What does this have to do with the covenant? Are other beings on the planet—animals in this case—parties to the covenant as well? If animals have rights, do they also have obligations? Does the covenant between researcher/healers and patients supercede any other covenant that other beings might enjoy? Might perspectives on covenant be helpful in resolving these disputes?

Ethical and Moral Views Differ

To those animal rights advocates who oppose animal research, covenant—or some notion like it—is precisely at the heart of the issue. They believe all living beings—trees, animals, fish, birds, and humans—enjoy equal rights to inhabit the world undisturbed. In the minds of animal research advocates, they do not.

Animal research advocates believe that because of the human being's ability to ascertain and behave in "higher" moral ways, human beings have greater authority to oversee all life. This authority extends to preserving and advancing life, even at the expense of sacrificing some lower forms of life for the good of humans. At the extremes, the lines are clearly drawn between the two camps—the animal research camp and the animal rights camp. It is easy to see that they hold different views.

The conflicts between these two camps have become deeply rooted in ethical issues with social and cultural biases. These issues have evolved over time. They also reflect economic realities. In 1860, for example, more than 90%

of all Americans lived and worked on farms, caring for and using animals to generate a livelihood. Today, that number is closer to 2%.[9] Any direct experience with the care and use of animals as sources of our food and clothing is virtually gone. In the experience of the average American today, food comes from the grocery already butchered, cleaned, packaged, and even pre-cooked; clothes come off the rack; and animals are not tools to be used, but furry companions with near-human qualities who are to be cared for, loved, and respected.

In the case of companion animals, views about their purpose and personalities are clear. We care for our companion animals very well. We purchase toys, clothing, and health insurance for them. We book appointments at salons for their grooming and pleasure. We use them as surrogates for children in childless marriages and companions in single households. Some have even become "healers" of a sort, visiting the sick and the elderly in Pet Partners programs intended to bring therapy, comfort, and companionship. They have become so important to us that we grieve their deaths and seek therapy to recover from such a loss.

Adaptations to a Changing Society

Other changes have taken place over the last one hundred years as well. Animals became less important for our livelihoods but more important to our life spans. As research methods and opportunities progressed, animals advanced human life by providing biological models to explore diseases and cures. Medical science, as it developed, began to use animals in much the same way as the family farmer, who acted on the belief that God—as reflected in the Judeo-Christian tradition—gave humans dominion over animals and plants for human welfare. Using animals to benefit humankind, therefore, was seen as the true and correct order of things in life, as ordained by a higher power.

The ideology of animal research supporters is based on traditional Western values: human beings are inherently good and have the moral authority to make decisions about natural resources; scientific advancement is positive; profit is desirable; and economic expansion is important for the continued evolution of the human race. This view does not condone needless pain and suffering, or even death, of the research animal, but it does not avoid the unpleasantness of such a task if the benefit is to save the life of a human. These views are in direct opposition to those in the animal rights camp.

The underpinnings of the animal rights supporters are traced to a different view of the world. In this view, human beings are not the pinnacle of creation, but are one of many creatures who are part of a balanced ecological system. Further, the very characteristics that make animals, and primates in particular, ideal research subjects are the same characteristics that should protect them from research risks. Primates, ideal because they are so like humans, deserve the same protections as humans. Specifically, animal rights proponents believe that the biblical approach of human dominance over nature promotes "speciesism," that is, preferring one species to another in the natural order of things, thus bringing nature out of alignment. They counter biblical notions with claims that Jesus was a vegetarian and would have granted animals their rights. Ingrid Newkirk, the most often quoted authority on animal rights views, has said: "Animal liberationists do not separate out the human animal, so there is no rational basis for saying that a human being has special rights. A rat is a pig is a dog is a boy. They're all mammals."[10]

It is not just in the area of research on animals, however, in which we have witnessed a change in attitude concerning research subjects. Over the past century, our views of research subjects have evolved into ethics in biomedical research. In the early days of this nation, for example, national racial attitudes shaped medical researchers' views concerning the tolerance of pain. This affected research on Indians and slaves. The European races were viewed as more "hypersensitive" and, therefore, poor research subjects in studies involving pain, while Native Americans and slaves were viewed as not perceiving pain until they became civilized. As a result, a famous gynecologic surgeon in the early 1800s performed experimental operations on slave women because "Negresses ... will bear cutting with nearly, if not quite, as much impunity as dogs and rabbits."[11] His view was common among those in the dominant culture of the day. Prior to our relatively recent ethical considerations of pediatric research, children, as well, were used as research subjects without the consent of their parents, exposing them to painful procedures, questionable experiments, and fatal diseases. Nazis performed human experiments without regard to the pain or dignity of their subjects—a fact that is positioned against animal research by artist Judy Chicago in *"Why Can't We Learn from the Past? Dachau/Silver Spring Study for Four Questions."* In this work, which is part of the artist's major project on the Holocaust, the high-altitude human experiments at Dachau are juxtaposed against experiments on primates at a Silver Spring, Maryland lab. Chicago states: "I keep asking: Where should the line be drawn between human experiments (which are generally unacceptable to most people) with animal experiments (which usually inflict intense suffering on the subjects but which most people accept, particularly if they 'save human lives')."[12]

Sophisticated Strategies Emerge

The animal rights groups promote their ideology in a variety of ways, and quite effectively so. Since animal rights groups tend to be more heterogeneous than the animal research groups, they can draw upon a wider variety of tactics for meeting their goals. This enhances the probability of their success. Some are peaceful, others are not. Those that are the most extreme tend to share belief systems anchored in socialist, equality-based views of the world. The more violent have links to the environmental movement and to terrorist organizations—something that is well documented internationally and followed by the Federal Bureau of Investigation. They share some traits with radical groups, as demonstrated by the statements of the most extreme of these activists. These groups view the use of animals akin to the abuse of humans. They see it as so entrenched that only a radical transformation of existing power structures and human consciousness can bring an end to it.[13] For these individuals, animal rights is a cause within a cause. Until the roots of the abuse are weeded from society, there can be no compromise.

Because the groups are so varied, some can act under cover of the others. Those that are violent can work with those that are peaceful to push the limits of their common agenda. Those that are peaceful can work with the animal research community to create incremental change. The general public, for example, believes that the Humane Society is a small, local operation of volunteers who shelter and neuter stray animals. In reality, however, the Humane Society of the United States (HSUS) is a powerful, politically active, national organization that is not affiliated with any local animal shelters or humane organizations. The HSUS operates nine regional offices and is the nation's largest animal protection organization, with more than 5 million members. HSUS promotes humane stewardship in the use of animals in factory farms, fashion runways, circus tents, rodeo shows, and local animal shelters.[14] But it also spends millions of dollars lobbying to eradicate a major segment of biomedical research that is dependent on animals. Although its activities are not violent, its leadership has grown more radical over the years, and some of the more extreme activists align themselves with HSUS initiatives.

Securing Public Support

Animal rights groups have positioned themselves as caring

---

individuals who are knowledgeable about the irresponsible practices of researchers. They also claim, and have been able to sustain due to the absence of compelling counter-claims, that there are alternatives to the use of animals in research. The decision to eliminate animal testing made by a consumer products company as significant as Proctor and Gamble confirms this view.

Animal rights groups have mastered the sound bites of modern communications. Further, and most interesting, they have succeeded in maintaining a favorable public image. Despite the presence of terrorists within their ranks, they are perceived as reasonable, compassionate individuals. Terrorist actions, such as threats against researchers and research lab break-ins, occur with relative frequency. Hundreds have been recorded over the last ten years, and in the last year alone militant activists have destroyed years of research and caused millions of dollars in damage to facilities. Yet animal rights groups have not lost favor with the public. In fact, they are very effective in securing public sympathy.

Animal rights groups are also effective in securing public policy support. They use litigation to increase lawsuits against animal research facilities. They use regulation to increase inspection of research facilities and reduce the use of certain species in biomedical research. They use state, local citizen, and parent participation in educational curricula to eliminate animals in science dissection lessons. They raise the barriers for the use of animals in public and private research centers, requiring ever greater care of those animals. They make communications about animal research increasingly difficult and risky. Though some tactics, taken individually, may seem trivial, collectively these incidents amass momentum and visibility and create precedents for new animal research barriers. Here are some examples:

- On April 21, 1999 the Supreme Court denied a petition appealing a federal appeals court ruling that gave human beings the right to sue on behalf of animals. This gives animals a standing in the judicial system.

- The Animal Legal Defense Fund ties up researchers' time and funds by suing the research community. The intention is to do this so often that researchers "won't know what courtroom they are supposed to appear in that day."[15]

- The Great Ape Project, backed by the Animal Legal Defense Fund, was a ballot initiative to give Great Apes human rights in New Zealand. Because New Zealand has no Great Apes, it was chosen as the location to initiate this change in public policy on the assumption that no interest or opposition would surface from the public. The initiative has failed so far, but if it succeeds it will create the first policy of its type and would create a precedent for similar policy efforts in nations that do have Great Apes.

- In England, animal rights activists orchestrated a campaign against Huntington Life Sciences, including abuse, intimidation, threats, property damage, arson, and physical assaults on people. A barrage of unwanted letters and packages was sent to employees' homes, company switchboards were jammed, and the financial backer of Huntington, NatWest, was targeted as well. Jail terms resulted for several members of the activist group, but not before Huntington lost its financial backers in the United Kingdom. The activism moved to the U.S. as activists targeted Stephens, Inc, a new Huntington backer, attempting to breach security at the office and blocking the street as workers attempted to leave for the day.

- Charitable groups have been targeted as well, attempting to stop donations to the March of Dimes because it is so dependent on public funds, fundraises over a short period of time, and hosts a major event—WalkAmerica—which is subject to easy disruption.

- In the United States, the 1966 Animal Welfare Act applies to all research facilities that use animals designated by the U.S. Secretary of Agriculture, including guinea pigs, hamsters, gerbils, rabbits, dogs, cats, non-human primates, marine mammals, farm animal species when used in biomedical research, and warm-blooded wild animals. Laboratory rats, mice (except field mice), and birds are not covered. The HSUS has petitioned the U.S. Department of Agriculture to add laboratory rats, mice, and birds to the list of designated animals. This would lead to annual inspections and detailed reports to account for each animal used in research. Since mice and rats comprise 90% of the animals used today, this expansion would create a substantial administrative and financial challenge for researchers.

- Finally, chimps bred in the early years of HIV/AIDS research are being phased out. Since they live up to 35 years past their time as research subjects and it is illegal to euthanize these animals, retirement communities or sanctuaries for chimps have been proposed. A task force of six animal rights groups has proposed The National Chimpanzee Research Retirement Act to advance this cause.

As radical as the actions of some animal rights groups might be, do they have a perspective that merits attention by the animal research culture? What steps should animal researchers take to resolve these seemingly intractable conflicts? Will the views of animal rights activists today represent yet another step in the evolution of human compassion? The attitudes and experiments performed on humans in the past one hundred years would be unimaginable today. Will we look back one hundred years from now and view this era as horrific for its use of animals? Is there a way to capitalize on the compassion, dignity, and humanity expressed in the animal rights views? Should there be greater protections for animals? Can we move deliberately to create alternatives to the use of animals in research? Can we protect animal research in the meantime? Can we find alternatives, not just for the benefit of the animals, but for the researchers and patients as well?

Defending Animal Research

Animal research defenders have so far proven to be no match for their opponents. In budgets they are outdone. It is estimated that animal groups collected more than $300 million in donations in 1998, while the two major animal research defense groups had budgets of less than one percent of that number. The efforts of the animal-rights opposition are successful and increasingly easy because the political landscape of the nation has shifted on this issue. The political environment has become more favorable toward the animal rights ideology as mainstream America has moved center-left on issues such as this. It is no longer easy to counterbalance the varied tactics of the animal rights groups within such a receptive environment. As a result, biomedical researchers supported by for-profit health care companies cannot be as vocal in defending animal research as they once were because the profit motives are suspect. Those supported by government grants and working principally in academia are also hampered, as the security systems that protect them and their research projects are inadequate for the potential threats from the more violent groups. The changed landscape makes researchers' politically incorrect views risky, especially in the context of today's disengaged public. The good intentions of researchers and even the clear, unmet needs of patients are not yet persuasive.

Animal research groups face other challenges also, and as a result they are no match for the tactics of their animal rights opponents. Communication plans are underfunded and are too diffuse to counter the specific targets of the animal rights groups. Animal research groups tend to be smaller, more homogeneous in their make-up, and more similar in their tactics than animal rights groups. They tend to focus on education and information about the value of research, science, and discovery. In the course of their educational messages they provide information about those projects that use animals, but because animal research is by no means their only message, the animal use components of the message are diluted. Academic, government, and private sector researchers are active in these educational and legislative lobbying projects in partnership with groups such as the National Association for Biomedical Research (NABR). They join state-based groups similar to NABR to educate school children and teachers on the importance of scientific discoveries in an effort to balance the anti-animal research messages now actively promoted to children by the animal rights groups. These activities are intended to help maintain whatever opportunity the animal research community has left, as the animal rights ideology progressively gains ground. Unfortunately, though, they distract researchers from a life's mission to discover cures and place researchers at even greater risks of retaliation.

Even these limited educational activities are vulnerable, however. Animal researchers are caring, compassionate, committed, and hardworking. Some are eloquent and passionate spokespeople. But most are afraid to speak out on the issue. Frankly, passion and commitment alone will not stem the tide of increasing barriers to animal research. The animal research community has attempted to identify and promote alternatives to the use of animals in research. Johns Hopkins Medical School houses the principal center for the study of alternatives, and numerous other groups in the private sector are seeking, albeit in limited ways, to end their use of animals. The NIH and a number of health care companies have provided funds for such purposes.[16]

Alternatives are emerging, and some are adequate replacements. There are not yet enough animal alternatives for use in the lab, however; nor are those alternatives adequate to demonstrate safety and efficacy to the FDA in compliance with its regulations for drug or device development and approval. Until the alternatives are accepted by the FDA, animal research must continue. Frankly, even the tangible products of their efforts—the medical discoveries, surgical procedures, pharmaceutical products, and insights into behavioral and physical mysteries—may not be enough. The balance between the rights of animals and the needs of patients has not been met, and the dynamics are tipping the scales away from research.

Engaging the Covenant
Unless a more productive dialogue is engaged between the animal rights and animal research communities, and unless patients and other healers become parties to the discussion, the animal rights effort is steaming ahead toward success in ending research on animals. The politics, the ethics, the economics, and the harassment will likely drive researchers and the use of animals out of the research enterprise. These threats to our national research endeavors have not ended with the September 11 terrorism experienced here—in fact, they have escalated. Animal rights extremism has continued with fire bombings, break-ins, and animal releases. As the Federal Bureau of Investigation is distracted on other fronts, addressing airline crashes, anthrax mail, and other national security issues, its resources have been diverted away from animal activist tactics.[17]

The result of such an outcome is not yet fully clear. Even today, animal research groups would like to reduce and, to the degree possible, eliminate the use of animals in their studies. Their long-term goals are similar to those of the animal rights groups. Animals are an expensive way to gain new knowledge and researchers are not, at heart, sadistic. It is the short-term goals of the researchers that are at odds with those of the animal rights groups. Researchers are not able to eliminate animals from studies at this time because there are not sufficient, legitimate alternatives. Regulatory agencies that approve products used by humans, and even by animals in their clinical care, do not sanction non-animal models as proof of safety and efficacy.

Given that both animal rights and animal research interests agree on the long-term objective, it seems that the issue is not one of whether science will end research on animals, but when and how. The HSUS initiative to end research involving unrelieved pain and distress in animals may or may not be met by its 2020 target, but the likelihood of ending all animal research within the predictable future is certain. It is likely that our children, or theirs, will live in a world in which researchers will not be using animals to explore health and disease. Alternatives will be sufficient, and regulatory requirements will be adjusted accordingly.

How will we continue discovery in the meantime? Will scientists continue to work under fire or will we come to peace? Who will tell today's impatient patients that they will not have treatments and cures for what ails them because the quality of an animal's life is more important than their own? How will we explain to our children that their diseases of middle and old age may not be treated for lack of knowledge and products? Conversely, how can we tell them that we allowed the research procedures that so many of them considered barbaric? How will new drugs be developed and proven safe for testing in humans if they have not yet been tested in animals? Can we accelerate the search for alternatives to animals? Will the nation provide better protection for its researchers/healers who use animals until alternatives are available? If animals have rights within the covenant, do they have responsibilities? If they join in the covenant, who will speak for them in creating and sustaining their reciprocal responsibilities to humankind? How do we engage the balance and seek the proper course within the covenant of care and discovery?

We in this nation have a covenant responsibility to those patients who are ill and with those researchers/healers who seek the cures to treat them. We also have a responsibility to the large segment of our fellow citizens who feel so strongly on this issue. As a nation, we have a responsibility to hear both voices—the one that calls for caring through discovery, and the one that calls for caring by ending research on animals. We have a responsibility to seek a peaceful resolution to the conflict. It would be a breakdown of the covenant of healing to allow these conflicts to threaten researchers and delay discoveries to cure disease. National leaders in research, clinical care, and government should create the forums, act as the arbitrators, engage the referees, and participate in the resolution. They should call upon those who are now activists to change their tactics, shift their focus, cease their violence, and seek peaceful solutions.

- It is through informed debates, rather than inflammatory rhetoric and terrorist activity, that this conflict should be resolved. In the meantime, in order to facilitate a resolution, it is time for a truce and a temporary cease-fire so that a real dialogue can begin. This dialogue must address how best to continue progress in discovery while we explore alternatives to animal research.

- Each side should acknowledge the concerns and views of the other, especially with regard to commonly held views. In this debate, the two sides have assumed polarizing positions and have hardened those positions over time. Demonizing the opposing side is not a productive road to resolution at a time when reason must prevail. The reality is that the goals of the "other" are not dissimilar and their common ground is big enough for both. Both animal research and animal rights advocates would like to end the practice of conducting animal research. Joint recognition of that fact should expedite their mutual goals to identify alternatives and to institutionalize them within the research and regulatory frameworks of discovery.

- Particularly with regard to the views of animal rights advocates, it is time for animal research supporters to listen carefully to the messages about humanity that are embedded in the ethics of animal protection. Here, in the new millennium, those views challenge the notions of who we are as a human species and may teach us important lessons about the value of life for the next one thousand years. Those views may lead to major social changes in the allocation of resources to programs that support children, the underserved, and the elderly in ways that we do not address comprehensively in this nation or on the globe today.

- Once the opposing sides have recognized their common ground and reached an agreement on the nature of the objectives, they should develop practical steps and a joint agenda for accomplishing the end goal. Doing so might include creating a timetable, a process, and increased funding for such activities to reduce any unnecessary use of research animals; developing alternatives to animals; ensuring the safety of researchers, their families, and their projects; and providing the most compassionate care of animals used in research.

- The groups should encourage responsible, mutually satisfying behavior among their members and should agree to monitor and police their own factions.

- Local, state and federal governments should assist with laws, regulation and enforcement actions that prevent and prosecute violence against researchers and property.

- Improper handling of research animals and known violations of lab animal standards by researchers should be prevented and prosecuted as well.

Years of hostility and opposition are not fertile ground on which to seek a truce, a compromise, and eventual peace. It will be difficult for the opposing sides in this controversy to work together, but it is the responsibility of both sides to do so. It will be difficult to call upon those activists who have been demonized and invite them into a covenant of caring for people through discovery. I believe that it is the community of healers who must make the first move, however, and do precisely that.

In fact, there is little other choice. When healers choose to embrace covenants, they must take all necessary steps to meet their obligations within the covenant. In this case, fulfilling those obligations entails engaging opponents who disagree with views about animal research. If healers today fail to take these steps, they will have failed within the most important covenant of all: the one that heals the patients that healers are sworn to help.

Chapter 5

Making Choices

Covenant in the Tradeoffs Between Privacy and Efficiency

Just like our free speech rights, privacy rights can never be absolute. We must balance our protections of privacy with our public responsibility to support national priorities—like public health, research, quality care, and our fight against health care fraud and abuse.

Donna E. Shalala, former Secretary of Health and Human Services, National Press Club, Washington, D.C., July 31, 1997

Making Tradeoffs

Are patients today willing to make sacrifices to reduce the cost of care? What kind of sacrifices would they be willing to make? Would they forego easy access to care? Would they do without convenient care? Comfort? Quality? Would they agree to sacrifice some loss of privacy or confidentiality in return for better quality at reduced costs? Would they be willing to share their health care data so that more research could be done on the problems of health care systems and disease? Would they be willing to have healers phone them to monitor their personal health practices and encourage healthier behaviors? Would they agree to be contacted by pharmacists, case managers, or medication compliance companies when they fail to renew their prescriptions?

Privacy and Confidentiality vs. Efficiency and Effectiveness

Questions about tradeoffs are rarely posed to the American public. Health care policymakers more often attempt to satisfy all of the needs of patients without asking them to choose from among desirable goals or limit wish lists. Health systems, for example, have attempted to provide high levels of access and quality at low cost, without sacrificing one for the others. When providers have been unable to satisfy all of the patients' demands, the result has been fairly consistent—anger and calls for patient rights and protections from the seemingly capricious actions of healers. This is the experience of managed care today, as it attempts to meet payers' demands to further reduce costs without sacrificing quality.

Without posing the question explicitly, the tough tradeoffs related to privacy and confidentiality versus efficiency and effectiveness are now underway. On behalf of the consuming public, legislation and recently promulgated regulations are making decisions about what information will be shared, how it will be managed, and whether patients will have the right to object and protect their health care information from disclosure. These decisions are being made in order to enhance the efficiencies and effectiveness of health care practices. Implied here is that patients will lose some acceptable level of privacy and confidentiality in return for some eventual financial benefits from better-managed health care systems. It is one of the most difficult tradeoffs that patients and their healers will face, and it is being done without a clear understanding on the part of patients—or their healers for that matter—of the implications and issues involved. Congress has made some attempts to deal with it, the Clinton Administration advanced regulatory proposals to do so, and the Bush Administration placed a clear stake in the ground by issuing regulations that were, literally, years in the making. None of these steps was entirely satisfactory to any of the stakeholders involved. This is not the fault of the regulations as they were constructed or those who have labored hard and long to see them issued. Whether policymakers opt for more privacy and confidentiality or for more efficiency and effectiveness, neither choice is likely to succeed in satisfying patients. The tradeoff involved is too deeply embedded in the Constitution and too deeply rooted in our wallets. We hold both our privacy and our finances dear, and we are not ready to choose between them when it comes to health care. Yet, the choice may require that we go beyond the values we have come to hold dear as a nation. This debate will produce agonizing choices and fearful solutions. Given its current course, this debate will also produce considerable consumer backlash as patients become more acquainted with how their data are collected and used throughout the health care enterprise without their knowledge and consent.

Health care providers today are searching for every possible way to reduce costs. As healing has evolved from a cottage industry of independent physicians and hospitals to major systems of clinical care, new ways to assess care, eliminate variations in practice, improve quality, and reduce costs have appeared. Data systems that track visits and billed payers are one of those ways that can be used to better understand the nature of the patients being served. Even in an era before electronic medical records, computerized billing data was a readily available source of information about the diagnosis, the patient's characteristics, and the services used to treat the condition.

Using Data to Create Efficiency and Effectiveness

Bills contain identifying information about patients: their names, addresses, telephone numbers at home and at work, Social Security numbers, insurance plan data, vital clinical history and physical information, diagnosis codes, diagnostic tests, interventions, and prognosis. The treating physician is also identified, making the source and location of the medical record clear for any follow-up inquiries about that provider that might be needed. This information is valuable for both the public and private sectors working to improve health care efficiency and data utility.

Government and employers were the first to need and

use this information in order to manage their own costs and understand the needs of their own beneficiary populations. They structured uniform bills and standards for collecting the information so that it could be collected reliably and analyzed across physician practices, hospitals, and regions of the country. Next, investors became important stakeholders. As those who provided capital for business growth, investors needed to assess their risks and likely returns to determine the performance of the firms using their resources. As utilization and prices changed and costs grew, so, too, did the need to understand the process of delivering health care and the ways to control and improve it.

The interests in efficiency never waned, and the importance of effectiveness emerged. There were heavy demands on data. It was through data, after all, that we expected our understanding of health systems to emerge. As an ancient healer might have explored the entrails of some animal for diagnostic clues, we searched the bowels of data, looking for information that would help to manage the increasingly uncontrollable nature of health costs. Health services research emerged as a new discipline of study. New investigative methods and data handling and warehousing systems were developed to provide the tools to assess care. Patients, physicians, hospitals, and regions of the nation were studied. An era of monitoring resources consumed against characteristics of the population and their diseases began. We looked for variations everywhere, not being sure what they meant, but hopeful that if we studied variations in practice patterns and utilization, the data would give up their secrets and inform us about the proper way to practice medicine. A federal agency was funded to conduct intramural and extramural research in the area of health services research and quality. It grew and became a significant player in understanding the nature of health delivery and quality in the nation.[1]

The billing data were useful in a number of ways.

Physician practice patterns were identified and monitored by third-party payers. Norms for physician practices were published and used to change clinical care. Slowly, but steadily over a number of decades, guidelines emerged from the data and were disseminated. At first, these guidelines were excoriated by the profession. Later, they were accepted and even expected. New patient intervention programs also emerged using billing data. Claims could be analyzed to determine which patients were not refilling medications so that they could be called and counseled to do so. Children who needed vaccines could be referred back to the doctor's office for shots at the appropriate times. Missed opportunities for mammograms and pap smears could be corrected. Physicians with low rates of preventive care could be educated to do better. Epidemiologists investigated patterns of disease and public health officials launched programs to prevent disease and disability. Quality committees studied hospitals and doctors to improve practice patterns. Medical science advanced, saving lives and dollars.

Patient medical records became useful for research and patient health care programs. This information was usually "scrubbed" so that the researchers would not know the identity of the patient. But not always. At times some users of health care data needed patient identifying information, and even when identities were removed, there was a chance that reverse engineering and merging of databases could identify a patient and, perhaps, bring them harm from lost privacy.

Certainly, patients knew that their bills and records were being shared with others in health care outside their physician's office or hospital room. A statement giving physicians permission to release medical information to secure payment was printed on each reimbursement form. Similar statements accompanied applications for health and life insurance. It is highly unlikely, however, that those patients and even many physicians understood the extent to which the data would be used for other purposes. It is also highly unlikely that they knew how data warehouses—similar to the bureaus for financial data—were developing and now reselling that information to researchers. And it is unlikely those patients realized that companies were using the data to conduct health economic studies and to develop new products and services such as patient marketing, compliance, and reminder programs.

It is for these reasons that privacy and confidentiality will be the sleeper controversy of the future for health care. The protections of privacy and confidentiality are taken for granted in the one-to-one healing encounter. Unfortunately, they are eroding in private practices and even more so in the corporate practice of medicine. As demands are made by patients and payers to control costs, the sale and use of health information becomes one strategy to deliver on the promise to do so. Health care businesses are taking risks with confidential data—sometimes on their own initiative, and sometimes under contractual agreements with employers and payers. As they do, they are at risk because they are acting ahead of the public's concurrence. Health executives believe they have the implicit, and sometimes the explicit, authorizations to share data, but they do not. They do not because the public does not know the full extent of these practices, and it has hardly been asked whether it is willing to sacrifice privacy and confidentiality in return for (eventual) lower costs and more effective care. The public does suspect, however, that some mischief is afoot. In a recent California Healthcare Association poll of 1,000 consumers, 60% trusted their personal physicians to keep information confidential, but only 35% trusted health plans to do so.[2] When the public finds out the full extent of the use of information, including how information is sold and used even by those they trusted most, they are likely to be angry. They haven't been invited to engage in a discussion of these issues or decide on this tradeoff. No issue in health care is more vulnerable to a widespread violation of the covenant today, and no issue is so vulnerable to consumer backlash as a result.

But back to the opening questions. Health care managers know that if they use the data from many individual healing encounters, they can do research, improve quality, and manage costs. Isn't that what patients want? Since patients rarely pay the full cost for their care, why not require that their encounter data be used as a *quid pro quo* for reimbursement? Over time, this would benefit the individual patient as well as other patients as a group—those treated by that particular healer, or with that particular therapy, for example. New knowledge would lead to new insights into care and cures. New methods of monitoring physician practices would lead to better fraud investigations. Costs would decline. Health care would become more efficient and more effective. Isn't that what patients and healers alike want? Perhaps not, as recent history has shown.

Privacy Goes Public

Recent public awareness of these issues flared after a front-page article appeared in the *Washington Post* on Sunday, February 15, 1998.[3] The story was a report—and an erroneous one at that—suggesting that CVS and Giant pharmacies had sold customer—that is, patient—lists to GlaxoWellcome, a pharmaceutical company. The story reported that drug companies were using those lists to persuade pharmacy customers to buy the company's drugs instead of the drugs prescribed by their physicians. It also reported that another company, Elensys, that sends compliance and educational literature on behalf of the pharmacies, had participated in a scheme that violated the privacy rights of the patients whose records were in the pharmacy computers. The *Post* articles reported that Elensys operated marketing and "switching" programs for pharmaceutical companies, and it reinforced that accusation in a February 18 editorial. Three days later the *Post* printed a retraction buried on page 18, explaining that GlaxoWellcome did not receive patient information. The damage, however, had already been done.

The *Post* story hit the pharmaceutical industry hard and should have reverberated throughout all of health care. It was not just a single blip on the radar screen, appearing and disappearing without notice. Rather, the story was one of several important events that drove home the challenges of privacy policy and practices.

Privacy concerns are real because privacy violations are real. The medical and mental health records of a congresswoman from New York were faxed to a local newspaper during her campaign. A Massachusetts HMO kept extensive notes of psychotherapy sessions on a central computer accessible to all clinical employees. Sales representatives of a managed care company in Maryland illegally purchased the computer records of Medicaid recipients from Medicaid clerks. A banker accessed that same database to check on the prognosis of loan customers with cancer. A medical student in Colorado sold hospital records to malpractice attorneys. In Florida, the names of over 4,000 HIV-positive individuals were obtained and sent to Florida newspapers. A purchaser of a second-hand computer discovered that the hard drive contained a grocery store's pharmacy records, including patient names, addresses, Social Security numbers, and prescription medicines. In a move that privacy advocates regard as "scary," Iceland's Parliament voted in December 1998 to draw blood from each of its 270,000 residents for detailed genetic research and sell that information to Roche Holding AG for $200 million. It also gave Roche the contents of its citizens' uniquely rich medical and genealogical records as part of the deal.

It took patient advocates in Iceland a few months to respond with their objections; Americans responded in a matter of days. Patients flooded CVS with complaints, causing CVS to terminate its patient education program and

Giant to halt one that it had planned. Newspapers and television stations around the country picked up on the *Washington Post* story, touching off a wave of negative media publicity. Within days, a CVS customer filed a class-action suit in Massachusetts Superior Court, naming CVS, Elensys, and GlaxoWellcome as defendants. That lawsuit has since spilled over to include other companies.[4] It did not matter that the media slant on this issue was not only misinformed, it was unbalanced. It did not look at the value of the educational programs or the necessity of working with patients to ensure that they took medications properly, all of which are intended to bring down the personal and societal costs of care and to improve the quality of the patients' lives. What the event did, though, was to demonstrate the volatility of privacy matters in health care. Policymakers and health cost-cutting program designers would be well advised to take note, especially as they pursue Internet and e-commerce ventures that will most certainly escalate privacy awareness.

These and similar events are beginning to create the political will to deal with the tough issues in protecting privacy, though success remains elusive. The Health Insurance Portability and Accountability Act of 1996 (HIPAA) required that Congress pass privacy legislation by August 1999. Although there were five major bills in the 105th Congress, none of them passed, and Congress missed its self-imposed deadline to act. During the Clinton Administration the Secretary of the Department of Health and Human Services issued draft regulations, despite requests from some members of Congress to delay action until they could reconsider the issues. The Administration moved ahead on this potentially contentious issue in the absence of a solid national understanding. The nation reacted, sending over 50,000 comment letters, some of which were signed by coalitions of sizable organizational members and most posing irresolvable policy and operational dilemmas. Despite promises to the contrary, the Clinton

Administration never finalized or issued those rules. To test the political waters, the Bush Administration again asked for comments about the "real world" implications of the regulation. This time 11,000 letters arrived, some of them with hundreds of signatories. On April 14, 2001, the final rule was issued and targeted entities were told to be fully compliant two years later, on April 14, 2003. To assist in the uncertainties in this rule, the Administration is promising a series of clarifications, which, to date, have been slow to emerge.

It is unlikely that the momentum on privacy regulations will continue—at least at the federal level—for some time to come. Privacy officials have been reassigned or their positions unfilled, and the nation's health officials are now consumed with the impact of terrorism on health. At the state level, however, action may well be anticipated, since there are more than 250 initiatives in state legislatures across the country to address patient privacy. Other action may well be prompted by privacy advocates, who recently released data on the implications of the rule for Internet sites. Their analysis demonstrates that the rules do not apply to most health web sites, that different rules apply to different sites offering the same services, and that some sites may not be covered even if they are offered by those organizations covered by the rule. National policymakers and health care businesses alike can anticipate that, even with a promulgated rule and promises of clarifications, we still face a complex patchwork of patient protections that, alone, would cripple the very efficiencies that data collection seeks to achieve.[5]

Involving Patients in the Tradeoff

Would patients really care? Would they be willing to allow data on their health care encounters with physicians, hospitals, home health agencies, and others to be used to study health care to reduce its costs? Would they want to restrict the use of the data to researchers? Would it be acceptable if entrepreneurs used the data to satisfy a health care market interest in lower-cost care? Would they trust those who collect, house, and use the data to secure it, protect their privacy and confidentiality, and use it only for healing purposes? Would they want a copy of the data? Would they want to correct errors in the records? Would they want to be paid for the data if others used it for some commercial purpose?

Frankly, we don't know the answers to these questions. The American public hasn't been asked. Someone had better ask them. Patient privacy and confidentiality is one of the most difficult sacrifices patients may be required to make as health care approaches the breaking point of cost control, and in an era of homeland-security concerns. The notion that we might lose it—and worse, that we already have—is shocking. Privacy and confidentiality, after all, was present at the birth of organized medicine. It was a tenet of the Hippocratic Oath, which states: "All that may come to my knowledge in the exercise of my profession or outside of my profession or in daily commerce with men, which ought not spread abroad, I will keep secret and will never reveal."[6] Few issues in medicine are more fundamental to the dignity of the patient and the trust required between patient and healer.

The consideration of privacy and confidentiality has so far been the turf of an elite group of attorneys and advocates who are protecting the patient's privacy rights against the corporate practice of medicine and the ever-present dangers of electronic communications. These advocates are doing a good job, to be sure, as are those wishing to use the data, but all of them together are only a small portion of the total players who should be engaged in the discussions. Few patients themselves have been involved, and few understand the implications for their jobs, their insurance, and their future. The likely outcome will be a loss of privacy and confidentiality rights for patients in favor of reducing the costs of care. As data-driven programs unfold and the devil in the details becomes more widely known, there will be hell to pay.

Some opponents of tough privacy legislation and regulation will argue that the issues are complex and that the public will not have the attention span required of participants in the debate. They may be right. Many public debates that engage the community are complex. This one will be even more so. That places an even greater burden on those shaping this policy and managing these debates to take the time and the care to do it right. A good place to begin on this issue is with the definition of the terms. The definitions are critical, and the terms are muddled. The definitions are especially important because the terms in this debate cannot be used interchangeably, though they frequently are.

Clarifying the Terms

Privacy is the right of the patient to have personal information kept secret and from others, including the health care providers involved in their care. Confidentiality is the protection of that information once it is disclosed from dispersal to persons not directly involved in providing care, both within and outside health care settings. Security encompasses the policy, procedures, and technologies intended to guarantee privacy and confidentiality.

Suppose that a patient seeks a diagnosis for an illness and gives permission for blood to be drawn and tested for a suspected condition like high cholesterol. The patient's right to privacy dictates that the healer test only for cholesterol level and not for other conditions, such as HIV infection, drug use, or genetic diseases, on its own or at the request of another party such as law enforcement, employers, or insurers. Confidentiality protections would ensure that the results of the cholesterol test, once known, are not disclosed outside the patient-healer relationship without the patient's permission. Security protections would dictate how the records of the test results would be stored and managed to ensure that they do not fall into unauthorized hands.

These are not esoteric definitional distinctions. Although these issues were once the territory of academics and scholars of constitutional law, average citizens now have a stake in them. The resolution of this debate in the public arena will affect quality of life in the future. People who lose their privacy, confidentiality, or security can suffer, and some already do. Some patients fear, and rightly so, that mental health records, HIV/AIDS status, genetic predisposition to health conditions, and disabilities will deny them jobs, health and life insurance, and even home mortgages. Some fear law enforcement surveillance of medical data in cases of drug abuse, spouse abuse, and child support enforcement. That is a realistic fear, as information becomes more widely accessible and electronically enhanced. It is no wonder, then, that a 1993 Harris-Equifax poll estimated that approximately 10% of health care is "off the books" in order to protect disclosure of medical information outside the healing setting.[7] Fear may well escalate if future Administrations, following in the footsteps of the Clinton Administration, propose that anyone receiving health care insurance reimbursement should allow their records to be used for purposes other than their own personal health care.

Framing the Covenant to Address the Tradeoff

Unless the tradeoffs between health care effectiveness and efficiency and personal privacy and confidentiality are addressed thoughtfully, both patients and healers will pay the price. Patients will suffer for the probable lack of privacy and confidentiality in their care. They will feel violated if confidential information is disclosed to others and that disclosure affects other aspects of their lives. If they cannot get jobs, health insurance, or mortgages, the consequences for them will be real. If they avoid care because they fear the implications for their lives, the consequences will be equally negative. Healers will suffer from the disruptions to their businesses. The costs of running a health care enterprise are likely to increase as privacy protections create new demands on medical record systems and procedures, and as patients sue for real or imagined losses of privacy. Negative press will tarnish the public image of healers, particularly those in corporate healing enterprises like managed care and pharmaceuticals. That negative press will further erode the trust in the clinical relationship between patients and their healers—and that trust is necessary for good clinical care. Legislation in this arena is critical, but to date it has been buttressed by incomplete and poor policy debates that are founded on too little data on the part of both patients and their healers. All of this is likely to impair the ability of the health care system to function optimally as it attempts to address the tradeoffs involved.

Former Secretary of Health and Human Services Donna Shalala developed a set of principles that will serve as the foundation for future debates on privacy. Those principles dictate that health data should be protected and used only for health purposes, patients should have control over their data, patients should be willing to share de-identified confidential information for improved understanding and care management, and providers who wrongly disclose data should be punished. These principles are a good starting point, and there is widespread agreement about them. But real questions remain. How long will this agreement hold up when the debate turns to writing regulations and requiring disclosure? Few in health care today are prepared to address the devil in the details of privacy and confidentiality. Nor are we prepared to address the devil in the dollars. Implementing the confidentiality and security provisions recommended by the Secretary will at least equal the cost of Y2K compliance. Physician practices, hospitals, and managed care companies already operating at low profit margins are under pressure to reduce medical errors and also facing the imperative to better prepare for bioterrorism. This creates tremendous competition within annual budgets for privacy provision costs, without the necessary capital to institute the variety of changes that will be required.

Regardless of the cost, the completeness and the soundness of the data sets will likely be questionable. For example, patients, in one instance in which they were asked, did not respond favorably to the sharing of their medical information. Mayo Clinic, a major, credible source of health care data, recently spent nearly $7 million to collect signed informed-consent forms from patients residing in a suburban county to satisfy a Minnesota state confidentiality law. Only 24% granted their consent.[8] The low response level may be the bellwether of patient willingness to disclose personal data. It may also erode confidence in the completeness of the Mayo database, but more importantly, it may indicate erosion in the level of trust between a significant number of patients and a well-known provider of high-quality care. If this is a challenge for one of the most respected healing institutions in the nation, what insurmountable obstacles might other providers face in the future?

Tough Questions and Dealing with the Details

To make any headway in the debate, patients and healers will need to answer difficult questions in six different areas of privacy, confidentiality and security. These are:

- patient consent and authorization
- data collection and use
- data management
- patient rights to view and correct records
- penalties for violations
- federal and state legislative autonomy

The first set of questions relates to the limits of patient

consent and authorization: How detailed must the patient's consent be for the disclosure and use of information? Should consent be required each time a patient's data are used, or is a blanket consent for any use adequate? Does it make a difference in granting consent if the patient information is "blinded" so the user does not know the identity of the patient? Should researchers and health plans pay patients for the use of their data? Should patients be required to "opt in," or simply allowed to "opt out" of case management and pharmacy compliance programs?

The second set of questions concerns how the data are collected and used: What data will be collected, and how will they be used? What patient identifiers will be used? Will patients be required to consent to the use of their data in return for reimbursement for care? Will every transaction between patients and healers be recorded, even if the patient pays cash for the service? Must patients consent to the use of their medical records for health systems management, public health studies, and medical outcomes research? Should law enforcement be allowed to use records for medical fraud or felony investigations? Should records be available for homeland security purposes? Will pharmacies and case management specialists be allowed to use information to improve compliance and educate patients? Can health insurers use the data to exclude patients with expensive conditions? Can lists of patients be sold to commercial companies for special promotions to patients?

The third set of questions relates to how data will be handled once they are collected: How will data be managed to preserve privacy, confidentiality, and security? How long will medical records be maintained? Like certain other records, must they be expunged over time? How can patients be sure that a researcher, or other user of "blind" data, has not merged the data with other data sets that could reveal their identity? Does a patient have a right to privacy on all medical matters, including communicable, fatal, and expensive diseases? Must all patient releases be in writing? Once a patient allows his data to be used, how long must confidentiality be maintained? Does it extend after a patient has died? Does the family of a deceased patient have a right to determine whether his data can be used? Can a child be protected against the disclosure of data about a parent, in instances where genetic information could be available and cause harm to the child or other family members? Should patients be required to disclose data as a condition for receiving public or private health insurance coverage?

The fourth set of questions addresses patients' rights to view and correct medical records: Should medical records be like credit records, and should patients have the right to view and correct them? Who will prevail if a patient and a physician disagree on the accuracy of the record? How will patients be allowed access to records? If uncorrected records are shared and the patient later learns of inaccuracies, must corrections be made through the entire chain of data users?

The fifth set of questions involves the penalties that will be imposed for violations: How will intentional and unintentional violations of privacy, confidentiality, or security be punished? Are individuals who violate privacy responsible along with their corporate employers? Should those who hold and use data be licensed and periodically inspected? Should data users be subject to criminal background checks?

The final set of questions covers which laws will win in a dispute between the national and state governments on these issues: The federal government is lagging behind the states in setting law, but will federal legislators claim superior jurisdiction and preempt state laws? Should federal laws create a "floor" over which stricter state laws can be imposed? How will conflicts between the state and federal laws be resolved? Which state laws will prevail as health care providers operate across state lines and face different standards in data management? How will Internet platforms be subject to state and federal law? If patients voluntarily place their records on Internet sites, which rules govern privacy?

Engaging the Covenant
The Congress, the rule-making process, and state legislatures are the forums where these privacy matters are already unfolding. They are also the same settings in which efficiency is being debated and demanded. Privacy and efficiency goals require the immediate attention of healers and patients in health care settings, since these are issues that must be engaged between the two most essential parties to the healing—the patient and the healer. Only then can privacy and confidentiality be addressed within public policy settings. Only then can the tradeoff be addressed. Without this step-wise progress—first, between the healer and the patient, and later, with others involved in payment and health care policy and management—the trust that is so essential to healing will be substantially eroded.

Medical oaths, as they were initially constructed, could not possibly have envisioned the uses of information and the imperatives of the tradeoffs we face today in modern health care. Only by addressing the issues squarely in the context of the healing relationships and articulating the tradeoffs we face today can we facilitate a public policy resolution. Without such a clear and open dialogue, the healing we seek in caring for patients will be at risk. Patients may become less willing to provide accurate and complete information to their healers and may be unwilling to have their data shared for the research purposes that improve care and create efficiencies. The potential to build, or conversely to erode, trust is very great in this aspect of caring and keeping covenants. There are a number of possible avenues for acting within covenant concerning privacy.

Whether in individual encounters, in union contract negotiations, in local town meetings or in contracting with health plans, the issue of tradeoffs between health care cost savings and privacy and confidentiality must get more of the attention it deserves. This is a complex issue that will be worked on for at least another decade, so we may as well start now to work together better. Making that investment in the dialogue will be well worth the time and effort required. There are a number of steps we can and should take immediately:

- Subscribe to the covenant. Privacy, confidentiality, and security issues call for the broadest possible recognition among healers of their status within the covenant. This means that not only clinicians, but all those involved in the payment, research, data management, and e-commerce businesses using data should subscribe to the same oaths that grew from the sacredness of the healing professions. Whether treating an individual patient, processing a payment claim for a single patient, or researching the patterns of disease for a group of patients, the goal is healing and the adherence to the covenant to serve those patients should be clear and unambiguous. These protections should be subject to laws and regulations to further reassure patients.

- Understand the uses of data. Healers who collect information from patients in the course of their work should become better acquainted with the various uses of that information as it flows downstream from their offices. This would include their knowing if insurance claim or patient encounter data are used solely for reimbursement or systems improvement within managed care, or if the data are also to be sold and used for other purposes. It would require that clinicians understand the role of Institutional Review Boards (IRBs) to assure that confidentiality is protected if records are accessed without consent. This is important for several reasons. First, such knowledge is necessary to fully inform patients how medical records might be used. Second, this understanding is important for assuring the accuracy of the data for potential users downstream. In recent studies of hypothetical patients who needed but could not afford care, significant numbers of physicians were willing to distort the clinical picture in order to secure payment.[9] Would they be so inclined if they knew the data were being used for other purposes in addition to payment? How might such distortions create problems in health services research, physician and patient profiling, and government investigations of fraud?

- Maintain privacy and confidentiality and address the tradeoffs. Those who are healers have a covenant responsibility to maintain privacy and confidentiality of medical records, to use the information only for healing, and to discuss doing so with patients. Those healers, whether they are individual clinicians or third-party payers mining data banks, should inform patients of the important and necessary uses of data for research, public health, disease management, and quality monitoring and seek their informed consent. This will lay the groundwork for a patient's own consideration of the trade-offs they are being asked to make. Today's consent forms are inadequate and do not describe the uses or users of a patient's information. Patients are not fully appraised of where, how, and by whom their data may be used, and this is a clear violation of the covenant.

- Participate in public policy. Flowing from the covenant with patients is an obligation on the part of healers to address privacy and confidentiality issues in public forums. Whether or not they are engaged in individual patient clinical care, a corporate-structured medical enterprise, or in data management, use, and sales, all healers are involved with data, even if all they do is collect the information. Public forums are one way to assure that patient stakeholders are involved in making the tradeoffs between the privacy they want and the health economic efficiencies they demand.

- Confront the tradeoffs. Patients, for their part within the covenant, should consider how their escalating demands for more care, more efficiency, and more effectiveness are at odds with their simultaneous interests in privacy and confidentiality. If it is not possible to "have it all," then what are the priorities? Which of the demands—access, quality, efficiency, or privacy—is the most important?

Americans appear to be willing to relinquish privacy in many ways. They do not object to background checks on nannies and child care workers, they use credit cards with impunity knowing that profiles are being created and used, and they disclose their unique Social Security number without a thought. But are they willing, as Bernadine Healy, former director of the National Institutes of Health (NIH), has asked, to allow the government and others to be trusted with such "sacred secrets" as sexual practices, impotence, abortion, suicide attempts, and other "potentially prejudicial" illnesses, procedures, and medications?[10]

Is gaining efficiency in health care enough of a reason to allow broader use of medical information? Is detecting fraud so important a goal? Is gaining new knowledge through research a compelling rationale? Are the richness of the available data and the power of technology to use this information too appetizing to refuse? Can the covenant between healers and patients be maintained, and even strengthened, while addressing privacy, confidentiality, and security of medical information?

As in the case of most challenges in the midst of an apparent crisis, there is great opportunity. The covenant can be preserved and enhanced if healers—those in clinical care, health care management, public policy and research—recommit to their obligations, if patients commit to theirs, and if both work together to make the tough choices in this emerging health care tradeoff.

Chapter 6

Pain and Suffering

Covenant in Conflict with the Law

We all must die. But that I can save him from days of torture,
that is what I feel as my greatest and ever new privilege. Pain
is a more terrible lord of mankind than death himself.[1]

Albert Schweitzer

If more people suffered visibly from the pain of terminal illnesses, it would no longer be a hidden public policy issue. Unrelieved pain would not be the unseen killer of the spirit that it is for so many people today. It would no longer test the resolve of the dying to live out the final days of their lives. It would no longer force families to confront the awful choices of the end days, including those choices of assisted suicide.

People today suffer, but they do not suffer visibly. They are most often at home or in nursing homes. Sometimes, but not always, they are in hospice care. Occasionally, they are in hospitals, where pain relief may not present any technical challenges, but will be fraught with social and legal hurdles. At any rate, those suffering among us are out of sight and out of earshot. They do not grimace as they pass us by in shopping malls, do not cry out at movie theaters, and do not shed their tears getting groceries. They and their families are most often alone and too often isolated, consumed with managing the hour-to-hour torment of unremitting pain along with the other aspects of the terminal disease, its frailties, fractures, and bleeding. If suffering people were visible to us, their pain would be front-page news. Their stories would stir action in larger numbers of important medical and policy centers of the nation. If their caregivers were not so overwhelmed with the task of easing the pain as they supported the dying process, they would be organized into effective, policy-changing groups. If their clinicians were not so burdened defending themselves before overzealous law enforcement as they attempted to prescribe, and defend their use of, adequate doses of pain-relieving medications, they would be more available to organize as well. These family members and clinicians could borrow a page from animal rights activist strategies and confront us with our lack of compassion. They would question our humanity toward our fellow men and women.

The Extent of Pain in Terminal Illness

Our best statistics are on cancer deaths and pain. An estimated eight million Americans will die from cancer, of whom 70% will have pain and fewer than one-half will be adequately treated for it.[2] Coping with the diagnosis of cancer and adjusting to the shocking news are challenges in the early stage of the disease. Coping with the fears of unrelieved pain comes soon thereafter. Becoming a burden on family members is the principal concern of dying people, and the fear of pain is the second most difficult problem they face. The fear itself exacerbates physical pain. Unrelieved pain leads to suffering.

Cancer is not the only terminal condition that creates pain, but it is the one for which we have the best statistics. Nor is pain associated with only terminal illnesses. Many people who are not terminally ill also experience pain.

In our society, many suffer from other causes of pain and rely—or should be able to rely—on our compassion and care. Chronic pain affects over 50 million Americans, and another 23 million experience acute pain from surgery and injuries each year.[3] Back pain affects over 26 million adults and is the leading cause of disability for people under age 45.[4] Arthritis affects one in six Americans[5], and 25 million suffer from migraine headaches.[6] Pain is estimated to cost $100 billion each year, causing over 150 million days of lost work.[7] A majority of people with pain cannot engage in the normal activities of daily living, such as grocery shopping, walking, or housekeeping.[8] Pain has been called the "silent epidemic," and for very good reason.[9]

If we as a society are unable to deliver pain relief—even to those among us who are dying—how can we expect to demonstrate compassion to the living? If we are unable to address the clear and unambiguous needs of pain relief in terminal conditions, how can we address those that are chronic? If we are helpless in the face of the conflicts that cripple our compassion in death, how can we expect any better in life? How can we ask those who suffer pain to bear it silently while we discuss public policy conflicts? How can we ask them to suffer endlessly because we cannot resolve our differences about the management of pain? How can we justify our failures when the covenant to relieve the pain of those who are dying should be so clear?

Addressing Pain: A Critical Test of the Covenant

The willingness to address pain should not depend on the visibility or invisibility of those who suffer, the number of people who are suffering at any given time, or what the cause of their suffering might be. Whether they suffer in our midst or alone, they suffer. Whether pain is common or rare, they rely on healers for relief. There should be no room in our healing enterprises for judgments about the cause of the nature of pain. Whether those suffering are children dying from cancer or elderly dying from the effects of life-long cigarette smoking, they need supportive and palliative care. Our healers have a covenant with them to relieve their pain, and our communities should share in that covenant by assuring that our public policies do not prevent the best possible palliative relief of their symptoms. All are deserving of compassion. Unlike beliefs common in the Middle Ages, pain is no longer viewed by large segments of society and within the healing professions as a signal of divine retribution or a requirement for eventual salvation.

There are some today who value the experience of fully embracing pain, and they should be supported in their choice to do so. But the vast majority of people today would rather have effective pain relief in order to be better able to put their personal affairs in order at the end of life. Regardless of the nature of their disease or the number who suffer or are isolated in their dying, those who are in pain require care. If that pain is not relieved, it creates suffering, and suffering is another matter altogether.

Beyond Pain: Suffering

The terms "pain" and "suffering" are sometimes used interchangeably, but they are actually quite different. Pain is "an unpleasant sensory and emotional experience associated with actual or potential tissue damage."[10] It can include aching, burning, numbness, loss of sensation, itching, and tightness. Suffering is a broader concept and goes beyond the sensations to encompass the hopelessness that some dying persons experience. In suffering, people feel a threat to their existence and to their "integrity as persons."[11] Suffering reaches into the heart of personal, family, and spiritual experiences and generates feelings of helplessness as well as hopelessness.

Regardless of how intimately we know a dying person or how remote they may be from our daily lives, the importance of this problem merits more concern. Those who are healthy and active have the means to reach for an analgesic to deaden our ordinary daily pains. Shouldn't we devote a portion of our efforts to helping people in our communities whose pain is more overwhelming and more compelling than our headaches, stiffness, and muscle strains? Society should be concerned that people suffer needlessly. Instead, we have made them and the pain in their terminal illnesses invisible and have refused to come to terms with our responsibilities to help.

There are many methods to relieve pain. Some require long-term efforts of caring individuals to teach meditation and relaxation techniques and to assist at the bedside to help patients change positions, remain comfortable, prevent fractures, and be free of sores and wounds. Doing this, however, requires devoting time and attention to these patients. Many people are not inclined or cannot be helpful in this way; and few participate as caregivers and volunteers in hospice and respite programs. Although approximately 500,000 patients use hospice services each year and the costs are covered by Medicare, most Medicaid, and many private insurers, a recent survey found that only 22% of all families who experienced a terminal illness used hospice services. Sixty percent of those patients had cancer, yet only one-half of all cancer patients used hospice services.[12]

Relieving Pain and Easing Suffering

The quickest method of relieving pain and easing suffering, and the one that demands the least effort, involves the use of medication. This method would seem to be best suited to those who cannot or will not take the time for the more personal forms of care that might be effective for many dying patients. Medication also appeals to the quick-fix inclinations and demanding lifestyles of those who are still healthy. Drug methods, however, are precisely at the crux of the controversies in caring for the pain of the terminally ill. Communities have negative biases about powerful drugs and have allowed fears to interfere with the relief of soul-crushing pain. Fear of powerful medications and the ways they can be misused increasingly prevents the compassionate care that should be given to the dying.

Ever since soldiers returned from modern-era wars with addictions to the pain-relieving medicines used to treat their physical and emotional wounds, society has become suspect and fearful of the power of legitimate medicines. Solving the problem became the task of law enforcement, which monitored the practices of physicians to ensure that they were not enabling addicts and creating new ones. These intrusions led to physicians' fears of prescribing these medicines for legitimate purposes and to regulatory barriers to make it more difficult for them to do so.[13] Special prescription pads were needed, special records were kept in pharmacies and forwarded to state authorities, and physicians could be questioned at any time about patients who were using these medicines.

Newer, more effective pain-relieving products became available. Physicians were not well educated about them because the legal barriers and risks to using these pharmacotherapeutics were so great that physicians preferred not to use them at all. Why engage in becoming expert in the value and appropriate use of new medicines one would be unlikely to prescribe? Old biases about the nature of the drugs and their effects on patients were therefore left to prevail. Even patients with terminal illnesses feared addictions, and many people avoided discussions about pain. Of all the families experiencing a death, only 2% had given any prior consideration to issues involving pain relief.[14]

Everyone—families, patients, physicians, and law enforcement—was ill informed and wrong. Patients treated with medications to relieve pain in terminal illness rarely become addicted.[15] Some physicians feared that increasing the dosage to the point necessary to relieve the pain would result in the patient's death. Research debunked that theory.[16] Others feared that, left in the hands of patients, overdoses would be common in suicide attempts. Again, the popular notions were wrong; patients would rather live than die.[17] It is the pain they wish to avoid, not life.

Families Seek Better Relief from Pain

The impact of unrelieved pain for patients and the loved ones they leave behind is profound. Only recently have we been able to document that family members giving care to seriously ill or disabled relatives suffer higher rates of mortality.[18] It is one of the most stressful times in family life, and one for which little financial or community support exists. Caregivers, who provide somewhere between $100 billion and $200 billion in uncompensated care, receive few returns from the communities that might otherwise support them with respite and other services.[19]

Beginning in the 1970s, this suffering led to the formation of a number of organizations dedicated to seeking a way out of the fear through political and legal solutions. Unable to find pain relief from healers and incapable of negotiating through the restrictions imposed by law enforcement intrusions into their care, families turned to politicians for intervention.

Their efforts over ten years of working with Congress brought their concerns to a head in 1982, when the National Committee for the Treatment of Intractable Pain succeeded in getting the attention of sufficient members of Congress. They were able to introduce legislation, force hearings, and even gain a vote on a bill to change national policy on the treatment of pain in terminal illness. The Compassionate Pain Relief Bill would have legalized heroin for the treatment of pain of the terminally ill and would have required the Department of Health and Human Services to manufacture and distribute it to pharmacies so that it could be prescribed for terminally ill patients with intractable pain. Advocates for the bill argued that on simple humanitarian grounds the pain of terminal illness should be relieved and the dying should not be required to suffer. They pointed to the use of heroin in England, which for one hundred years had provided effective pain relief. They argued that the British model of pain management should be copied because some patients, especially those with terminal cancer, could not be treated effectively with currently available analgesics in the United States.

At the time, the Reagan Administration officially opposed the bill on scientific grounds. Well-controlled clinical trials of the day demonstrated that morphine was just as effective as heroin in pain relief and newer (at the time) and more potent analgesics had just become available.

The debate had one positive effect: It exposed the

nature of the problem. The dilemma in the United States was not that there were not adequate medicines, but that the way in which physicians managed pain was inadequate. Physicians in this country medicated for pain in a more limited and ineffective way because of their unfounded fears of addiction and well-founded fears of law enforcement intrusions into their practice. With no such fear abroad, physicians in England used more medication more often on a routine schedule intended to anticipate and prevent the recurrence of pain. It was not, in fact, the heroin they used, but the way they used it that made the difference. The patient advocacy groups were right, but for the wrong reason. We needed change in this country, but not in the pharmaceutical arsenal. We needed a change of law and of heart that would allow for the use of appropriate medications that were already on the shelf.

The Reagan Administration feared that the use of heroin, even in medical circumstances, would signal that its use for other purposes would be tolerated. In addition, it feared that the presence of heroin in communities would increase the rates of pharmacy and drug-seeking crime and cause its diversion into the illegal drug markets. The bill was defeated. Families, desperate for a solution, forced a vote in Congress. There was not yet adequate consensus at the time about the need for a change in pain-management policy, and anti-drug-abuse forces won the debate. This brought defeat to years of effort to create change. However, the effort did not die. The families were effective in setting the stage for more attention focused on the treatment of pain. The Department of Health and Human Services and the American Medical Association embarked on a campaign to educate physicians in practice. These efforts prompted major policy and educational discussions within the clinical community. Have they been successful?

Healers Respond to Patient Needs
Nearly twenty years have passed. In some ways the situation has improved. New research has produced better pain

management strategies. Media coverage of pain management has increased. Recognition of pain as a clinical issue has expanded, its own set of side effects and sequelae are understood, and pain has been acknowledged in other previously undertreated groups, such as newborns and children.[20] The National Cancer Institute turned its attention, though less than 1% of its budget, to the issue of pain management for cancer patients. Congress requested that the Medicare Payment Advisory Commission (MedPAC) study inpatient and outpatient reimbursement barriers to appropriate pain management. A number of new pain management societies formed within the medical profession. Two of the most important groups, the American Academy of Pain Management and the American Pain Society, issued a joint statement recognizing pain relief—including with therapies that may hasten death—as the ethical obligation of all health care providers. They concurred that pain is often treated inadequately, despite available medicines.[21]

Patients, families, caregivers, and physicians continue to struggle with the task of caring for the dying and how best to relieve their suffering. The debate on the moral and medical challenges of care for the dying requires a response. That response demands extraordinary efforts to improve end-of-life care and optimal management of pain and suffering. We have the knowledge and ability to deliver skillful and effective control of pain and suffering at the end of life.

The JCAHO escalated the concern for health care facilities on matters of pain. Its new long-term care manual gives residents the right to expect a quick response to reports of pain and calls for statements to be posted in every patient room that notify patients of this right. In JCAHO-accredited facilities, patients are told they can expect that their reports of pain will be believed, that they will be given information about pain relief from concerned staff, and that pain will be responded to quickly and effectively. The JCAHO standard recognizes pain as common, as having serious consequences if not relieved, and as an important part of the ethical care of patients. It encourages education and involvement of the family.

Some State Medical Boards and legislatures have also recognized the problems of overzealous monitoring of pain medications and have initiated pain study groups and educational efforts. A majority of states already protect physicians from disciplinary, criminal, or civil action for prescribing medications to relieve pain through laws, regulations, and Medical Board Guidelines.[22] Most recently, the North Carolina Medical Board ruled that physicians will not be subject to disciplinary action, even if the medications they prescribed or administered to relieve a patient's pain hastened death. Ten states have passed legislation protecting medical professionals and family members who prescribed or administered medications for the relief of pain, even if the medications hastened the death of the patient, as long as the intent was not assisted suicide.[23] By 1999, another seven states had sought to protect physicians and families and had introduced similar legislation.[24]

Have these efforts been effective? A number of physicians, and a significant number of medical organizations, studied this issue and are on record as agreeing that despite the legal and regulatory protections offered them by their states and Medical Boards, law enforcement still intimidates physicians in their actual practices.[25] Actions, like that of the North Carolina Medical Board, were intended to respond to those physicians' concerns. In the words of Hospice for the Carolinas President Judi Lund Person, "I think this is sending a message. What we have all been trying to do is to quell real or perceived fear that if doctors prescribe what they think is enough pain medication, the medical boards may go after them."[26] Even other healers have "gone after" clinicians. Harvard Professor of Medicine Jerome Groopman, tells a compelling story of a physician who, with the consent of a dying patient and her husband, administers pain-relieving morphine that all knew might have the effect of reducing breathing or lowering blood pressure. The respiratory therapist attending the patient objected and accused both the treating physician and the patient's husband with hastening her death. Both the hospital review board and district attorney found the charges unfounded, but what impact will this experience have on the next such case that the clinician confronts?[27]

Have we gone far enough in reassuring physicians? Can we assure patients that actions such as these will help to relieve the pain of the illnesses that devastate their loved ones?

Suffering Continues

The family of William Bergman filed a complaint with the Medical Board of California against his physician after Mr. Bergman's death. The complaint requested that the physician be disciplined for failing to prescribe the medications that would have relieved the lung cancer pain he was suffering as he died in his daughter's home. The Board agreed that the pain management for Beverly Bergman's father was inadequate, but they rejected her request and declined to discipline his physician.

Subsequent to the Medical Board action, the family sued in court. Since California law prohibits awards for pain and suffering after the death of the patient, the family sued under "elder abuse" statutes and was awarded $1.5 million in damages. Since the failure to treat was not malicious, there were no punitive damages, and the award was subsequently reduced in a higher court to $250,000, but the impact at the time of the trial was predicted to be far reaching. It has been. Since that time, pending legislation in California would require physicians to receive continuing education in pain management in order to renew medical licenses.

Few families have made such disciplinary requests and even fewer have resorted to litigation, but family support and lobbying groups are currently recommending this as a strategy for driving change. This may well be the harbinger of a new trend in patient and family activism and empowerment. If so, it may also prove to be an unfortunate one.

Physicians practicing today, regardless of whether they are educated and experienced in pain management—and most of them are not—are caught in the middle between drug abuse and pain management tensions. Claims similar to those of the Bergman family were recently successful in Oregon, where the Board of Medical Examiners disciplined a physician for grossly undertreating pain in six patients. As a part of the disciplinary action, the physician must complete an extensive educational and counseling program.

Although some will hail this as the right prescription for bringing doctors into the proper practice of pain management, it is not. Healers who fail to act within their oaths and according to the standards of practice should be disciplined, but witch-hunting will not solve the dilemmas we confront in managing tough issues such as pain management, which are more social and legal than technical and clinical. Actions such as this, if they are abused, will place healers, patients, and families in an increasingly tenuous position. To subject those who prescribe and administer medications to the tensions between law enforcement and medical boards without a community-based policy and political resolution places both the healer and the patient at even greater risk. It encourages the physician to abandon the patient altogether. It encourages the family to limit whatever medicines are prescribed. As in ancient days, if physicians are made to walk clinical and regulatory tightropes and risk retribution for their attempt to treat the most needy of the sick and dying, they will be inclined to select their patients carefully. Left with no other choice, they may decline to treat those in greatest need of palliative care. If, at any time, healers might be called to defend their practices to drug enforcement agencies and medical boards—neither of which treat patients and both of which are charged with limiting drug use—they might become reluctant to provide that care. If, at any time, families are questioned about their methods and motives for using medication, they, likewise, will be reluctant to do so. The inevitable result for patients will be the painful deaths so many of them fear.

If these actions become witch-hunts, a cycle of fear will be created that will become even more deeply embedded in the care of the dying. Physicians' fears about prescribing important and necessary medicines would exacerbate the undertreatment of patients' pain, which causes unrelieved pain and in turn creates fear among patients and others who watch them suffer. Fear comes full circle. It is the greatest irony of all when patients suffer because the two gifts from the gods—the law and the healing arts—cannot resolve the tensions between them for the benefit of the mankind they were intended to serve.

Congress Muddles the Issues

Unfortunately, healing and law enforcement clashes were renewed when Oregon voters sanctioned a law allowing assisted suicide under some circumstances. In 1994, and again in 1997, the voters in that state approved a "Death With Dignity Act," which allowed patients to seek the assistance of their physicians to end their lives. Unrelieved pain was one, but by no means the only, aspect of dying that was cited by those who encouraged adoption of the voter referenda.

After Oregon passed the law, the federal Drug Enforcement Administration (DEA) informed physicians in the state that they risked losing their federal license to prescribe controlled substances if they used controlled drugs to assist in a suicide. The letter impacted physician practices and the number of prescriptions for controlled substances declined. Physician/healers, obviously concerned about the implications of being accused of misusing powerful, pain-relieving medications wrote fewer prescriptions for pain relievers. In June 1998, United States Attorney General Janet Reno issued an opinion that the DEA could not prosecute a physician who acted in compliance with the Oregon Death With Dignity Act. As a result, some members of Congress decided to act, launching another round of volleys in the conflicts over medical use of these medications for the pain of terminal illness.

The first was the Lethal Drug Abuse Prevention Act, introduced by Senator Don Nickles (R-OK) and Representative Henry Hyde (R-IL) in 1998. The act was intended to stem the tide of assisted suicide, fueled not only by the developments in Oregon but also by Dr. Jack Kevorkian's challenges to laws in other states. The act would have given the Department of Justice the authority to review the medical decisions of physicians with regard to prescribing drugs that relieve pain. More than 30 respected national organizations representing physicians, patients, nurses, cancer survivors, and pain specialists opposed the legislation. The positive aspects of the bill to improve palliative care were more than undone by the fears that federal investigations would create. As a practical result of the bill, not only would the actions of prescribing physicians be investigated, but their motives as well. The legal burden of proof, even in a drug abuse-paranoid society, would have remained on the investigators, but the impact on the physician, left to demonstrate that his or her motive for prescribing the medication was not assisted suicide, would have been extremely disruptive. It was widely feared, and rightly so, that it would have the chilling effect of creating even greater fears among physicians. The most compassionate and technically competent healers, who chose to stand by and assist dying patients in pain, would most certainly have been at greatest risk.

The legislation died. However, it rose again in 1999 under a new name. The Pain Relief Promotion Act of 1999 retains the essential components of the 1998 proposal. A third bill, the Conquering Pain Act, was introduced in response to the other proposals by Senator Ron Wyden (D-OR) and Senator Connie Mack (R-FL). It improves education, develops community resources for pain management, and requires studies to determine how government-funded programs can better manage pain. It calls for a study of pain management by the IOM, a highly respected and visible advisor to government. It will not resolve the problems we have created over the past five decades, but it will be a step in the right direction. The Pain Relief Promotion Act of 1999 passed the House and has been endorsed by a number of clinical groups, pain societies, and patient interest groups. It has redeeming features, particularly related to funding authorizations for education in pain control. However, it also continues to promote the second-guessing of clinical intentions of prescribing physicians. Mr. Wyden threatened to filibuster the bill in the Senate and it eventually failed. It would not be long before the Bush Administration would reverse the position of Attorney General Reno, however, and decide to "target" physicians who prescribed drugs that could have pain-relieving—though lethal—effects. Is this the best step we can take to aid the dying?

Communities in Conflict

At the root of the dilemma is America's drug abuse problem. We know from public service advertising that drugs fry your brain, and a majority of the kids who use drugs don't live in big cities. Full-page ads tell parents how to talk to their kids about drugs and show them how to plan their child's funeral if they don't. Some employers require pre-employment drug screening; others conduct drug tests on a periodic, and sometimes surprise, basis. Statistics from the Drug Abuse Warning Network (DAWN) report on the level and type of drug abuse activity. Local and state police and the federal DEA arrest dealers and users and display their conquests of these illegal networks with pride. There is no doubt that drugs are a problem that both law enforcement and health care experts need to address. Recent awareness of the abuse of Ocycontin® brought abuse issues to the fore once again.[28]

Preventing and treating drug abuse in this country is a valid objective, but it cannot be the only one. It is necessary, but it is not sufficient. We must also prevent and treat pain in terminal illness, and we know that is a problem for this country as well. It is a part of our lives and of our arts. It is portrayed in *Terms of Endearment* and the Pulitzer Prize-winning play, *Wit: A Play*. In these portrayals, we, as humans who ought to know better about how to care for each other, do not fare well. We speak, in our culture, as if we care about both the drug abuser and the terminally ill patient, and yet we act as if we care only about one to the exclusion of the other. What happens when law enforcement and medicine are at odds? What happens when they clash? Why is it that when some of us abuse drugs, the rest of us, our clinicians, and our caregivers become suspect if we use that same substance for medical reasons? Can we reduce the suspicion about the valid use of medicines to treat pain? Will we ever correct the tragedy of underprescribing the medicines that patients need as they die in pain?

How can we better resolve the tensions between law enforcement and the practice of medicine? How can our communities better balance the need to keep the streets safe from illegal drugs and yet ensure that patients in pain get the medications they need for relief? How can we protect physicians and nurses from harassment and provide patients with medicines while we sort out our differences about drug abuse prosecution and legitimate prescribing? How can we come to agreement more quickly so that more of us do not suffer needlessly as we die?

Confronting the Challenge of Compassion Within the Covenant

"Compassion" means "to suffer with," and we do precious little of that in the United States today. Dealing with the pain of some terminal illnesses and relieving suffering at the time of death have been among the most sacred responsibilities of healers for thousands of years. It should be no less the case for us today. In fact, the burden of the covenant should be even greater because in this era, unlike in earlier times, we have a panoply of medicines and better methods for accomplishing the goal of pain relief. If we apply those methods well, we can assure virtually all patients that virtually all pain can be relieved.

Compassion for the pain of illnesses that cause death should be the hallmark of a civilized society and a central tenet of the healing covenant. In undertreating pain, we do violence to patients at a critical time in their lives. This problem is not a new one and is in no way related to the proliferation of managed care or other reimbursement changes in health care systems. It is, instead, the result of factors that have their roots in denial, ignorance and conflict—all of which create fear and, in turn, allow pain to rule in the final days of terminal illness for too many people. It is clear that we are at loggerheads in this country on this matter. Law enforcement agencies, and recently some members of Congress, have ignored the very real suffering of the dying. They draw hard lines around the use of pain-relieving drugs and neglect the fact that healing entails the soft side of compassion. Healers, though they have recently become more effective in engaging in the policy debates, remain too silent on the challenges of pain management. We have failed to resolve our differences, and while we are deadlocked in conflict, our dying suffer.

The issues are clear. Should we, as a society, formally invite Congress and law enforcement into the covenant between the dying patient and the healer? How would that be accomplished? What experiences of caregiving would serve to educate them on the realities of pain? What remedies would we ask they pursue if these experiences commit them to caring? Are we asking the dying to disengage from the covenant and suffer because we fear our addictions and doubt our ability to manage them? Are we asking them to suffer in isolation because seeing their pain makes our communities wince? How can we balance the needs of our covenant to care for both the dying and the addict? Can we protect healers from bearing the brunt of the conflicts?

Creating a Covenant to Relieve Pain at the End of Life
Today, we have the most extensive arsenal for the management of pain in the history of medicine. No era has had such powerful pain-relieving technologies. Our medicines, surgery and complementary methods of pain relief are more developed now than at any time in history. Our understanding of the nature of the terminal illness and dying process has never been richer. Each pharmaceutical product is researched, manufactured, and licensed as safe and effective for working its miracles. Today's methods rarely fall short. Yet no healing responsibility has been so severely tested. Even those within weeks or days of dying are frequently denied the pain-relieving medicines that could ease their suffering, enable them to put their personal and spiritual affairs in order, and deal with the grief of their impending death with family and friends.

There are important ways that healers and communities, acting within their covenants with patients, can address these conflicts. The covenant between the healer and the patient was reinvigorated within a new paradigm with the work of Dr. Elizabeth Kübler-Ross, who brought us a new appreciation for the value of living embodied in dying and showed us ways to support the process of living until the end. That work extended through the hospice movement and has been institutionalized by health care reimbursement, patient demand, and volunteer service. The hospice movement has created a critical mass of patients and healers who, working together, have improved care and pain-management options. They entered into a covenant of obligation. The healer provided the supportive caring of human touch and palliative medical technique. The patient allowed the healer into his personal life, shedding intimate and protective boundaries and disclosing the seriousness of his pain and dependence on others. This covenant has not yet succeeded, however, in achieving a final resolution to the intractable conflicts that leave so many in pain, because communities have not yet been engaged to participate. Communities must now enter into a covenant of obligation with their own who suffer and with the healers who relieve that suffering. A number of additional steps are needed to achieve a resolution.

- Those who work in the fields of cancer care, terminal illness, and palliative care are in the best position, because of their knowledge and their standing in their communities, to call for a special covenant with the dying. In the style of all covenants, they are the superior parties who can grant the healing pain relief and who can create the obligations that will sustain the covenant. In the context of their own covenants with the patients they care for, they should lead the way to crafting a solution that can assure pain relief for those who need it.

- Congress and communities, for their part, should enter into this covenant, because it is conflicting public policy objectives that created the tensions that have resulted in so much unnecessary pain. This will require an intensified dialogue at the national, state, and local levels among clinicians, families, law enforcement, and policy officials who deal with both concerns—those of drug abuse and those of pain. It will also require extensive education of all parties— and particularly national, state, and local law enforcement agencies—about the nature of pain management in terminal illness. Finally, it will call for those of us in communities to trust our healers to practice the arts and skills we empowered them to use to our benefit. We can no longer explain away our lack of compassion for the dying and lack of trust in our healers with our fears of addiction and abuse.

- Any individual who holds a position of responsibility or influence in policy, clinical care, communications, or law enforcement should be required, as a part of this dialogue, to participate in the care of those who suffer from pain in terminal illness. They should see for themselves what has been hidden. They should learn the value of the medications that have been denied to suffering people. They should understand the consequences of their failure to act quickly.

- Each existing and new legislative initiative or regulatory control to prevent or manage drug abuse must be examined in the context of how best to accomplish not only abuse prevention, but also pain relief.

- The new clinical care groups and study centers, formed in the last several decades to heighten the awareness of pain management and conduct pain research, should be more widely acclaimed for their work. The work of groups such as those who have received "The Circle of Life Awards" should be placed in spotlights by the national media.[29]

- The press should heighten the awareness and knowledge of the public and the professions about the availability of safe and effective means of managing pain and should work to dispel the myths that prevent good palliative care for the dying. Further, the press should avoid sensational reporting about the illicit use of legitimate products, which only creates an increasingly hostile climate for product development and supply.

- In the context of a worldwide covenant of healing, we should recognize that the problem of treating pain is a global challenge. The World Health Organization (WHO) estimates that more than half of those suffering from cancer worldwide have unrelieved pain.[30] The U.S. should enter into projects and participate in efforts with the WHO and the International Narcotics Control Board to ease suffering everywhere, not just in this country.

- Finally, having addressed the most obvious of pain management issues—that is, the relief of pain in terminal illness—we should turn our attention to the relief of the chronic and sometimes unremitting pain endured by many people in this country and throughout the world. Herein lies an obligation created in our covenants with those who are dying. Through their stories and the willingness of their families to address these issues where they cast the sharpest shadows and draw the sharpest lines in public debates, we may accomplish a goal to relieve their pain and those of other dying people like them. Calling us to more compassion, however, may help healers and the nation to deal with the even tougher issues of pain suffered by those who are not terminally ill, and who pose even more difficult questions for medicine and society to grasp.

These are simple steps, but they may be difficult to take. The attitudes of everyone involved have been ingrained through years of practice. The suffering of so many is silent. The denial of death is so great. It is a task that must be embraced with greater energy and attention.

Can it be done? I believe so, and I draw my optimism for the future from my brother, Jim, and his wife Nancy, who for more than twenty years have volunteered their time to a hospice group. Jim wants to write a book. He'd call it, "You *Live*, Until You Die." It comes from his experience of seeing the old and the sick die well, living—and often laughing—right up to the last moments. It would be a book of warm, tender, and funny stories. His stories echo the words of one cancer patient who helped us understand the importance of pain management back in the 1980s. She said, "I found that when I didn't have the pain, I could forget I had cancer."[31] As healers and as communities, we should offer that to all our dying patients. To do less is to diminish the living of everyone, especially the ones they leave behind.

Part 3

GLOBAL CHALLENGES AND OPPORTUNITIES

The terrorism that struck the nation on September 11 shattered the safety and security most Americans felt within the borders of this country. That day, and the weeks and months that followed, heightened our anxiety and led us to consider what new steps would be required to enhance national health security. The first steps, predictably, were domestic. Subsequent steps, however, must be international. The U.S. will never have true national health security unless the health and disease realities of the world—particularly the developing world—are addressed.

Those nations—regardless of how poor they are or how distant they may seem—are neighbors. This is not a poetic illusion; it is a travel fact. In the early days of our country, wagon trains assembled in the nation's capitol to head west. Most often, these were comprised of families who, taking great personal risk and spending most of their financial assets, made their first night's stay just ten miles away in what is now Bethesda, Maryland. A statue of a pioneer woman and her child commemorates the spot. In that same length of time today, a traveler can depart Washington's international airport, and for a fraction of his or her wealth and virtually without risk, arrive at nearly any destination in the world.

This same access to safe and efficient travel is likewise available to those who travel from other nations to ours.

When they arrive on our shores, these travelers bring with them the diseases that are prevalent in their countries. These disease conditions do not respect the laws of international travel or commerce. Diseases do not respect national boundaries. Diseases do not seek passports or tickets to travel. Diseases hitchhike indiscriminately, whether in coach class or first class, whether by air or by boat. Diseases, unlike currencies, are not "changed" in some way to be more "acceptable" or "compatible" with the new host at the new destination.

As a result, serious and deadly conditions that are rare in the United States but common elsewhere in the world can arrive on our shores. We are not ready for these conditions today. Will we be ready tomorrow? Do we understand the nature of the problems in the world and how they impact the lives of others and, ultimately, our own? Do we comprehend the risks to our own health if the health of those around the world deteriorates? Can we grasp the political and economic consequences—not just to other nations, but to our own—of the crushing blows that diseases can deal when they overtake a society?

How will we use our resources to assist the global community and protect ourselves? What do we have to offer? How should we act, and what are the responsibilities of those in other nations who, though they may truly be poor, are nonetheless partners in health and healing with the wealthier nations to whom they look for assistance?

Chapter 7

Global Clinical Trials

Covenant in the Global Search for New Knowledge

New knowledge is the most valuable commodity on earth. The more truth we have to work with, the richer we become.

Kurt Vonnegut, Jr., *Breakfast of Champions*[1]

If the quest for new knowledge brings riches, nowhere is that more true than in health care, where new knowledge brings riches not only for those who seek the knowledge, but also for those who benefit from the resulting research discoveries. Our search for the truth about health and disease and about the causes and cures seems a thirst that cannot be quenched. Each new discovery brings yet another opportunity for new learning and begets new tools and new enthusiasm for pursuing the unknown. The American public is remarkably supportive, with more than 85% saying that the U.S. should maintain its place as a world leader in medical research.[2]

Increasingly, this is not solely a domestic venture for Americans. It is, more and more, a global endeavor. We have sought knowledge in and on foreign soil, to the benefit of all parties involved. Companies have entered into agreements with governments of tropical nations to catalog forest life in search of plant species and soil samples bearing potentially life-saving organisms or properties. Newly identified compounds are being screened against known diseases in hopes of identifying treatments and, better yet, prevention methods or cures.[3]

It is not just the natural resources of the forests that are important to today's research, however. It is people themselves, who form a reservoir of human subjects for research. With greater and greater frequency, investigators are looking to the developing world to identify the subjects who will participate in the development of the new human clinical knowledge that leads to innovative health products. This search is by no means a one-way street. The other nations where we seek human subjects are the same nations that seek our help in times of disease crises. We request research subjects to probe the mysteries of health and disease; they request disease detectives from the Epidemic Intelligence Service of the Centers for Disease Control and Prevention (CDC) to probe the mysteries of epidemics. In addition, those nations and ours collaborate in numerous other ventures. We maintain global disease surveillance systems, share medical education assets and participate in global health ventures through the WHO and its regional offices. Each of these ventures faces challenges. Some are under-funded. Others confront language and cultural differences. Still others must perform under adverse weather, geographic, and time zone conditions. The most contentious aspect of this international collaboration, however, concerns the use of human subjects for biomedical research studies.

How did the search for human research subjects turn outside the borders of the U.S. and other developed nations? Is the research conducted according to the same standards as research in the U.S.? Should it be? What is the covenant between the healer, the patient (or, in this case, the research subject), and the community in determining the appropriateness and conduct of the research? How can research studies be done in areas of the world where access to even the most basic clinical care is not the norm? When clinical trials are coordinated across several nations—as they often are—is it unethical to allow local standards and norms of care and of human subject protection to prevail, or should researchers adhere to a single international standard? How is the covenant tested in situations in which the cultural perspectives of the healer/researcher and patient/research subject differ to a great degree and language and ethical standards are widely divergent? Can global clinical trials rely on informed consent as the keystone in the covenant relationship among those involved? Is a covenant possible in global human research? Should we allow standards of research in clinical trials conducted in developing countries to be determined purely by economic considerations? Should we focus on procedures or on outcomes in our attempts to protect research subjects? Is it ethical to pursue biomedical research on subjects in developing countries for diseases common in the developed world? Or should human studies in the developing world be confined to diseases rampant in those countries?

Oaths

Each of the major medical oaths prescribes that healers will seek new knowledge about the workings of the human body and the nature of health and disease. In each, healers invoke all they hold sacred to assist them as they pledge, not only to care for patients, but also to learn more in order to care for them better. It is a sacred duty of the healer. They agree, as part of their obligations to the Divine, their patients, and communities, to study, learn, and share that information with other healers. The Oath of Hippocrates included research by implication in this commitment to learning and teaching, swearing:

> To consider dear to me as my parents him who taught me this art ... to look upon his children as my own brothers, to teach them this art if they so desire...[4]

Maimonides was considerably more explicit about research in his prayer:

> Thou hast granted man the wisdom to unravel the secrets of his body, to recognize order and disorder; to draw the substances from their sources, to seek out their forces

and to prepare and apply them according to their respective diseases.

And also:

Grant me contentment in all things, save in the great art. Permit not the thought to awaken in me: You know enough...[5]

And the Islamic Medical Oath was unmistakably clear:

... to strive in the pursuit of knowledge and harnessing it for the benefit but not the harm of mankind.[6]

That healers would also be researchers and develop new knowledge was therefore clear. *How* healers would do that was less prescribed in the oaths. For certain, the oaths speak generally to ethical conduct in encounters with patients. Patients are to be helped, not hurt. They are to be respected and privacy protected. They are to be granted the best that healers have to offer in terms of time, effort, and skill. Do those same standards of ethical conduct also apply to healers who are not involved in the clinical care of the person, but only in the pursuit of new knowledge as researchers? How should researchers balance the obligations between the quest for knowledge and the care for the human subject, who, in many cases, is a person—a patient—with a disease condition seeking treatment?

Human Clinical Studies

There are many ways to address the requirements of the oaths to develop new knowledge. Epidemiology and other population-based studies yield insights into health and disease states. Not all of these require the time or cooperation of human subjects. Computer simulations and models have certainly contributed to medical knowledge, but even today's sophisticated mathematical models and high technologies are not sufficient to tease all the mysteries from the human body. To fully comprehend the nature of the body and the impact of disease upon it, other methods are required as well. Regardless of the insights from simulations and models, eventually healers must conduct "tests" or "trials," first, using *in vitro*—test tube—techniques; next, with animals; and, finally, on human subjects. Studies conducted in human subjects are called "clinical trials." They are the final phase in the development of drugs and devices that diagnose, prevent, and treat disease. Without these tests, it is impossible to know if the product will be safe and effective for its intended use. Without the costs incurred by the developer and the risks incurred by the patient/research subject, the benefits of the promised therapy will never be clearly known or realized.

While there is no doubt that the techniques of clinical trials existed long before modern medicine, we in the West trace the beginning of clinical trials to the eighteenth century, when six treatments for scurvy were studied in twelve patients.[7] The immediate need of the sailors was not the concern of the investigators; rather, it was the nature of the intervention to prevent scurvy that was important. Although the trial lacked the rigor of modern research, it was the first recorded Western instance of a documented scientific approach comparing the effect and value of a group of interventions in humans.

A modern clinical trial is much more sophisticated than this early instance, but essentially has the same purpose—a *prospective* study to compare the effect and value of an intervention against a control in human beings.[8] This means that an intervention is planned and used selectively in humans to discern whether it will have an impact. When properly planned and conducted, clinical trials are a powerful technique for assessing the effectiveness of an intervention,[9] and they have been called the "most definitive" tool for evaluation of new products and treatment approaches. They are usually viewed as the research activity with the greatest potential to improve the quality of health care and control costs because they carefully compare alternative treatments.[10] In conducting clinical trials, investigators employ one or more intervention techniques and compare the results to a control group in which no intervention is made.[11] It is from this comparison that conclusions are drawn about the impact and value of the intervention. It sounds simple, but in practice, it is not.

In the earliest days of clinical research in the U.S., human subjects were drawn from pools of patients within this country. Research endeavors were small and initially were funded privately by philanthropists supporting individual researchers. As federal funding grew, starting in the 1950s, the need for research subjects grew as well. These subjects were increasingly drawn from institutions that housed large numbers of accessible research subjects: prisons, schools for the retarded, and the military. By the 1960s, the demand for research subjects grew even more as pharmaceutical companies faced stiff new research requirements under the Food, Drug and Cosmetic Act Amendments of 1962 to demonstrate safety and efficacy of drugs. The skills to conduct these studies also developed and expanded. Paradoxically, over the next twenty years, as the need for clinical research subjects grew, the supply of research subjects gradually declined as local access to new health care technologies improved. This is because prior to the 1980s, many patients sought to participate in studies as a way to access the best medical centers and clinicians in the country. As health care technologies reached local communities, it was no longer necessary to participate in trials to get high quality clinical care. When they could, patients opted to receive care closer to home rather than travel to major medical and research centers where, in addition to receiving care, they would most likely also participate in research.

These factors were already creating competition for human subjects for research in the 1980s, when the nation was stunned by the appearance of HIV/AIDS. As the disease took hold and the search for therapies progressed, the HIV/AIDS community influenced the nature of clinical study participation, creating a research-subject empowerment movement. HIV/AIDS patients became more influential in the conduct of research than any group before them. They participated in the structure of protocols and, as research subjects, even tested their experimental compounds in laboratories to determine if they were getting the active drug or the placebo. Some demanded changes in research design to assure that all patients, at some point in the trial, would have access to the active, hoped-for-therapeutic compound.

A decade later, the research pipelines of federally funded investigators and pharmaceutical developers exploded not only with new HIV/AIDS therapies but with other disease-target products as well, producing an even greater demand for research subjects. In addition, the regulators became more sensitive to the needs of an increasingly diverse American population and sought better balance in gender and ethnic age representation in clinical trials. The National Institutes of Health (NIH) developed web-based communications to attract patients to research trials.[12] Pharmaceutical companies even engaged advertising firms and partnered with practicing clinicians to recruit human subjects. Disease-based patient groups maintained registries of members willing to participate in studies. In the end, none of these efforts succeeded in recruiting a satisfactory supply of human subjects.

By the turn of the century, pharmaceutical companies were anticipating a 65% increase in the number of new compounds coming from their labs, and over 41,000 clinical trials were being conducted by private and public sector researchers. Of clinical trials underway, 80% were not meeting their enrollment deadlines for patients, and 27% of clinical development time was spent enrolling subjects. Industry was incurring losses of up to $1.3 million per day in incomplete trials in the U.S., though it was spending an estimated $1 billion just to recruit patients.[13] Government-funded research was increasingly addressing disease problems of the developing world and pharmaceutical companies were increasingly serving global markets and needed access to patients in those countries that would eventually be markets for their drugs. It should come as no surprise, then, that researchers began in earnest to look abroad for human subjects, particularly in those developing nations that had not already saturated the available clinical trial population with their own research.

It should also come as no surprise that with increased activity came greater scrutiny of the effort. The DHHS Inspector General (IG) studied patient protections in global clinical trials, noting a 16-fold increase in the number of foreign clinical investigations between 1990 and 2000, while the number of countries in which clinical trials were conducted grew from 28 to 79 during the same period. The IG recommended increased attention to foreign IRB capacity building and monitoring, improved sponsor monitoring, and tracking of studies and leadership from the U.S. to ensure patient protection.[14] An Office of International Activities was created within DHHS to monitor government studies. In the private sector, a new non-profit organization, the Association for the Accreditation of Human Research Protection Programs (AAHRP), was formed by a number of medical education and research organizations to develop standards to accredit and guide academic research policies and procedures.[15]

Clinical Care vs. Clinical Research

Whether the research is conducted here or abroad, one of the challenging issues faced by researchers is that clinical *research* is fundamentally different than clinical *care*. Clinical research may occur within clinical care settings, but it has traditionally been viewed as having an entirely separate and distinct purpose. Is it important to distinguish one from the other in order to discuss the ethics that should be present in each?

Clinical *care* is the activity of a healer to improve the patient's well being and attain a desired state of health. Clinical care can take a variety of forms—it can be diagnostic, preventive, convalescent, or supportive. Clinical *research* is the activity of a healer in carefully applying an intervention (as determined in the research protocol) to the patient and monitoring its effects on health or disease. Even though the clinical care provided to individuals involved in clinical research may be the same as provided in clinical care absent research, the respective purpose is different. Should the roles and expectations of the parties then be different as well? Clinical care is guided by a set of clearly-defined medical ethics. Can and should those ethics now be applied to clinical research, even though care of the patient is not the ultimate goal? What are the appropriate ways to ethically conduct research abroad, particularly in countries where the language, notions of disease, economies, and culture are radically different from those in the U.S.? These questions are challenging, and they are made all the more so by a history in which the ethics of clinical care were not applied to clinical research. As these lapses were often to the detriment of the research subjects/patients, this history has eroded confidence in the ethics of the research enterprise, making the consideration of global clinical trials dangerous waters for the unwary.

Ethical Lapses in Clinical Research

There are notable examples of dangerous and harmful experiments performed on non-consenting patients. In the most egregious cases, nonconsensual experiments have been performed on captive people in institutions, particularly those regarded as "lesser humans," such as Jews in Nazi concentration camps, the mentally retarded in institutions, persons of African descent, and indigent patients. Most often, these were people who were unable to decline or reject their participation in the research study.[16] In some

---

cases, informed consent was not sought or obtained, although the consequences for the patient were potentially harmful. In some cases the researcher, often a physician, fraudulently described an experimental procedure as either a diagnostic procedure or a treatment for the patient's condition, including cases where there was no reason to believe that the patient might benefit from the experiment.

Our modern perspective on research ethics came about largely because of these revelations, particularly those regarding the medical experiments conducted by doctors in Nazi concentration camps. However, abuse of human subjects was not confined to the Nazi regime, nor were abuses confined to prisoners. In 1963 American researchers injected live cancer cells into elderly debilitated patients in a Jewish chronic disease hospital.[17] In another incident, intellectually disabled children were injected with hepatitis in a New York State public institution.[18]

One of the most widely known incidents of its type, the Tuskegee syphilis study, came to light in the 1970s. From 1932 until 1972, nearly 400 African-American men from the rural south diagnosed with syphilis were left untreated—and were actively discouraged from seeking appropriate care—as part of a study designed to observe the natural course of untreated syphilis. The study was no secret among physicians who worked on sexually-transmitted diseases, and results from this experiment were published in medical journals for over thirty years. It was not until 1965, nearly twenty years after penicillin was demonstrated to be effective against syphilis, that clinicians objected to the experiment on ethical grounds. It was 1972 before a reporter from the Associated Press (AP) was tipped off, broke the story, and brought the study to the attention of the public.[19]

It is no surprise that the Tuskegee study continues to affect attitudes about clinical research within the African-American community, 81% of whom are familiar with its history (as compared to only 28% of whites). As a result, just over half of African-Americans who know about the study are now reluctant to participate in clinical trials, versus only seventeen percent of whites.[20] It is astonishing that mainstream American medicine was so blind to the ethical issues involved in withholding care—especially after penicillin was discovered to be an effective treatment—and that these studies could be allowed to continue for such an extended time. The medical research community clearly failed in its ethical responsibility to these men, and others who were research subjects without their knowledge and consent.[21]

The Tuskegee study was, unfortunately, consistent with other studies and was typical of practices in clinical research prior to our relatively recent concern for human subjects. In the Tuskegee study the issue was informed consent.[22] In other studies, prisoners were subjected to malaria, typhoid, and cholera. Given that most reasonable healthy persons would be unlikely to subject themselves to such risks, ethicists have since questioned the extent to which their consent was voluntary and recently have wondered if prisoners, given their dependent circumstances, can give their consent at all.[23]

In another study, the issue was compassion: a famous gynecologic surgeon conducted surgical experiments on African-American women without anaesthesia, because he believed that they did not suffer and would "bear pain" better than white women.[24] These practices, unethical by today's standards, were by no means only an American phenomenon, nor were they solely historical. A high-profile report questioning international clinical trials raised concerns and attracted the attention of Congress in the year 2000.[25] In New Zealand, a hospital ethics committee and IRB approved a study that denied treatment to women suffering from cervical cancer. The women were not told of their diagnosis or of the research study, though they were repeatedly brought back to the hospital for observation. Many died when timely treatment could have saved their lives.[26]

By the time the U.S. National Commission for the Protection of Human Subjects on Biomedical and Behavioral Research issued its report in 1979, it was clear that the risks, burdens, and benefits of research were out of balance. The risks and burdens of research subjects were falling largely upon the poor and the disadvantaged, while the benefits of improved medical care were being granted primarily to the more advantaged of society.[27] Might that be true today as we seek to conduct clinical trials overseas? How do we, in this nation, respond in ways that support the development of new knowledge while accommodating the complexities of global clinical trials?

Setting Ethical Standards

The global community responded to the research conducted by Nazi doctors, calling them crimes and crafting the Nuremberg Code. The Code constituted the first international normative framework to regulate standards in clinical research trials.[28] This document was subsequently superseded by the Declaration of Helsinki, which became a code for research and experimentation endorsed by the World Medical Association (WMA) in 1964. The Declaration of Helsinki has since been revised on five occasions to keep pace with the progress of science and ethics[29], and it is one of at least a dozen national and international standards directing ethics in research. What medical oaths lack in specificity, the scientific, regulatory and clinical communities now provide.[30]

Informed Consent as the Keystone of Ethical Research

For many years, the informed consent of the research subject was the key factor in assessing the ethics of the study. IRBs were created to assure that investigators take research subjects' interests into consideration, particularly those related to consent. Authoritative guidelines for research defined informed consent as a process by which an individual voluntarily expresses his or her willingness to participate in a particular trial, after having been informed of all aspects of the trial that are relevant to his or her decision to participate.[31]

The mechanics of informed consent for human research protocols have been carefully defined and detailed by institutional, governmental, and global organization regulations. Because these standards emphasize the *process* of obtaining consent and not the *documents* produced, securing valid informed consent is a complex process that involves multiple, interrelated elements. Valid consent comes only when the research subject has the capacity to understand and decide whether or not to participate and authorizes that decision voluntarily. That decision can be made only when all of the necessary information is disclosed.[32] In the U.S., while the burden of ensuring informed consent lies with the physician, the ethical standard recognizes informed consent as shared decision-making that involves the patient, physician, nurse, family, and all those with an ethical interest in the patient.[33]

In an ethically sound consent process, a member of the research team provides information to the potential subject and determines that the subject understands the information. The subject then must voluntarily agree to participate. In the documentation of the process of informed consent it is essential that the subject signs or otherwise indicates his or her agreement to participate. Many settings also require that the investigator who obtains the consent signs the consent form or other related documents and a witness (or person designated by the participant) attests to the process. The disclosure requirements in the U.S. are codified in the Federal Policy for the Protection of Human Subjects at 45 CFR 46.116(a).[34] The "basic elements of informed consent" set forth in these requirements for clinical trials include:

(1) A statement that the study involves research, an explanation of the purposes of the research and the expected duration of participation, a description of the procedures to be followed, and identification of

any procedures which are experimental;

(2) A description of any reasonably foreseeable risks or discomforts;

(3) A description of any benefits to the subject or to others, which may reasonably be expected from the research;

(4) A disclosure of appropriate alternative procedures or courses of treatment, if any, which might be advantageous to the subject;

(5) A statement describing the extent, if any, to which confidentiality of records identifying the subject will be maintained;

(6) For research involving more than minimal risk, an explanation as to whether any compensation and an explanation as to whether any medical treatments are available if injury occurs and, if so, what they consist of, or where further information may be obtained;

(7) An explanation of whom to contact for answers to pertinent questions about the research and research subjects' rights, and whom to contact in the event of a research-related injury to the subject; and

(8) A statement that participation is voluntary, refusal to participate will involve no penalty or loss of benefits to which the subject is otherwise entitled, and the subject may discontinue participation at any time without penalty or loss of benefits to which the subject is otherwise entitled.

Challenges to Informed Consent in Global Clinical Trials

American investigators are bound by American ethics requirements if the data from a study are to be used in the approval of therapies regulated by the FDA for the U.S. market. Although those standards allow for modifications based on local circumstances in developing countries, there is little guidance concerning how adaptations should be made. This makes the informed consent process as potentially uncertain from a regulatory perspective in the U.S. as it can be daunting from other perspectives in the foreign land.

Some of the challenges are economic, with some of these nations lacking the basics in even housing, food, transportation, and energy. It is no wonder, then, that the public health and clinical care infrastructures in these countries are also fragile. There are few systems for collecting data on the health of the population or the prevalence of diseases in the nation. Facilities are not readily available for identifying and screening study participants. Clinics lack basic medical supplies and are understaffed, even when the most basic conditions are being treated or researched. Despite such barriers, however, ethical clinical research can be conducted. Even many of the poorest countries have an educated class of clinicians, ethics committees, scientific peer reviews of research protocols, and local scientists and governments that are qualified to determine if the research may ultimately benefit the country.[35]

Some of the challenges are cultural. In some countries, for example, individual consent on many matters important to life is not a commonly held value; hence, the notion of individual consent in research must be imposed upon the citizens by the government and the participating research teams. In those nations, it is acceptable for consent to be granted by the community-of-the-whole, by tribal leaders, or by some other person, such as the husband of a female subject.[36] The age of majority also varies around the world. In the U.S., the legal age for consent is 18, but in many other countries it is much younger.

Some of the challenges are technical. Even though informed consent is legally viewed as a *process* rather than a *document*, the process is usually accompanied by a document that is signed by those involved in the research. This can be problematic in countries with low rates of literacy[37] or in countries where citizens fear that signing a document may place them or their families at risk of reprisals from an oppressive government.[38] Informed consent is also problematic in countries where the language has no words for "research study."[39] Host country representatives can translate consent forms, but agreeing on a form that is both culturally acceptable in the host nation and consistent with U.S. regulatory agencies is no small undertaking.[40] In some cultures, research subjects' belief systems about science, health, and disease are so divergent from those of Western nations that the nature of the research intervention cannot be explained accurately.[41,42] Some regulatory requirements common in the U.S. cannot be adopted overseas. Requiring the name and telephone number of a research contact and a human rights contact, for example, is impossible in a country where people do not have telephones.

Increasingly, the challenges are political as well. Even in the developed world, researchers encounter subjects who enter the trial in order to receive health care, not to be part of developing new knowledge. Patients, trusting in their physicians in clinical settings, believe that the investigators are acting as their physicians—in other words, as *clinician* healers, rather than as *researcher* healers.[43] This phenomenon, known as "therapeutic misconception," is widespread throughout the world. It is at the cutting—and bleeding—edge of research ethics today.[44] Therapeutic misconception rests on the confusion between the aims of research and the aims of medical treatment of patients. It is by no means a developing-world phenomenon, though it is likely to be more prevalent in developing countries for several reasons. First, patients may rarely receive care at all or may receive care only in government-controlled settings in which other forms of consent and individual choice are not the norm. The trust, dependency, and power in the patient-physician relationship transfer to the research encounter. Second, international advocates, acting as surrogates to promote the interests of the research subjects, often intervene to ensure that care is provided in the context of the research study.

Informed Consent Not the Sole Ethical Touchstone

Current federal regulations in the United States require IRBs to determine that "risks to subjects are minimized by using procedures which are consistent with sound research design."[45] The regulations further require that "risks to subjects are reasonable in relation to anticipated benefits, if any, to subjects, and the importance of the knowledge that may reasonably be expected to result."[46] While the federal regulations do not tell IRBs to review the scientific merit of a research design, research with flawed methodology will not generate valid or reliable data about the efficacy of the experimental intervention. In such cases, participants will incur the risks, inconveniences or discomforts of being involved in research that lacks the potential to produce general and beneficial knowledge. Thus, the scientific merit of research is an ethical issue because it would be unethical to put people at risk or even to inconvenience or discomfort them through participation in a poorly designed study. IRBs, therefore, assess both the scientific and the ethical aspects of the protocols they review.[47]

At long last, these considerations—which go beyond those of informed consent—are being addressed by ethicists now working to detail additional ethical requirements for clinical research.[48] Their continued exploration of these issues greatly enriches the notions of covenant that should be embedded in the pursuit of new knowledge using human subjects today, in all places on the globe. These new elements suggest that the study should have social or scientific value and should be conducted in scientifically valid ways because scarce resources (financial or human) should not be spent on projects that are unlikely to benefit mankind. They suggest that justice requires that subjects be selected in ways that are fair and do not stigmatize, or make vulnerable, someone who may be a participant. They propose that the poor and powerless should not be chosen for more risky (or less beneficial) research, while the rich and powerful are chosen for less risky (or more beneficial) studies. They also suggest that there be independent reviews of the research in order to assure public accountability and minimize potential conflicts of interest. Finally, in addition to informed consent, they believe that respect for human subjects should be demonstrated by allowing them to withdraw from the study, by protecting their privacy, by informing them of study results—including both risks and benefits—and by maintaining their welfare during the trial.

This last issue is at the cutting edge of ethical considerations in global clinical trials. In 1991 and 1993, the Declaration of Helsinki was supplemented by international research ethics guidelines produced by the CIOMS in collaboration with the WHO. This set of documents proposes new protections from exploitation for participants in research, and a critical new benefit as well. In this iteration of the global standard of ethics, sponsoring agencies are called upon to ensure that, at the completion of successful testing, any product developed can be made reasonably available to those in the developing nations in which the research was conducted.[49]

The importance of this proposal, as well as the minefield of ethical issues, became apparent in a recent controversy regarding global clinical trials. A North American company prepared to study a surfactant product in premature infants with idiopathic respiratory distress syndrome (IRDS).[50] Since a product for this condition was already approved in the U.S., testing against a placebo—no therapy—in the U.S. would have been an ethical breach. Likewise in the U.S., it would have been unethical to select infants for an experimental—unknown—therapy when a known therapy was available. As a result, the company turned to Latin American countries where products were not available in some locations, proposing to do the research there. The company and its advisors reasoned that infants receiving the experimental product would actually receive a higher standard of care than what was otherwise available. Significant objections from critic groups were raised with the FDA on the grounds that infants in Latin America deserved the same standard of care as those in the U.S., making the research company a party to the delivery of care. In its response, the company exposed its design committee makeup, ethics advice, clinical trial plans, and subsequent marketing and medical education plans. Beyond that, this example demonstrated the degree to which conducting research in the developing world is not only a matter of good clinical and ethical design, but a matter of equitable access to care on a global scale, enforced through public pressure and politics, to ensure current and future clinical care.

Maturing Covenant in Global Research Ventures

There is little doubt that the advances in medicine since the early seventeenth century when modern biomedical research began have greatly extended average life span, reduced morbidity and improved the quality of life in both the developed and developing worlds. There is little doubt that health care will continue to require human subject research in order to continue to make progress in addressing both the prevalent and emerging diseases of the world. We owe a great debt to the scientists and clinicians that created innovative and dynamic experiments for the advancement of medical technology and science.

However, any progress made in developing new knowledge depends on the willingness of those individuals who participate in studies as research subjects and who risk pain, disability, and even death as they face the unknowns. We owe a great debt to them as well. It seems clear that most people will acknowledge that a covenant exists

---

between those who conduct clinical research—the healers—and those who participate in it—the patients. It is time, now, to include in that covenant those who benefit from research—the community. The time has come to construct a covenant that can address the complexities of a research enterprise that is no longer confined to one nation, but that covers the globe in an attempt to better address all the diseases of the world. This covenant would find ways to deal with the complications of this global scale, where the communities within which research is conducted and the communities where the researchers are based have many cultural, socioeconomic, and political differences.

The challenge for U.S.-based researchers lies in satisfying many masters. One of those masters is the imperative for sound clinical trial design. Another is the need for adherence to sound ethical principles in research that have been described here. Another is adherence to U.S. regulation. Yet another is sensitivity to local and global cultural differences.

The major driving force among those is U.S. regulation. In essence, the United States bundles its research regulations, its ethical principles and the commitments that underlie them as part of the research projects it exports. Consequently, collaborative research protocols conducted abroad need approval not only of officials of the host country and local research institution, but also of the IRB at the investigators' or sponsors' home institutions. Protocols also need the approval of the FDA that will rule, ultimately, on whether the research can be used for product approvals. Yet existing rules and regulations governing the conduct of U.S. investigators (and others subject to U.S. regulations) may impede international collaboration and unnecessarily complicate or frustrate research projects. Just as ethics is not a trivial matter, neither is the delay in important research. How do we find a balance between the need for new knowledge and the imperative to treat human subjects in the most ethical ways? How do we balance the hunger for new therapies in a wealthy nation like ours with the contributions that the poor of the world make to our health as they agree to participate in studies that develop products they may not be able to afford? Where do the responsibilities of the healer/researchers end, and those of the American community begin?

It is difficult to reach the answers to those questions from purely research, economic, or bioethical discussions. These questions call for the participation of more parties—parties to the covenant of research. Complexities abound, yet there is little doubt that despite complex realities, ethical precepts, and multinational interests the end result will still focus on the relationship between individual healer and patient—even if in this case they are called researcher and subject.

- The patient has two faces—the one participating in the trial and the one whose fate that trial could ultimately affect. Both are important. For that reason, perhaps it is no longer ethical to speak of "therapeutic misconception." Perhaps the time has come for all *research* to also *care*, not just for the patient who will receive the research-demonstrated therapy from pharmacy shelves, but also for the one who agrees to place his or her own life, health, and comfort on the line to get the proof. The research covenant exists first within its own microcosm, where only the relationship between healer and patient exists; where the abilities of the healer nurturing the patient, and the reciprocating trust and compliance of the patient, should be the sole litmus test of what is, and is not, appropriate.

- The researcher has two faces as well. He or she is both healer and investigator, caregiver to a patient and objective monitor of a research protocol. Particularly in the global research arena, wearing both faces across cultures that may differ greatly from one's own will require guidance from the local

community. Principles, dictums, and ethical guidelines are all helpful, but there will never be a substi-
tute for making the global, local.

- It is for this reason that the dialogue with local communities, however they are defined in other nations,
must be frequent and careful. In many global studies, the diagnostic, educational, and therapeutic
interventions exceed the standard health care practices of the host nation, but are still inferior to those
offered in the U.S. Only the local community can
determine whether this is tolerable. Research subjects
and their national regulators and researchers should
be given the opportunity, if they so choose, to participate in trials that are incremental steps toward better care in their nation. The perfect, in some nations,
might well be the enemy of the good. Decisions
about when this is the case can be made only by the
people and the nations involved.

- When the studies are feasible in the host country in
terms of cost, public health infrastructure and cultural norms, but inferior to those of the U.S., are they
unethical? Though federal regulations clearly state
that a country's cultural standards and norms should
be taken into account, little guidance is provided
concerning how to do that.[51] Efforts to do so should
begin. The American public, if it desires an acceptable ethical standard that matches what it would
anticipate in this country, should also be prepared to
provide the funding, through public resources or
product purchases, to ensure that the necessary
resources are available when the trials are undertak-
en.

- Oversight of international clinical research should
apply to all research, regardless of source of funding
and purpose. Further, oversight should entail consultation, education, and consensus-building about the
value and methods of the research project and not

just regulatory restrictions and delay-causing requirements.

- Americans, too often unwilling to participate in clinical trials themselves, should increase their participation in research as subjects. Today's plentiful treatment options are the result of the participation of past generations in research. We, who now benefit so greatly, now owe it to future generations to join forces with researchers today in the search for new knowledge.

The world today faces a large number of unresolved health and disease concerns and a rapidly emerging set of new research methods. The needs of the poor in the developing world for health care will continue to run headlong into the American frontiers of biomedical science. This should sound a call for a dialogue among those who design, conduct, and participate in the quest for new knowledge, and, increasingly, this dialogue should involve the rest of us who will benefit from their efforts. It is a positive sign, indeed, that concern for research subjects in other nations has emerged as a public policy issue in the U.S. It is, in some small way, an indication of our rightful stewardship over U.S.-based research ethics. Now is the time, however, to consider the consequences and to own up to the complexities and costs as we move forward to adhere to the standards we promote and hold dear.

Chapter 8

Infectious Diseases and Bioterrorism

Covenant Within a Shrinking Globe

Be fertile, then, and multiply; abound on earth and subdue it.[1]

God

Noah, his family, and the animals had just landed on dry ground and left the ark. This particular story may be of Judeo-Christian origin, but, in actuality, it is only one of the "great flood" myths of the many cultures on this globe. Legend and literature tell of what happens next. YHWH—or in the case of other traditions, the creator-god of the myth—promises never again to destroy the earth by flood. The survivor Noah and his crew of humans and animal cargo are told to repopulate the earth. The organisms that cause illness in those humans apparently heard the command as well. They've done well, these many millennia. They've adapted to the climates of the globe and circumnavigated it as hitchhikers, as we traveled. They have survived nearly all of the attempts of eradication by us, their hosts.

This tongue-in-cheek commentary on the presence of disease-causing life forms on the globe today may be humorous, but the truth of the devastation caused by them—and those who use them as weapons of terror—is no joke. We should not minimize the challenges that lie ahead as we address the very real threats to human life from our inability to live side-by-side with so many organisms that cause the infectious diseases that maim, disable, and kill. Some of us have been protected with healthy immune systems, safe food and water, good housing, sophisticated health care, and preventive vaccines. In this new era of terror, some of us will be able to rely on security and intelligence forces to monitor, detect and prevent bioterrorist acts. But not nearly enough of us have received the benefits of those measures we know protect humans from the ravages of threats we cannot even see. All of us, regardless of how privileged, are at risk of becoming ill and suffering from a substantial number of diseases for which there are no preventive or curative medicines.

How will we choose to address the disease conditions that so threaten the health of the world's population? Will we continue to invest in public health and take the social and economic steps necessary to improve the living conditions of people on the globe? Will we support the diplomacy and peace-keeping efforts that prevent wars and the disease consequences they bring as refugees flee their homelands? How will those of us in the nations of wealth and privilege support infectious-disease prevention efforts in the developing world? How can we best develop the technologies and reform the health systems to bring vaccines and medicines to those who need them? How can we best prepare for the anticipated global pandemic that the influenza virus so reliably causes? How will we address the horrors that can result when these organisms are used to wage war? Will we find our way to global cooperation and true public-private partnerships?

Infectious Diseases Span Time and Cross Borders

Infectious diseases cause disruption of the world's economic well being. Diseases take life and cause disability. Diseases interfere with trade, tourism and foreign investment.[2] This, in turn, can further destroy a country's economic viability, as it is required to spend more of its GDP on health care during times when diseases are causing morbidity and mortality in the nation's workforce, keeping workers from their jobs. The more economically deprived a nation, the more widespread disease can destabilize governments, particularly newly democratic governments, as dissatisfaction with leadership creates reversions to oppressive regimes. In the past, these scenarios were playgrounds of fiction writers[3]; now they are ground zero of public health and safety officials.

Many of the infectious diseases that create these disruptions—plaguing plants, animals and humans—may be as old as the earth's earliest-formed microorganisms. Although they may have first attacked humans, it is believed that some we know best today—tuberculosis, for example—probably originated as zoonotic diseases; that is, in animals. When humans lived and worked in close contact with animals, were scratched or injured by animals, or when they ate poorly cooked or raw animal meat, the diseases carried by those animals may have mutated to adapt to these new human hosts.[4] The apparent transformation of bovine spongiform encephalopathy in cows into Creutzfeldt-Jakob disease in humans may be a modern example of that phenomenon.[5] A similar theory has been used to explain HIV/AIDS, which may have adapted to humans when people ate the sooty mangobey monkey (green monkey), a carrier of a simian immunodeficiency virus (SIV_{sm}) that closely resembles HIV2.[6]

There is little information about the infectious diseases of prehistoric humans, but we do have information from the study of Egyptian and South American mummies[7], along with medical case reports from early physicians.[8] Tuberculosis, caused by *mycobacterium tuberculosis*, is believed to have originated around 15,000 years ago, possibly by crossing the species barrier from cattle when humans drank milk from cows with *Mycobacterium bovis*.[9] A pre-dynastic Egyptian mummy from 3400 B.C.E. showed DNA evidence specific to the mycobacterium that causes Pott's disease (tuberculosis of the vertebrae), and studies of a 900-year-old Peruvian mummy indicate that tuberculosis existed in the New World long before Europeans arrived.[10] Early written evidence of pulmonary tuberculosis was found in the library of Assurbanipal, an Assyrian king (668–626

B.C.E.).[11] Tuberculosis was documented by Hippocrates in his "Of the Epidemics," written around 400 B.C.E. Hippocrates called the illness *phthisis* and identified it as the most widespread disease of the time, noting it was usually fatal. Similar documentation comes from the Roman physician Claudius Galen.[12] Shakespeare mentioned tuberculosis in his plays, as "consumption" in *Much Ado About Nothing*, and as "scrofula" in *Macbeth*.

Malaria is another ancient disease. The malarial *plasmodium* parasites probably originated in Africa, possibly before the dawn of man, since fossils of mosquitoes up to 30 million years old have been found.[13] References to deadly fevers that were probably malaria, can be found in Indian Vedic writings of 1600 B.C.E., and again in the writings of Hippocrates from around 2,500 years ago. Since the medical texts of the early Mayans and Aztecs make no reference to malaria, it is reasoned that it came to them with the European military and civilian settlers who came to colonize the New World. That form of disease transmission would not be uncommon. Malaria is mentioned in military accounts as devastating troops more than battle injuries, and it is believed that Alexander the Great spread malaria during his various far-reaching military campaigns. One of the first military expenditures of the Continental Congress was for $300 to buy quinine to protect the troops of General Washington. During World War II, when General Douglas MacArthur commanded troops in the Southwest Pacific, he complained that it would be a long war if only one of three divisions could face the enemy while the other two were either in the acute or recovery phases of the disease.

Measles can be found in references as far back as the seventh century C.E. In the tenth century, Rhazes described the disease as more dreaded than smallpox, and there is mention of measles often occurring along with other epidemics. A smallpox and measles epidemic from 1530–45 killed nearly 1.5 million people in Mexico.[14] Diarrheal diseases caused by several different and distinct organisms—cholera, typhoid fever and dysentery—killed many and created major problems for soldiers in numerous battles throughout history.[15] Pneumonia and other acute respiratory diseases—particularly influenza—have killed millions of people worldwide through the centuries. One influenza season alone in 1918–19 killed 20 million people.[16]

It is no surprise, then, that man has attempted to control these diseases. Within the covenant of obligation created at Sinai, community public health measures were detailed to prevent and control the spread of disease. Some were drastic, calling for homes with mildew to be sealed for a time, replastered, and, if the mildew did not disappear, to be dismantled and taken to a dump outside the town.[17] People were cleansed in prescribed ways and their clothes burned if they contracted infectious diseases.[18] Other methods have been mounted since that time, such as public health measures to provide safe food, pure water, uncrowded housing, and vaccinations, and many of these measures have been successful. Medicines have been used to treat the overwhelming infections caused by the offending organisms. Hospital care and oral rehydration are also used to support patients as they suffer and recover from the malady.

Mankind has attempted, as well, to eradicate infectious diseases altogether, and several are on their way out. It is projected that polio and leprosy may be conquered by 2005, and measles and hepatitis B by 2010.[19] A campaign for global eradication of malaria was initiated by the WHO in the mid-1950s, but by 1967 it was clear that eradication was impossible and the focus shifted to a more modest goal: control. In one of the most notable private-sector endeavors, The Carter Center embarked on a number of projects in the developing world to improve health and survival. It attacked river blindness, *trachoma*, *schistosomiasis*, and *lymphatic filariasis*, and it achieved a 97% eradication of Guinea Worm in Asia and Africa.[20]

Man has been able to eradicate only one disease so far: smallpox. Though the Chinese may have attempted to stem the tide of smallpox over a thousand years ago, we in the West credit Edward Jenner, with his first vaccination in 1796, as the beginning of immunization science. It would be many years, however, before smallpox eradication would be attempted, and the successful achievement of that goal would not be announced until 1979.[21] With any luck, the announcement will not be premature, as some public health experts wait to see if icecap melting from global warming will lead to a renewed exposure to the smallpox some scientists believe may be trapped within the ice[22], and as national security experts wait to see if smallpox will be used as a weapon in the post-World Trade Center terrorism era.

Even in the absence of extraordinary circumstances, mankind today continues to confront virulent diseases. Together, six diseases cause 90% of global infectious disease deaths: tuberculosis, malaria, diarrheal diseases, acute respiratory diseases (including pneumonia and influenza), measles, and HIV/AIDS. While most of these diseases are very old, some are quite new, which means that we must also confront the reality that new diseases can emerge on the globe and strike us at any time. In the past three decades alone, thirty new infectious diseases have been identified, including rotavirus, a cause of infant diarrhea; Human Immunodeficiency Virus, a cause of HIV/AIDS; *Borrelia burgdorferi*, a cause of Lyme disease; Ebola virus, a cause of acute hemorrhagic fever; *Legionella pneumophila*, a cause of Legionnaires's disease; *Helicobacter phlori*, a cause of peptic ulcer disease; Hantavirus, a cause of adult respiratory distress; and Nipah, a cause of severe encephalitis.[23]

The "Big Six" Take Their Toll

Tuberculosis was thought to be under control until it reemerged in recent years—with a vengeance. It is the largest killer of women of childbearing age, and altogether kills nearly 1.5 million people a year. Two billion people—one in every three worldwide—have latent tuberculosis, giving the disease a large potential reservoir. Adding to the human reservoir of disease is bovine tuberculosis, which is endemic, as children and adults drink contaminated milk in many parts of the world.[24] What is even more frightening is the widespread emergence of drug-resistant tuberculosis strains, created when people do not take medications consistently or stop taking them altogether midway through treatment.[25]

Malaria is endemic in sub-Saharan Africa, where the disease accounts for one in five childhood deaths. Pregnant women are more likely to suffer miscarriages, give birth to low weight babies, or die from the disease. It is estimated that 300–400 million people are infected with malaria yearly, and it kills over one million people annually. After some years of control, it is currently rebounding in many developing nations.

Measles, the most contagious disease known to man, infects 42 million children annually. It spreads easily by wet droplets from sneezing or exhalation, and infection is immediate. Measles is a major childhood killer in developing countries and a leading cause of death among refugees and displaced persons. It kills nearly a million people every year, mostly children.

Diarrheal diseases also strike children and are a major cause of death in the children of developing nations, especially under the age of five. Pathogens such as *Salmonella typhi* (typhoid fever), *Shigellosis* (bacillary dysentery), *Vibrio cholerae* (cholera), and *Escherichia coli* can be contracted from contaminated water and food, usually a consequence of poverty in areas where waste disposal and facilities for hygiene are inadequate. Periodic epidemics of typhoid fever and cholera are also killers of adults, particularly the elderly and those with compromised immune systems.

Acute respiratory infections (ARIs), such as pneumonia and influenza, are highly contagious and kill mainly the very young, the elderly, and those with compromised immune systems. It is estimated that these ARIs are responsible for 3.5 million deaths yearly. The misuse and overuse of antibiotics contribute to growing bacterial resistance to the most common drugs used to treat these infections.

HIV/AIDS is the most well publicized of the major infectious diseases. It is a true pandemic. While its devastation of sub-Saharan Africa is now well known, it has also spread in other populous areas, such as China, India, and the former Soviet Union.[26] There are estimates of the number of HIV/AIDS-infected people worldwide, but many within the health professions believe the numbers to be much higher than what is reported. The majority of those infected with HIV/AIDS are working-age adults. The disease is fatal. While there are medications that will prolong life, the death toll and the consequences to family life and national economics and stability will be staggering in developing nations that do not have the infrastructure to promote prevention and education, provide HIV testing and clinical care, afford the medications, and ensure patient compliance.

Causes Are as Old as Mankind

Before the late Neolithic period, acquiring disease in any way—either from animals or plants, or from other humans, for that matter—was not a major problem for mankind. Hunter-gatherers lived mainly in small clans of 25 to 50 people that were well dispersed from each other. Even if an infectious disease spread within a clan, the rest of humanity was safe. As people adopted an agricultural life, however, clans grew into larger tribes, providing more human hosts in which the disease could spread and creating a more substantial impact on the economics of the community and the survival of the people.[27] Today, the population size and density are beyond what early man could have imagined. The worldwide population is currently six billion and is expected to rise to nine billion before it stabilizes. But population size alone is not the only driving factor in the spread of infectious diseases; other human behaviors and cultural dimensions help enable these devastating diseases to spread all the more rapidly.

Human travel is one of those behaviors. Travel has always spread infectious disease, and more of us are traveling today than ever before. Two million people cross international borders each day. Each week, a million people will leave a developing nation to travel to the industrialized world, principally to find work. In a year's time, fully 10% of the world's population will leave one country to travel to another[28], and few will understand their risks of contracting disease or take precautions to prevent acquiring a transmissible disease.[29]

We not only travel more, we travel faster and connect more remote locales directly to the most populous areas. In 1850, there were fewer than one billion people in the world and it would take nearly a year to circle the globe. Today, any one of our more than six billion "neighbors" can travel from their home to ours, arriving on our doorstep in less than one day. In the case of our North American continent, of the 350 and 500 million visitors each year to the U.S., more than a million come each day from our closest neighbors—250,000 from Canada and 800,000 from Mexico. In less than the incubation period for many diseases, an infected person can travel across our borders, or across the globe. An infected patient or treating doctor could easily leave the area of an Ebola outbreak in Africa and arrive in another country halfway around the world before the first symptoms became evident. Likewise, one person can infect others across their own country. This happened recently within the U.S. when a patient infected airplane passengers on a flight from New York to the Midwest,[30] and when teenagers returning from a summer mission in Mexico spread pneumococcal pneumonia through five states, causing both illness and death.[31] Air travel has also made it easier for animal and insect disease vectors, such as mos-

---

quitoes, to spread over an increasingly larger area of the globe. Malaria-carrying mosquitoes have been identified in industrialized country airports "hitching" on commercial flights. Mosquitoes carrying dengue virus or yellow fever can do likewise, as can other disease-carrying insects, such as tsetse flies, which carry *trypanosomiasis*, or sleeping sickness, and sandflies, which carry *leishmaniasis*.[32] Ships and their commercial cargoes of equipment and food multiply the possibilities for transporting the vectors that cause disease into areas that previously had little or no incidence of the condition.

Even travel within a nation spreads disease. Every year, people leave rural areas to migrate to cities, principally for employment. Over the last century, cities in both developed and developing nations have seen major growth and overcrowding. In developing nations, the infrastructure of these cities has not kept pace with population growth, and public health measures, such as clean water and effective waste removal, have deteriorated. Making matters worse, many of those who emigrate are poor and live in overcrowded and substandard housing, where airborne diseases spread rapidly. Poverty and the physical environment surrounding the poor are prime areas for the growth and dispersion of harmful organisms. Open and stagnant pools of wastewater are perfect breeding grounds for insects and parasites.[33] But diseases are transmitted from person to person in the developed world as well, where those of us with adequate housing and sanitation frequently neglect the important, well-known and simple preventive measures, like sanitary food handling, hand washing, and vaccines.

As the population migrates to cities, economic development and land use choices have disease consequences. Destroying forests and grasslands for agricultural use forces disease-carrying animals and insects to come into closer contact with humans. Lyme disease-infected deer, therefore, are no longer distant in forests, but are forced into suburban backyards. Rabies-infected animals search for food in neighborhood waste bins. Building dams for recreation and irrigation encourages the spread of water-breeding vectors, like mosquitoes and snails, and when grasslands are destroyed for farming, disease-carrying field mice come into closer contact with farmers and their animals. This same migration has created a market for trafficking in young girls and women who, lured by promises of factory employment or sold by families for the value of their labor, become sex-workers forced into brothels in cities, contributing to the spread of HIV.[34]

Each year in the past decade, there were 40–59 wars on the globe.[35] Refugees fleeing fighting zones bring their diseases to new areas. The crowding and poor nutrition and sanitation in refugee camps add fuel to the fire by allowing diseases to spread rapidly. Tuberculosis, malaria, cholera, dysentery, and HIV are abundant in many refugee camps in both sub-Saharan Africa and the Middle East.[36] Peace-keeping troops spread disease also, as the prostitution that accompanies any military presence results in an attendant increase in sexually-transmitted diseases.[37] In the face of the budgetary strains of war on the nation, military spending is high and health care spending is low, even though far more people die from infectious diseases than from the consequences of combat. In the past fifty years, wartime spending globally exceeded $864 billion. Twenty-three million people died. In that same time period, prevention spending for only three infectious diseases—AIDS, tuberculosis and malaria—was only $15 billion, despite the fact that those diseases took the lives of more than 150 million people.[38]

War not only spreads disease; disease is a weapon of war.[39] Mongol soldiers in the 1300s used bodies of dead plague victims as cannon balls. Shot over the walls of a fort in Genoa, they infected the retreating troops, who carried the disease back to Sicily and from there to the rest of Europe. Lord Cornwallis attempted to spread smallpox throughout New York during the Revolutionary War.

General George Washington ordered letters received from Boston dipped in vinegar to kill germs he suspected were being used to contaminate fighting forces. One hundred years later, a Southern sympathizer would attempt to spread yellow fever through northern cities using clothing infected with the disease from an epidemic in Bermuda. Smallpox was also used by Spanish conquistadors and the U.S. army to subdue Native Americans.

Mankind has attempted to manage these disease conditions. Public health measures to assure good sanitation, housing, and vaccines are essential to disease control, as are surveillance, reporting, and management of outbreaks, including measures as drastic as quarantine. There is no better way to start—after these basic public health measures are in place—than with education, though this is lacking in many parts of the world. The best contemporary example can be found in HIV/AIDS. Even today, misinformation, bias, and ignorance about its transmission exist in the developed and developing worlds alike. This causes discrimination and violence against persons with AIDS, sometimes resulting in the denial of care. Sometimes—as in Africa, where it is believed that sex with a virgin will rid a man of HIV—ignorance has resulted in violence and rape of young girls, which actually further spreads the disease.[40] Sometimes—as in the case of Buddhist monks in Myanmar, who share razors to shave heads[41], or in rural areas of China, where the sale of blood contributed to the growing HIV epidemic[42]—ignorance hampers efforts to prevent practices that are not intended to be harmful, but are.

Frequently, education is minimal because the infrastructure for communicating with the nation is poor. Health care system weaknesses cannot do other than mirror the poverty and economic conditions of the region. Government leadership is sometimes lacking and native healers, long trusted but rarely able to stem the tide of the severe infectious diseases attacking the population, cannot fill the vacuum left by inadequate facilities, limited caregivers, and unavailable medicines. An exception is the currently widespread use of anti-microbials, where the cure might someday be worse than the diseases due to the increase in resistant pathogens caused by the misuse and overuse of drugs. In many developing nations, these drugs are available over-the-counter and can be used at the discretion of the patient. Sometimes they are used as replacements for vaccines that are intended to prevent the diseases. Further, these drugs are misused in both the developed and developing worlds when patients do not take a full course of prescribed treatment. Both misuse and overuse can lead to the emergence of resistant pathogens, a factor in nosocomial (hospital-acquired) infections. This problem is increasing globally and has serious national defense implications.[43]

Bigger Challenges Need Expansive Covenants

Those of us in the U.S. can no longer enjoy the illusions that we are protected in this country by our wealth, public health systems, and distance from these diseases. Health isolationism is, frankly, an unhealthy practice. In addition to the moral issues, there are practical ones. Even with the best that medicine has to offer available to us here, diseases that circumnavigate the world will show up in our cities and visit our schools, theme parks[44], homes, and hospitals. They will stress our health care system, deprive us of productive work and school time, cost us money, and, in some cases, take our lives or leave us with short- and long-term disabilities.

Intrigue surrounds the specter of bioterrorism today. Which nations have the capacity to spread anthrax or smallpox to the U.S. or throughout the world? Who might contaminate the food supply with botulism? From where might the next threat emerge? Might it be from a domestic source? Or are our only enemies those of hostile nations?

In many cases, the enemy is the disease itself, and one that we have, for too long, ignored is influenza.

Misperceived as a "mild" and "unimportant" disease, it is truly a killer of many. Influenza—commonly called "flu"— is one of the oldest and most common diseases known to man. It may also be one of the fastest killers. Influenza was first described by Hippocrates in 412 B.C.E. The disease today still affects large sections of the population each year. Its ability to kill stems from the fact that the virus can mutate quickly, often producing new strains against which humans have no immunity. Influenza epidemics occur nearly every year and in most countries. In the United States, annual influenza epidemics and associated complications are associated with 4 million to 24 million healthcare visits, 314,000 hospitalizations, and 20,000 to 40,000 deaths. These effects, in turn, drive the estimated $4.6 billion in spending each year in the United States on influenza-related direct medical costs, with the total costs upwards of $12 billion per year.[45]

There are two major types of influenza viruses known: *type A* and *type B*. These are further classified into subtypes on the basis of two surface antigens: *hemaglutinin [H]* and *neuraminidase [N]*. Both types of the virus undergo continual antigenic change (antigenic drift), resulting in new strains. The constant development of antigenic variants through *antigenic drift* is the basis for the seasonal epidemics and the reason why the influenza virus is carefully tracked worldwide and the vaccine updated annually. In addition, *influenza type A* viruses are more unstable than *type B* and can undergo a more dramatic, abrupt type of antigenic change called *antigenic shift*. In antigenic shift, which occurs when there is an exchange of genetic material between two different influenza viruses, a large proportion, or even all, of the world's population lacks the immunity to the new virus. In this circumstance, a pandemic can result in which disease spreads quickly and causes even greater illness and death.[46] An epidemic is bad, but a pandemic is far worse. The first well-described influenza-like pandemic occurred in 1580.[47] Since that time, 31 influenza pandemics have been documented, with three occurring in recent memory: 1918, 1957, and 1968.

When pandemic influenza occurs, mortality rates can be staggering. During the "Spanish Flu" pandemic of 1918–1920 *(A/Spain/[H1N1])* at least 20 million people died from influenza, including 500,000 in the United States. In addition, 20 to 40% of the worldwide population became severely ill with a virus that was especially quick to kill. Many people who felt well in the morning became sick by noon and were dead by nightfall. Those who did not succumb to the disease within the first few days often died of complications caused by bacterial illnesses, such as pneumonia. During the Asian flu pandemic of 1957 *(A/Asia/[H2N2])*, more than a million people died worldwide, about 70,000 in the United States. The Hong Kong flu of 1968 *(A/Hong Kong/[H3N2])* also killed more than a million people worldwide, including 34,000 in the U.S. These last two pandemics together caused an estimated $32 billion in economic damages worldwide due to medical expenses and productivity losses.[48] Another pandemic is highly likely, if not inevitable, according to the experts.[49] The Spanish Flu of 1918 circled the globe in a number of months, but any new pandemics are predicted to spread much more quickly given population density and rapid travel.

Based on rates of illnesses and complications observed in the previous pandemics, preliminary estimates from the CDC indicate that the next pandemic could kill as many as 60 million people worldwide.[50] In the United States, the potential impact is estimated to be between 89,000 to 207,000 deaths; 314,000 to 734,000 hospitalizations; 18 to 42 million outpatient visits; and 20 to 47 million additional illnesses. The estimated economic impact would be $71.3 to $166.5 billion, excluding disruptions to commerce and society.[51]

One of the most recent and worrisome influenza events occurred in Hong Kong in 1997. The virus infected eighteen people, killing six of them—a high death rate for an infectious disease. The outbreak highlighted the success of the global influenza surveillance network at the time, which is one important indication of a global covenant.[52] It all started in May, when a three-year-old boy with influenza-like illness was treated with salicylates and later died of complications consistent with Reye's syndrome. The laboratory diagnosis included the isolation of *influenza type A*, but the specific strain or subtype could not be further characterized with reagents distributed by WHO for diagnosis of human influenza viruses. Within days, infectious disease experts from around the world converged to investigate. Within weeks, tissue samples were forwarded to the CDC in Atlanta, to England's National Institute of Medical Research (NIMR) at Mill Hill, London, and to the Dutch National Institute of Health and the Environment (NIHE) in Amsterdam, the Netherlands. By August the virus was characterized as an H5N1 sub-type.

It was the influenza surveillance and warning system that noted the occurrence and alerted public health officials. In conjunction with the French *Institut National de la Santé et de la Recherche Médicale*, WHO maintains a global surveillance system, FluNet.[53] This system runs 24 hours per day via the Internet and links 110 WHO Influenza Centers in 83 countries. The centers communicate electronically, allowing each one to enter data remotely and to access real-time epidemiologic and virologic information. In addition, there are four other Collaborating Centers for Reference and Research on Influenza located in Australia, Japan, England and the United States. The global influenza surveillance monitors how influenza viruses vary within and between countries and continents during an influenza season, and it ensures both the collection of viral isolates for rapid characterization and the assessment of the epidemiological activity in the participating countries. This surveillance is critical in monitoring antigenic drift and shift.[54] Using this information, governments determine which strains require protections within the supply of the country's influenza vaccine and companies manufacture, in very short timeframes, the vaccine to those specifications. Vaccine in hand, public and private health care providers immunize susceptible groups.

Although the disease has occurred in chickens in subsequent years, officials have taken the appropriate actions, and the world is fortunate that the Hong Kong outbreak has not spread, initiating the long-anticipated, much-feared pandemic. Still, a pandemic is predicted and planning for the event is underway within this country and in international health care settings.

Managing Bioterrorism: Disease as a Weapon of War

In 1997, experts from around the world arrived in Hong Kong within days of the alerts about the new influenza strain. Their responses were prompt; cooperation was evident. A global infrastructure was in place and succeeded in alerting all nations to the possibility of the anticipated pandemic. Political will, public health readiness, and press coverage—perhaps generated by the impact of prior pandemics—has helped us achieve better global health protection from influenza. Does influenza pandemic planning now provide us with a road map for considering global covenants regarding infectious disease—and particularly those that are intentionally inflicted? If we are going to respond now to threats of uncontrolled, serious disease—whether induced unintentionally or intentionally—can we use influenza as a model to address the seriousness of the challenges that lie ahead?

Perhaps influenza is the best of all models. On one hand, the experts say that a pandemic is a near-certainty, and so on those grounds, the effort to plan, protect and educate the public is a worthwhile investment to make. On the other hand, the unknowns of an intentional spread of disease are speculative, and securing the political will to plan for and fund the necessary infrastructure will therefore be difficult. Influenza pandemic planning with bioterrorism in mind may be the best and most successful alternative.

Engaging in planning for the intentional infection with deadly disease will require substantial education of the public and policymakers. Bioterrorism has yet to take its toll in modern times, but its potential is not new to the public health and safety community. Historical public health studies have charted the course of plagues through Europe and Asia, going back thousands of years. The experts are well aware of infectious diseases and their consequences. However, the notion that these disease epidemics could have killed 25 million people in the mid-1300s—which was 30–50% of the European population at the time—is staggering to the modern imagination. Even those in political and leadership positions who may deal with similar scenarios today are unprepared for the types of disruption in economics, politics, religion, agriculture, and science that was caused then by the Black Death.[55] Yet, we will inevitably face some of those same consequences in our time—if not from bioterrorism, then from HIV/AIDS.[56]

Understanding how diseases can be transmitted, how they have been used in wartime[57], how they have been used in domestic terrorism already, is key to grasping the urgency of addressing bioterrorism today. Since attempts at bioterrorism have been foiled[58] and incidents have been rare, they seem too remote for serious attention. As time passes and memories of Postal Service anthrax incidents of 2001 fade, it will be difficult to maintain the momentum needed to successfully plan and prepare for possible future attacks. What today seems *possible*, tomorrow may seem *improbable* and next year may seem *impossible*. Because of their planning, experts today know about the most likely diseases that would be employed in an attack. They also know our current national vulnerabilities, have created scenarios to anticipate the impact on the nation's health, and have proposed programs to improve our readiness.

Despite these plans, it has been difficult, unfortunately, to secure the funding necessary for the infrastructure required for readiness. As a result, public health surveillance and communication systems are weak, laboratory facilities and manpower are insufficient, vaccines are not available in adequate types and supply, and coordination across the myriad of local, state, and national agencies had been untested—at least until September 11. The WHO encouraged world leaders to plan, Presidential Decision Directives guided federal agencies, and the CDC coordinated with states, but, in the opinion of many experts, we are still woefully unprepared for an attack. The execution of the Postal Service contamination might have been a surprise; our failure to adequately respond to it was not. If there is a positive side to this event, it is that the nation's political leaders and the public now know what public health experts have known for decades about the risks of serious infectious disease. Will the nation now be more willing to invest in those services and systems at a level sufficient to protect us in the event of a future attack?

A truly global covenant to protect and care for the world's people as they live, work, and travel more often and in closer proximity to one another is needed. If one is to emerge, then we in the U.S. and other developed nations must become more aware and take more definitive action. If we cannot respond out of compassion and social justice, then enlightened self-interest will do. But act, we must. There are no "developing-world" diseases. There are only global diseases. Despite our wealth, education, and privilege, we and our children will be exposed to these diseases through global commerce, education, and entertainment. Despite our immigration and border controls, we will suffer the consequences of the presence of these diseases in other countries. Despite our own relative domestic tranquility, the harsh realities of disease-driven destabilization in other countries will impact our lives. Despite our best efforts, bioterrorism may be the most devastating weapon our enemies will use against us—or others—and the impact will be felt in our own communities.

The Global Village Needs an Expanded Covenant

The *New York Times* recently reflected on the dilemma of our living side-by-side with microbes:

> Microbes, are, after all, members of the most ancient, zealous and Darwinically gilded 24-7 delivery consortium. They travel by land, sea, air, nose, blows, glove, love, sewage, steerage, rat backs, hat racks, uncooked burritos, overlooked mosquitoes.[59]

The poetry of this statement should not distract us from the deadliness of the illnesses cause by microbes. We will certainly face them as a nation—and a world—in the coming years. So what actions should we take? Charting the course is underway in government and private sector groups, and a consensus is emerging. To better prepare for the future, we need to learn from simulations like *Dark Winter* and from the reality of outbreaks as they have occurred.[60] What these lessons have taught us is that our public health infrastructure—at local, state, national, and global levels—is tattered and our lost confidence in its ability to protect us is justified. It needs improved communication systems, more laboratories and personnel, additional disease surveillance capability, and stockpiles of drugs and vaccines for at least the most predictable of our needs. We also need improvements in public education and awareness about the appropriate use of antibiotics, and encouragement for the wider acceptance of vaccines. Health care professionals need education to better diagnose infectious disease and identify unusual patterns of illness, even in small populations, and clear protocols for treating patients when these diseases strike. Additional research on infectious diseases is needed to develop control strategies, drugs, or vaccines as a national defense strategy. Since many of the disease killers today are caused by organisms that can be controlled if we make the appropriate investments, eradication is also a necessary component of any strategy.

Not all our needs lie within the purview of the health sector, however. The policy, ethical, and legal foundation must be laid now, during these times of heightened awareness and relative tranquility, to address the complex issues of personal rights in an era of disease and bioterrorism. In 1893, Muncie, Indiana, suffered a suspected smallpox outbreak. The diagnosis of the disease, and therefore the government recommendations for quarantines, were questioned by the local community. Army guards patrolled neighborhoods, violators were jailed, and several public health officers were shot.[61] In Boston in 1902, public health officers ordered smallpox immunizations, fined or jailed those who refused to comply, and forcibly immunized others using squads of special police.[62] Is this our likely future as well? Now—not when the crisis is upon us—is the time to consider what we will require of the public in terms of quarantines and what rights to personal choice and privacy they will have. Likewise, we should consider now the implications for post-crisis malpractice and product-liability litigation in the context of treatment administered by overtaxed clinicians with incomplete information and resources.

Those of our healers who work in public health will plan for, and respond to, the challenges of global infectious disease and bioterrorism acts within their current environment; and herein lies another challenge. Health care today—here and abroad—is stressed. Much like a physician uses "stress tests" to detect the weaknesses in the patient's body, infectious diseases and bioterrorism are the "stress tests" of the health infrastructure. The limits of knowledge, information, surveillance, personnel, facilities, and treatments are, now more than ever, clear to us. This is true of our mental health care systems as well as those for our physical health. Our vulnerabilities are showing, and they promise to worsen over time.

How will it be possible to address these issues? It will be possible through a sustainable effort of both public and private sectors. It will be possible through the coordination of local, state, national and international alliances of health and other sector leaders. It will be possible if all the parties involved—patients, healers and communities—embrace a global covenant.

- For patients, this will mean becoming educated about, and practitioners of, those behaviors that prevent the spread of disease. We will have to wash our hands, use antibiotics correctly—and only when necessary—and be willing to take vaccines. We will have to take curative medicines—such as those for tuberculosis—in compliance with recommendations.

- For healers, this will mean developing and maintaining the capacity to deliver services and supplies when epidemics strike. Collaboration is one avenue to success, and there are models that point the way. In the case of tuberculosis, the WHO championed and initiated direct observation therapy (DOT), for example, wherein a health care provider actually observes patients taking tuberculosis medicines to be sure it is done correctly, thus working to prevent further treatment-resistant disease.[63] In the case of malaria, the WHO developed the *Roll Back Malaria* program, encouraging the use of bednets impregnated with mosquito repellent to protect from mosquito transmission of the disease. At a cost of a few dollars per bed, malaria transmission will be cut by 50%. ExxonMobil contributes to *Roll Back Malaria*, as well as to several other malaria projects investigating antimalarial drugs.[64] Mothers in Ethiopia, trained by a Johns Hopkins School of Hygiene and Public Health project, have reduced malaria in young children by 40% in a program to diagnose the disease, treat it with chloroquine, and detect adverse reactions.[65] This collaboration requires that agencies resolve infighting[66], corrupt leaders not use national needs to amass personal wealth[67], and tensions are resolved between the public and private sectors.

- For communities, this will mean financially supporting public health tools so that they are ready when disease disasters strike. The effective methods to address infectious disease are too numerous to list here. But some examples are indicative of the approaches to protecting health. Public funding is one way, private investment is another, and philanthropy is an increasingly important way. In recent years philanthropists have directed their efforts at global health causes. Bill Gates' donation of $21 billion to The Bill and Melinda Gates Foundation to improve health care in the developing world is the single largest of its type, and since 1998 the foundation has contributed $845 million[68] to tuberculosis projects. Ted Turner has likewise made notable donations. They are among the richest people in the world, and their philanthropy, as well as the donation of others, is on the rise, particularly among Americans, who are the most generous of all the nations.[69] Their efforts, though criticized by some, are laudable and more should be encouraged, not only here, but abroad. Our tax-deductibility measures are one way that the social objective of giving is supported by national policy. Other nations, most of whom do not support giving with tax incentives, might well consider doing so. Even Americans, however, can afford to be more generous as a nation. Despite being the most generous—in both real dollar and GDP terms—we still donate a scant one percent of our national GDP. It is estimated that up to half of the health care provided in many developing nations is funded through donations, and so the maintenance and growth of these programs is critical to the future of health.[70]

- For the developed nations, this will mean addressing the underlying causes of disease by assisting with development projects that bring safe water and food and adequate housing and sanitation to those who lack them on the globe. It will also mean addressing other root causes of conflict. The public health community was recently criticized for positioning infectious disease and bioterrorism in the context of the wider social issues of global power shifts, poverty, and injustice. When it advocated that seeking ways to alleviate poverty and negotiate peaceful settlements to disputes was an essential part of prevention, the American Public Health Association leadership was jeered in some quarters. In fact, those healers who ply their skills in the public health arena are calling our attention to a very important fact: that the best way to assure health over the long term is to reach the social roots of disease conditions. They are calling for the interdependence that covenants entail. They are warning us that, while depending upon them for assistance when we need them is within their covenant of caring, it is also expensive and should be unnecessary. They are inviting us into a covenant of obligation and pointing the way to the social, economic, and cultural issues that must be addressed in order to exercise that obligation. If public health officials can succeed in accomplishing the action steps they intend to take, they may well be able to restore and strengthen confidence of the public in the health care system—and the government—to care for the nation's needs. In return, political leaders and the general public should respond by not only supporting the needed resources, but also with mandates to work toward resolving the political and economic conditions causing intentional and unintentional epidemics.

There is a simple reason to accomplish these goals: no one is safe. Pathogenic microorganisms do not respect man-made national borders. As people cross borders, they bring diseases with them. Whether their know they are carriers or not, whether their intentions are innocent or malevolent, too many of these diseases can kill. We in the U.S. might think we can ignore the actual death toll in other nations, but we cannot. Aside from the human impact, there are the social, economic, and political impacts of disease on those nations, and ultimately on our own. Gro Harlem Brundtland, Director General of the World Health Organization, has said, "With globalization, a single microbial sea washes all of mankind. There are no health sanctuaries."[71] Not even here, in this most prosperous of lands.

Chapter 9

Healing Beyond Our Borders

Covenant and Medications for the Global Community

> *Suffering today is because people are hoarding, not giving, not sharing.*[1]

Mother Theresa

Recognizing Need

The world beyond our borders is a globe romanticized by television's *Discovery Channel* and *National Geographic*. It is a fantasy of *Arabian Nights* and jungle princes cartooned by Disney. It is a world of poetry and adventure tourism.

The developing world is altogether different, and since September 11, we in America have become more aware of its realities. It is a nightmare of child labor, child soldiers, starvation, death, slavery, and war. It is a world with few hospitals. Clinics are a thirty-mile walk from home. That is, if the person has a home: far too many people are refugees from wars, persecution, and natural disasters, living in unspeakable conditions. Parasites live in the drinking water. Most of the people do not have access to health care as we know it. Health care spending may be as low as $10 per person each year—or less—and millions die annually from diseases that could be treated with modern public health measures and medical care. People, especially children, die from pneumonia, malaria, diarrhea, tuberculosis, and vaccine-preventable diseases. If they do not die, they may be left orphaned when their parents or grandparents die—11 million are orphaned worldwide from AIDS alone.[2] Blood is not safe from HIV, hepatitis B and C, and syphilis contamination. Government corruption is common. Public health and disaster relief systems are stressed beyond capacity.

Some of these developing world diseases do not cross the oceans and continents easily to threaten the United States, but some do. Tuberculosis is one of those diseases, particularly as it becomes increasingly drug resistant. Declared a global health emergency by the WHO, tuberculosis is spreading around the world at faster rates than public health experts anticipated and at much faster rates than they can control. Dubbed by the Institute of Tropical Medicine as "The Real Millennium Bug," it is spread easily by coughing. A passenger from the Ukraine recently infected 13 people on a flight from Paris to New York, and a child from the Marshall Islands living in North Dakota infected 56 people at home, school, and day care settings.[3] They join the growing number of cases in the United States that are caused by recent arrivals to this country.

Even in the presence of the emergency and global attention, fewer than 20% of people infected with tuberculosis are receiving even basic treatments. Public health experts today estimate that 1.9 billion people currently have active disease, and it spreads to 8 million new people each year. As a result 1.9 million people die annually. Even with newly recommended treatments in place, the next generation of public health experts is predicted to see between 171 million and 249 million new cases of tuberculosis and between 60 million and 90 million deaths from the disease during their careers.[4,5] Future scenarios for a disease so easily transmitted are horrifying.

Reaching Out and Responding

Clean water, sanitation, reliable supplies of food, economic development, and democracy would go a long way to improving the lives and preventing the diseases of most of the developing world's population. It would also protect those of us who live in privilege in the developed world.

That is not the only reason to reach out, however. An even better reason is that there are people in poor countries around the world in such need and we should live in covenant with them. They live at levels of poverty and disease unimaginable to even the poorest in this country. It is so shocking, in some cases, that even travelers to those places can become numbed from the immense needs and forgetful about what they have witnessed once they arrive home. As health care practitioners and healing enterprises in the United States, we have the technology, the insight and, occasionally, the personal and political will to assist in these ventures. Some healers in this country act within a covenant to care for others in these distant places. Clinicians spend their vacation time overseas doing surgery and treating patients; medical centers send their consultants, journals, and books to mission hospitals that can use them; churches sponsor exchange programs and summer trips abroad for teens to build sanitation systems and shelters to help families. Those in health care cannot do it alone, nor do we need to. Tackling immense problems such as these requires the efforts of more than just a few.

International aid from North American, European and Japanese governments supports development projects and makes contributions to the improvement of living conditions. Private firms, foundations, and service organizations also contribute. For example, The World Bank provides $800 million annually to HIV prevention programs.[6] Private non-health care firms doing business in the developing nations of the world contribute to the economy and to health care as well. ENI, an Italian firm, gave the World Health Organization $750,000 to fight malaria in Azerbaijan. BP Amoco financed child nutrition programs in Vietnam. De Beers contributed $2.7 million to the WHO to fund polio eradication and used its own employees to help in the immunization campaigns. Eskom contributed $5 million to develop a vaccine for AIDS.[7] The Bill and Melinda Gates Foundation contributed $50 million[8], Ted Turner

contributed $28 million[9], and Rotary International commit-
ted $500 million to eradicate polio.[10] The Gates
Foundation is also contributing $750 million over five years
to other child vaccination programs and $50 million to pre-
vent maternal mortality.[11] Kiwanis International has
pledged $75 million for salt iodization programs spon-
sored by the United Nations International Children's
Emergency Fund (UNICEF) to prevent the iodine deficiency
disorders that impair the mental health of children.[12] There
is no tally of the total value of donations such as this, but it
is large. Even in the face of expansive philanthropy, the
need is still overwhelming—especially for pharmaceuticals.

The World Health Organization estimates that 30% to
50% of the world's population does not have access to
needed medicines.[13] Recent litigation focused attention on
the need for the sophisticated AIDS drugs in the developing
world, and the outcome was predictable: regardless of the
availability of the medicines, it is difficult to get them to the
people in need. Another outcome was less obvious: the
reality that even many of the basic vaccines and medicines
are unavailable to many people around the world.
Developing nations are too poor to purchase them on the
world market, even when they are available at low prices.
The professionals who can prescribe or dispense the products are not accessible in many countries, and the infrastructure to deliver the products to the clinic or hospital sites
often does not exist. Roads are not passable. Trucks don't
have fuel. Land and water barriers prevent easy passage.
Refrigeration is not available for products requiring special
handling. Wars and natural disasters interrupt the supply of
necessary goods and services.

To assist in meeting the needs for medicines, some very
inexpensive products are made available through loans
and purchase programs of the WHO and other international agencies. A number of countries are attempting to
develop their own local pharmaceutical industry to manufacture generic products and to make them available for

export. Some medicines are donated by the research-intensive industry in the United States, Europe, and Japan in order to make the most modern medicines available to a wider group of people who need them. As in the case of the total health or economic assistance to the developing world, there is no precise estimate of the volume of this assistance, but it is substantial. Those who donate medicines provide the products and, frequently, the technical assistance to assure their correct usage. Working with not-for-profit agencies, donor companies arrange for shipments of large volumes of products overseas. In some cases they also provide the trucks, pay the import duties, and provide the healers in order to get the products to the people. Lately, they also combat the public relations fallout of their well-intentioned efforts.

Healing in the Absence of Explicit Covenants

Healing has always been a risky business. If not tampering with the power of the gods, the healer might have been viewed as bargaining with the devil. Fail to cure and the consequences could be great. Lose a patient in surgery and a doctor could be fined—or worse, could lose a hand. Attempting to provide healing services in the absence of an explicit covenant carries great risks as well. This was true of secular healers in the Middle Ages who practiced medicine without benefit of holy orders. It proved true as well for American pharmaceutical companies who donated products to private relief agencies whose mission it was to bring them to people in need around the world. One particular story is notable and provides a clear example of how the lack of an explicit covenant among all the players involved in the healing process can create problems. This is a story of "good deeds punished." It is a story of the unreasonable and outrageous backlash that can befall a healer who acts in the absence of an explicit covenant with the patients and communities they seek to heal.

It required some hard work in 1994 for pharmaceutical

company Eli Lilly to donate 25 million doses of Ceclor CD®, a potent antibiotic, to Rwanda to treat the wounds people suffered in that country's civil war.[14] The product was a newer, more potent version of an antibiotic already on the market, but it was not yet approved for sale in the United States; and, therefore, could not be donated to help the people of Rwanda, either. Lilly learned of the need for the drug and recognized that it would be of particular help in treating the machete wounds suffered in the war because the company's research showed it to be particularly well suited for treating skin wounds. The company approached Commissioner of the Food and Drug Administration David Kessler with a request to approve the medicine in order to release it to Rwanda. Dr. Kessler and his team worked nearly round the clock over a weekend to review the company's studies and to release the drug for the donation.[15] Rwandan agencies, hospitals, clinics, and ministries of health received the drug from the private relief agencies who partnered with the company in making donations such as this. The result should have been public acclaim for the company, kudos for the quick action of the FDA, and international thanks for the generosity of Americans. Instead anti-industry activists unleashed a public relations disaster on everyone involved.

What went wrong? Eli Lilly believed that since the product was needed and requested, it would be accepted when it arrived and used quickly to help the people in need. The company, which was not interested in public relations coverage, was unprepared for the public relations disaster that followed. It was interested in helping. Should Lilly have been prepared for the backlash? How could it have known that the attempt to do good would be punished in the press? What are the motivations for mounting public attacks on donors of products and services? Is there a way to structure the international relationships to accommodate the objectives of all the parties involved? Who speaks for the patients in poor countries who need but will not receive these medicines unless they are donated? What is the best way to help those patients? Can we come to peace with profit and allow those companies that discover and make these medicines—and make profits on some of them—to give them away without such public relations disasters? How can we encourage, rather than discourage, generosity from a nation and an industry that has produced such abundance? How, in the face of such international need, can we not support the efforts of those who are trying to assist? Could the existence of an explicit covenant have prevented the conflicts that ensued?

Dealing with Public Relations Disasters

In the case of the Lilly donation, the United Nations High Commission for Refugees (UNHCR) miscalculated the flow of Hutus back to Kigali, where the medicine was waiting for them. When Lilly and the relief organizations learned of this, they attempted to recover the drug supply from the warehouses where it was being stored and to redeploy it to other locations where it could be used. They also offered to provide the country with fresh supplies of medicine, since the first shipments were now close to expiration in the warehouses. Rwandan government authorities blocked those efforts, held the drug until the Ceclor CD® expired, and then made claims that Lilly had donated expired drugs. The government's version of the story was published by *TIME* magazine, criticizing Lilly and leaving readers with the impression that expired, unnecessary drugs were "dumped" so that the company could enjoy a tax write-off for the donation. In its handling of the story, *TIME* blackened the eye of Eli Lilly and similar corporate efforts to assist people and nations in need.[16]

TIME magazine was trying to make a point. It was a point that needed making, because in the past there have been problems in donations of all types and from all donor sources. Unfortunately, the magazine selected the wrong example. In the witch-hunt to find and punish an errant healer, the magazine's reports oversimplified the complexity of donations and stimulated unproductive conflicts in the international health community. In doing so, it risked a substantial portion of the donations from the U.S. companies who were swept up in the wake of the Rwandan *cause célèbre.*

TIME assumed that only the pharmaceutical company could have been held accountable. It neglected the facts that drugs are donated from a variety of sources, for a variety of reasons and may pass through many hands on the way to the patient. Some donations come from pharmaceutical companies directly, but others come from physicians, hospitals, pharmacies, drug wholesalers, churches, and individuals. Many donations come from the United States, but they also come from other countries. The donations may come in shipments of drugs and medical supplies, or they may be consolidated with shipments of food, clothing, and materials to build homes. The shipments are rarely delivered directly by the groups making the donations. Rather, they are shipped and delivered "in-country" by private groups with experience in managing the complexity of delivering donated goods. Shipments also pass through the hands of local government officials at customs offices and other stops along the delivery route. These stops incur delays and risk diversion into the black market. The private relief agencies generally manage the problems of war-torn areas, the challenges of tribal conflicts, and the problems of transport where no roads exist or trucks can travel. They are familiar with these conditions because their local operatives are often native to the country, or are long-standing missionaries with credibility. They have influence in addition to years of experience. Having trouble with a customs official who will not clear a shipment, for example? Then perhaps this official's third-grade teacher, the nun in the religious order partnering to receive the goods, can place a call to him and expedite the clearance. Unable to land a plane in one country? Then arrange with your field operations to land in a neighboring country and truck the materials across the border, where the customs officials are more favorably inclined to let you pass through. Can't donate what the recipient needs, but something else instead? They'll take what you have and use it to barter for something else on the long wish lists they keep. Sometimes that's how it works.

Relief on a Massive Scale

Natural disasters and changes in political systems—such as those in the former Soviet Union, Eastern Europe, and Africa during the last decade—have escalated the demand for donated products. In the face of growing international needs, the number of relief organizations and donation transactions is also growing. Yet despite the complexity and size of the donation process, the players are independent, autonomous groups and individuals. They include domestic and international, private, not-for-profit relief agencies, foundations, churches, pharmaceutical companies, hospitals, medical schools, pharmacies, wholesalers, governments, shippers, private practitioners, and individual citizens. Some of these groups have decades of experience; others are entrepreneurial start-ups, particularly those serving regions of the former Soviet Republic. Some groups are large multi-million dollar operations, some are single individuals with not much more than a passion to save their homelands. This group of varied players has no commonly agreed-upon vision, no mission statement, no standard policies and operating procedures, no accountability structure, and no ongoing monitoring. They also have no explicit covenant, either with each other or with those they serve. Given the complexity of the operations, the number of transactions involved, and the troubled regions of the world served, it should be no surprise that there have been problems.

In recent years, published reports indicated that problems have sometimes occurred with drug donations and that some donations have failed to serve the needs of the organizations and people receiving the products.[17,18,19,20] With increased scrutiny by the WHO and, more recently, the U.S. Congress, it would be no surprise if more major crises were to surface. Donors, frequently unfamiliar with local needs and circumstances, have created problems in areas they intended to assist. During the Armenian earthquake in 1988, 5,000 tons of drugs arrived, of which 22% were expired or damaged. In 1989, during the 30-year war for independence in Eritrea, seven truckloads of expired aspirin were received. It took six months to burn. One unsubstantiated report claims that half of the drugs entering Albania during the Kosovo refugee crisis were found to be unusable, probably because the products had less than twelve-month dating.[21] Between 1992 and 1996, over 17,000 metric tons of drugs donated to Bosnia and Herzegovina had to be destroyed, at a cost of $34 million.[22]

A number of different types of problems have been prevalent in donations: Shipments have included expired drugs and drugs that had not been requested by the relief agency. When this occurs, local medical teams, who are already stressed with patients and strapped for cash, must arrange for destruction of the products. Drugs not relevant to the diseases in the country have been sent, again creating destruction problems. Drugs have arrived unsorted, poorly labeled, or labeled in a language not understood in the country. This makes use of the drugs difficult in what are already difficult treatment situations in field clinics and hospitals. Drugs have been improperly packaged, exposing them to temperatures and moisture that degrade the products and expose the environment to contamination from the drugs.

These problems have occurred when those involved are well intentioned, but ill informed or ill prepared for the tasks of delivering and using the medicines. In some cases, the donors are local church and service groups, unfamiliar with pharmaceuticals, who purchase and collect medicines and treat them like other commodities, ignoring the needs of dating, refrigeration, and humidity controls. This also occurs in cases where medical missions are so desperate for any products that they accept whatever is given to maintain any supplies they can and to have pharmaceutical products to barter for other goods. It is also a problem when hospitals, clinics, and wholesalers send about-to-expire products in order to make their products available for others in need. Finally, the problem is created by new relief organizations targeting particular war-torn or natural disaster areas of the world, reacting to the crisis needs of the nation but short-cutting the precautions needed for medicines. As a result, countries and clinics receiving the drugs have been left with problems of good intentions and bad operations. This further stresses their already stressful national situations.

Most pharmaceutical companies and relief agencies have policies and procedures that minimize the chance of ill-informed donations. Questionable donations have rarely been traced to particular companies in the past, but U.S.-based companies take the brunt of public outrage resulting from problems, as was the case for Eli Lilly. It is easy for a company to be in the line of fire. Ultimately, donated product is imprinted with the company name. Find a tablet disintegrated, damaged, or outdated in warehouses in troubled regions of the world and the only certainty is the name of the manufacturer emblazoned on the product. The others involved in supplying the products more easily escape scrutiny and accountability. Even when companies do not donate the product themselves—as when relief agencies purchase medicines for donation or when hospitals, wholesalers, and others donate inventory—companies can be forced to accept responsibility for the final disposition of products that have long since left their control. Finally, companies' philanthropic gestures are drowned by accusations of corporate welfare. Anti-industry activists have claimed that donations are nothing more than inventory dumping in exchange for tax deductions.

Seeking a Solution

It should have been no surprise, then, when in 1995, the WHO, along with a number of international organizations, drafted *Guidelines for Drug Donations*.[23] These guidelines were intended to facilitate the movement of scarce medical supplies to the most needy areas of the globe. The pharmaceutical industry was a significant target for the guidelines. It was also no surprise that the American companies were under the most scrutiny and took the most direct hit at that time.

In draft form, the guidelines were widely circulated and adopted by a number of countries to improve the flow of donated medicines into their countries. The guidelines promote four core principles: maximum benefit to the recipient, respect for the wishes and authority of the recipient, uniform standards of drug quality, and effective communication between the donor and recipient.

In practice, the guidelines state that:

- Donations should be based on need, relevant to the disease pattern of the country, and sent only with prior clearance from the recipient, except in emergencies.

- Products should be registered for sale in the recipient country, donated in the formulation and strength similar to those used in the originating country, and appear on the WHO Essential Drug List (EDL) or the drug list of the country.

- Products should be from a reliable and quality source, complete with labeling in the language of the country and in large quantities. Products should have at least one year of shelf life upon arrival in the country, unless the recipient knows shorter-dated product is arriving and can properly use it.

- No products should be donated if they have been issued to patients and then returned to the pharmacy (a common practice among European donors), nor if they have been given to doctors as free samples (formerly a common practice among U.S. donors, particularly those associated with physician groups).

- Recipient nations are to be informed of all donations, with transportation, port clearance, storage, and handling paid by the donor, and the declared value based on the wholesale world-market price.

Developing Covenants

The guidelines were an attempt to solve the problems associated with donations and have resulted in a covenant, of sorts. They could have resulted in a true covenant if all the players in the drug donation process had been involved in developing them. They were not. Neither the product donors nor many of the relief agencies were involved in the early drafting. Nor were patients involved. In fact, the guidelines, when they emerged in draft, came as a complete surprise to most of the American donor companies and relief agencies involved in making and facilitating donations.

It is not possible to craft a covenant without the full range of parties involved. Attempting to do so from the start would have required substantially more effort, and it would have been difficult. Defining the nature of a covenant in global ventures will never be easy, but in fact, doing so is essential. The complexity of managing operations such as those embodied in donations across different cultures, languages, medical systems, political boundaries, infrastructures, and players makes defining the covenant all the more critical.

The guidelines also could have been more covenant-like if the value of the healing efforts of donations had been acknowledged and if the guidelines had not been used as a weapon to attack the donors. Instead, the international dialogue required to achieve the resolution was conducted against a backdrop of controversy. After several years of contentious debates, accusations, and counteraccusations punctuated by the *TIME* story, the guidelines were finalized in 1999 and are now supported by significant parties to the discussions. At long last, the covenant discussions were initiated.

Significant in this resolution was a meeting held at Notre Dame University in 1997, which should stand as a model for covenant development ventures. The Notre Dame meeting was the occasion of the first global, comprehensive, and candid public discussion of the issues involved in donations. Recipient countries described the loss of national pride from having to provide care for their countrymen with donated goods and expertise. The WHO noted the problems of donations that did not fit the profile of planned health care needs of the developing world.

The Notre Dame meeting was also the first forum in which pharmaceutical companies disclosed the challenges of dealing with negative publicity. Saddled with the burden of proving that they did not cause donation problems, companies have been forced to conduct their own investigations of frequently unfounded allegations. All too often they have been left to manage the cleanup of negative public opinion. It was in this context that some drug company representatives admitted that under continued, burdensome threats to company operations and image, they might consider terminating product donation programs. Workers in the medical mission field acknowledged that would present a crisis of unimaginable proportions.

The dialogue that took place at Notre Dame changed the landscape of the debate and began the first, tentative steps toward reaching a compromise that would create a true covenant. It was the first time in anyone's recollection that donors, relief agencies, missionaries, and recipient countries discussed their common interests. It was the beginning of fruitful discussions about the best methods to manage a global, multiorganizational, multicultural effort in easing suffering and saving lives with donated pharmaceuticals. It was also the catalyst for donor companies and relief agencies to form relationships that improved each of their separate and joint donation operations with refined policies and procedures. But all parties did not yet agree to a covenant, and so, to political observers, the response was predictable. Attacks against industry continued, taking on a different tone. By late 1997 and into 1998, industry critics opened fire in a new direction. This time, they took aim at the tax deductions for donations. They claimed that the deductions were the driving force in company decisions to donate and, in the case of problem shipments of drugs, were examples of corporate welfare gone wrong.

Managing the Domestic Spin

Those who deal in global healing must be prepared for domestic consequences. In the midst of the international debates, claims concerning irresponsible international donations reached the readership of the *New England Journal of Medicine* in a December 1997 Sounding Board article on problems in Bosnia and Herzegovina. The article reported that as much as 50% to 60% of medical supplies sent to Bosnia and Herzegovina between 1992 and 1996 were "useless or unusable." They cited the discovery of World War II medical supplies and expired and inappropriate drugs among the thousands of tons of humanitarian aid deployed to the site. They stated a common view among some groups that the relief effort may have been used to dump outdated supplies.[24]

This article sparked Congressional reaction in January 1998, when Representatives Dennis J. Kucinich (D-OH) and Fortney H. "Pete" Stark (D-CA) requested an Internal

Revenue Service (IRS) investigation into drug companies and other medical suppliers whose goods landed in Bosnia and Herzegovina during the crisis. The threatened IRS investigation served as a wake-up call to donor companies, alerting them to the fact that their philanthropy was being questioned. The IRS did not immediately respond to the Stark and Kucinich request for an investigation, but the major U.S. pharmaceutical companies were eventually exonerated. Dr. Philippe Autier, a researcher who examined the drug donation records on site, confirmed that at least the large U.S. pharmaceuticals could not be blamed for the donations. He did eliminate the big companies, such as Eli Lilly, because "big names don't play that game; what can they gain?" Instead, he named direct retailers, consumers, hospitals, and charities as the guilty ones.[25]

This wake-up call was not entirely a false alarm, however. Although it appears that no IRS response will come, other actions may result from Capitol Hill initiatives. The House and Senate considered a Joint Resolution, introduced by Kucinich, to adopt the WHO guidelines. The rationale for the resolution is based on a recitation of the type of anti-industry accounts that characterized the initial WHO guidelines document.

Obligations to the World's Needy Patients

Donations of pharmaceutical products and medical supplies—whether they are shipped from surplus inventory or manufactured specifically for donation—are laudable endeavors that are consistent with an American impulse toward philanthropy. But they are also complicated by an interplay of international political agendas and activists. In the wake of anti-pharmaceutical industry activity at the World Trade Organization meetings, beginning in Seattle in late 1999 and continuing through 2001 in Doha, these activities are likely to intensify. Unfavorable press concerning donations is an international health activist tool to erode the image of the pharmaceutical industry and limit its participation in public policy discussions. The activists condemn Americans and the industry for their donation policies and interests at a time when the industry is also vulnerable to criticism on other fronts at home. This adds to the risks that companies will consider limiting donations altogether, a most unfortunate necessity, should the controversies not be resolved. If donations are to continue, three challenges within the world's health care network must be addressed: (1) marrying donations policy with other international drug policies, (2) balancing power among the players, and (3) limiting international activist incursions into U.S. tax policy. Covenants can be helpful in this regard because they can encourage each of the parties to move beyond limited, self-interest agendas.

The first challenge of linking donation policy with other international drug policies is related to the two-fold strategy to make drugs available to more people on the globe. The first component of the strategy is to eliminate, or at least severely limit, intellectual property rights for drug developers. The second is to entrench the WHO EDL, which forms the basis for acceptable donated products in the guidelines.

It is well established in the developed world that patents provide the opportunity for drug companies to gain returns from the risks of pharmaceutical research and development. Without the ability to gain a return on investments made to discover a medicine, no private firm would be able to engage in drug development. Those nations with the best patent protection have been the sources of the most innovations for precisely that reason.

While eliminating or limiting patent life—either directly through law, or indirectly by allowing parallel trade—might seem a reasonable short-term solution to the problem of the availability of medicines, it is unwise from several perspectives. First, it will rather quickly limit the supply of new drugs for the entire world coming from research pipelines because companies could no longer realize the returns that draw inventor risk-capital and would therefore be unable to sustain research costs. Second, it ignores the reality that many of the disease problems of the developing world will not be treated with current medicines. The companies whose research resources would be lost to patent infringement are today exploring those developing world diseases most in need of cures. Third, companies have demonstrated in the past several years that, informed of the need for drugs, they will manufacture medicines for the specific needs of the relief agencies.

A much older issue is that of the EDL. First developed in 1977, the EDL was initially intended to reflect a minimum list of medicines that should be available in every country of the world, regardless of the level of poverty. It provided guidance to assist poor countries in purchasing the most cost-effective products. In recent years, however, the EDL has increasingly been promoted as a restrictive formulary and now is used to regulate the movement of donated drugs. Since the guidelines restrict donated drugs to EDL-listed products, the EDL is further entrenched as a normative formulary rather than a "minimum list." Applying EDL restrictions to donated products is a distortion of the intention of EDL that unnecessarily limits the availability of products to people who may need them. Strict interpretation of the EDL also restricts U.S. philanthropy, since the list includes only older, generic drugs which, by-and-large, are no longer manufactured by American companies.

If a company wishes to exercise its philanthropic intentions—and many do—they, their partners, and recipients in the donations must clear special hurdles to send the proprietary, state-of-the-art products that companies produce today. When these hurdles become barriers, they defeat the purpose of the covenant relationships that should be the foundation of the guidelines. Working together to make these guidelines support, rather than prevent, the movement of necessary medical goods, is the goal of a new coalition of companies and relief organizations, The

Partnership for Quality Medical Donations.[26]

The second donation challenge relates to the fact that donation policy discussions are hampered by an underlying imbalance of power and accountability. This is a covenant issue as well. It is important to resolve the issue of power among the players. Unfortunately for people in need, and wholly inconsistent with a covenant, the guidelines, as they have been implemented, provide a mechanism to "balance" the power. They give the recipient countries the "power" to refuse donations for downstream users. This has resulted in some unfortunate lost opportunities to provide care to needy people. Medical missions of surgeons, on one-week trips overseas, have been denied entrance at the border because the drugs they were carrying and would use in surgery in the coming week lacked twelve-month dating. In 1998, entire shipments of requested medicines to Haiti, Kenya, and Egypt were denied acceptance because a portion of the products had less than twelve-month dating. As a result of the strict interpretation of the guidelines, the people in these countries were denied access to an estimated 200 to 400 cartons of antibiotics, pain relievers, and vitamins, among other basic products.[27]

Additionally, donor companies—usually large pharmaceutical firms in the case of medical supplies—exercise great and independent power, because they choose whether or not to donate. Some relief agencies and others purchase the products they donate in the United States or in other markets, but the bulk of the donated products comes directly from the manufacturer. The relief agencies that deliver the goods are intermediaries between the companies and the recipient nations. Since the relief agencies are dependent on the companies for products, some of them, particularly the smaller operations, at times feel obligated to take any product, regardless of need, in order to ensure that the pipeline of donations remains open.

On the other hand, some relief agencies exercise power over the recipient governments and clinics that receive products and distribute them to other health care providers or patients. The recipients are wholly dependent on both the companies and relief agencies, and they must work to maintain good relations with upstream suppliers. Products flow from the companies out to the relief agencies, then to the recipient countries and to health providers, and finally to the patients. The companies appear to exercise the greatest power in the transactions, and they operate within a covenant of grant. They are, therefore, held to the highest level of accountability among all other players and are frequently held accountable for actions over which they have no control. Many donors today, however, are calling for relationships of mutual responsibility and accountability—a covenant of obligation, though they do not use that specific term. In so doing, all parties would work more cooperatively to ensure the desired goal. In the course of refining donation operations in recent years, this is beginning to happen. Many of the donors and larger relief agencies have worked to ensure that communications are improved and good records of transactions are kept. As a result, donations have actually increased, even in the face of negative publicity. These policy and procedural changes enhance and operationalize the growing covenantal relationships among the involved groups.

In reality, since donations advance the agendas of all the players, donations should be managed within a set of interdependent relationships bound in healing covenants. It is an optimistic trend that, increasingly, they are. Donors receive the satisfaction of meeting philanthropic objectives, improving corporate image, and seeding future markets. Relief agencies meet their organizational missions more efficiently. Recipients care for the needy with the benefits of free, developed-world technologies.

The WHO guidelines take some steps in distributing power among the players, but they could do more to create true accountability and interdependence among them. For example, the guidelines briefly address the responsibility of recipient countries to distribute the products efficiently to meet patient needs, but they do not yet require any substantial accountability of the recipients to the donor through reporting of treatment programs and their impact on health. As these final guidelines are implemented, and in subsequent revisions, new discussions can create a forum among equals in which each party would recognize the value of donations to the others and reach toward mutually beneficial solutions to problems. More relief agencies and recipient countries would then be free to follow the lead of most responsible groups today, who refuse unneeded products without fear that they will lose future donations. Companies, in turn, could require information concerning the use and impact of their donated products and could be better prepared to deal with any negative consequences of the donations.

The third donation challenge relates to the fact that international activists are critical of American tax policy that rewards personal and corporate philanthropy with deductions. As a result of their disagreement with our national policy, they intend to lobby for the elimination of tax benefits for donations—at least for pharmaceutical donations. Non-U.S. players and activists view donations as mere tax strategies, since ours is the only country in the world that encourages private philanthropy through its tax code.

It is unlikely that their efforts will be successful, though any debate could be damaging to the climate for pharmaceutical donations. The U.S. Tax Code has supported the deductibility of donations of all sorts since the enactment of the first U.S. Income Tax in 1913, which allowed for deductions for charitable contributions. Through donations, major educational, artistic, and charitable ventures have provided services to millions here and abroad. Public support for individual and corporate philanthropy remains high in this country. Not only is there a support for the policy, but there is action as well. More than three-quarters of all U.S. households donate to charities and, in the past 25 years, the not-for-profit sector in the United States has grown at approximately four times the rate of the economy as a whole. That makes the United States unique in its private approach to giving. Other countries promote care of the poor through direct taxation of corporations and individuals. This difference in national cultures and policies creates suspicion of U.S. companies' motives.[28]

The resolution of this debate will be particularly important given that, in reality, pharmaceutical companies receive tax deductions whether they donate or destroy products in inventory. The exact calculation depends on a number of factors and each situation is unique, but it is fair to say that deductions do not drive the decision to donate. In fact, although the calculation has never been made, it is probably the case that if the total costs of donations were tallied, in some cases companies would find that their donations are actually more costly than destruction of the products. This is because companies pay for much of the costs associated with making most of the donations—not only those in their internal operations and recordkeeping, but also those external costs associated with shipping and handling and import duties on donated products. In the final analysis, for some companies the tax deductions may be an incentive to donate, while for most others, deductions merely remove some of the disincentives to becoming involved in this type of philanthropy.

Sustaining the New Covenant
The Notre Dame conference, the guidelines, and all the other communications among the participants in the donation of medical products and services are important steps toward developing a global covenant of obligation to care for those in need. Other steps will be necessary to refine the covenant, to further develop the systems to support the caring, and to bring other donors to the table. It is critical for the health of people around the world that we continue to reach out to each other to ensure that the flow of devel-

---

oped-world technology not only continues, but becomes a torrent of giving. It is critical not only for health, but for peace and prosperity globally.

To that end, donations of all types are important and greatly underappreciated for the contributions they make to the lives of the people in developing nations. This is especially true for the pharmaceutical products that reach the most remote places and the neediest people. Aside from the safe water and environments, and the food and housing that the developed world can lend, there is no more important, cost-effective donation than that of a medicine to prevent and treat disease.

Working cooperatively with the industry can result in new programs to create solutions to tropical diseases, as recent experience has demonstrated. Merck developed and now donates Mectizan®, which prevents river blindness with only one tablet per patient per year. Over 250 million tablets have been provided to 31 countries in Africa, Latin America, and the Middle East.[29] SmithKline Beecham pledged to donate albendazole for lymphatic filariasis, to treat the 120 million people in 73 countries who suffer from that intestinal parasite.[30] The company has committed to continue the donations until this public health problem is solved. GlaxoWellcome committed to one million courses of treatment with its drug Malarone®, which will cure over 98% of the patients who receive it and will assist in reducing the suffering and death from malaria.[31] Bristol-Myers Squibb has committed $100 million over the next five years in its Secure the Future™ program to find sustainable solutions to HIV/AIDS for women, children, and communities in sub-Saharan Africa.[32] In all, ten major disease conditions are the subject of global philanthropy: African trypanosomiasis, HIV/AIDS, leprosy, lymphatic filariasis, malaria, onchocerciasis, polio, trachoma, and vitamin A deficiency disorders.[33]

The impact of some of these programs is still too new to quantify, but the size of donations from major donors overall has recently been calculated at nearly $2 billion between 1998–2001.[34] This figure does not fully capture the contributions of smaller donors, who are numerous and make substantial efforts to relieve suffering through their programs. The types and numbers of donors and relief agencies are so varied that a complete list would be difficult to compile. The evidence of the value of the products is largely anecdotal. A recent study by Harvard University Professor Michael Reich is a testament to the complexity and value of even a limited sector of the donation community's effort to get products to people. Even after years of study, this expert in international public health could not quantify the impact of more than a small segment of the donated products.[35] But we do not need to fully quantify the value of the donations to know that philanthropy from the developed world has value.

Few would disagree with the statement that poor nations and disaster areas have needs that exceed the capacity of local governments and international health agencies, such as the World Health Organization. We know that there are people in need and there are people who are willing to help. The most crucial thing we can do to address these needs now is to return to our values as healers and Americans. Will we isolate ourselves and refuse to see the needs beyond our own shores? Will we support or hamper the efforts of those who are the donors? Can the philanthropic intentions of companies prevail in the face of international condemnation? If a resurgence of attacks were to occur, would donors decide that destroying products is a better alternative than donating them? Will the public, once it learns that companies are making international donations, force them to redirect drug supplies to the needy population within this country?

Robert Davies, head of the Prince of Wales Foundation, notes that in workshops to teach WHO and other UN officials to work with the private sector, the tensions mount as the teaching proceeds. Frequently, shouting erupts on both

sides. Government officials view the private sector with suspicion and see it as corrupt and immoral. Business people
view governments as corrupt and inefficient. In fact, the
only thing they agree about is each other's corruption.[36]
Coming to peace across the public-private table will not be
easy, but it must be done. Coming to peace with the presence of a for-profit sector within the global health care
enterprise, likewise, will be fraught with challenge. Lives
are at stake as we debate. Coming to peace will involve
engaging new partners and learning new skills. Coming to
peace will require developing new operations and elevat-
ing the concerns for health care in the developing world at
a time when America is struggling with its own health care
crises. The most recent set of revised guidelines is a start,
but more steps must be taken by all parties in order to
secure even more comprehensive standards.

One of those steps was taken recently in a milestone
effort. A number of organizations, including the World
Bank, the World Health Organization, Agence Européenne
pour le Développement et la Santé (AEDES), and The
Partnership for Quality Medical Donations, jointly conducted a study of drug donations in four national emergency
situations. This joint effort represented an unprecedented
collaboration between formerly hostile players in the donations arena. The results of the study produced helpful relationships, and data, for future endeavors. The critical need
for drugs in emergency situations, the value of the donation
guidelines, the need for effective coordination, and the role
of the media in alerting the world to needs were evident. In
addition, however, it also became clear that no major U.S.
pharmaceutical manufacturer or donor partners had made
inappropriate donations. Aware of the guidelines, they
operated within them, unlike some of the smaller, less-
experienced governments and organizations that now must
be educated in their value and application.[37] The organizations are working cooperatively to acquaint the small, well-
intentioned but unknowledgeable, donors about the impor-

tance of the guidelines to assure their donations are in compliance. They will also offer small donors effective and efficient alternative pathways for the donations they wish to make.

Similar steps must continue if the donation effort, a decade from now, is to be even more substantial than it is today. To help, national policymakers should allocate some time to engaging in the substantial additional dialogue that will be required among the WHO staff, U.S. Congressional staff and members, pharmaceutical companies, recipient agencies, nations, and activists. Some of these discussions might address questions such as:

- Who should take the lead in ensuring the quality of donations? Should it be pharmaceutical companies themselves, who have so far borne the burden of bad press? To keep the pipeline of donated medicines open to developing nations, companies should maintain impeccable donation operations, select relief agencies carefully, and respond to the political backlash that some donations will likely create. Whether for commercial, philanthropic, or image objectives, no company donating medicines today can ignore either its own operations or those of others who may be handling, receiving, and even donating their products. Goodwill can be generated through targeted and controlled donations; disasters can be created out of unmanaged philanthropy. The reality is that when donations go bad, it is the company that takes the heat. Should that be the case, or is the donation effort ready for shared responsibility and should others also be accountable on the world stage?

- Who should develop and manage the complex infrastructure required to ensure the quality of shipments under these most extreme circumstances? With a worldwide enterprise at least as large as any Fortune 100 corporation (in terms of transactions, international regulation, staffing, budgets, and volume), it is unwise to assume that donations can be managed with anything less than a common mission statement, operating procedures, extensive communications, and accountability. Perhaps common sets of forms, policies, and procedures should be developed across the entire supply chain, modeled after those used by large, sophisticated, and accountable relief agencies today.

- How should the responsible donors, recipient countries, and agencies make the effort to eliminate the (usually) smaller, local, irresponsible players in donations, who through their efforts disrupt the internal health care operations of the recipients? Though well meaning, they are often uninformed and uneducated in the policies and procedures that guide good donation practices. Their misadventures threaten the entire legitimate donation effort of the responsible players.

- How can non-health care players be brought into the discussions of health care needs to support infrastructure development? As companies like IBM, Dell, AT&T, and Microsoft enter the American health care market, should they be invited into the global donation effort? How can those in the fields of education, communications, and economic development be engaged for the good of people's health? Where can their resources be spent to improve the living and working conditions of local employees? What are the best incentives local governments can provide to increase their involvement?

- Can we bring an end to demonizing profit in the health care sector? Is the greed we perceive just a misunderstanding of the commercial imperatives of businesses that rely on private sources of capital? Is there an alternative to current revenues that will pay for research, or can we come to terms with the need for profit? Do governments want to increase their own levels of research effort to discover the drugs for the developing world, or should companies be allowed to proceed? How can local generic industries be developed to expand the availability of important products without harming progress toward innovation worldwide? How can we recognize that differential pricing of products actually supports access to medicines and that a single worldwide price would spell disaster for all nations?

- Can we stop demonizing government regulators and bureaucrats? Is the inefficiency we perceive just a misunderstanding of their operating constraints? How can those in the for-profit sector support the imperatives of governments? How can the public and private sectors work together to meet their mutual goals of providing care to the needy?

- How can the parties to this debate best understand each other's separate agendas? Can we develop a global research agenda that, coupled with incentives for public and private sectors, could result in new solutions to tropical diseases? Can we find our way through issues as complex as this in a nation (the U.S.) which until recently had been isolationist in the perceived safety of the post-Cold War era?

In the end, the enemy is disease, not the parties to the debate. The weapons will be cures, not rhetoric. Maintaining the covenants that supply donated products and services and creating new covenants of obligation will require that the most powerful player in the process of drug donations—the American pharmaceutical industry—bear the lion's share of the effort. It will require that the industry work to ensure quality donations through its own donation channels and through the contacts of others, that it weather the storms of public image attacks, and that it continue to offer a wealth of products and talent to the developing world. It will not be easy. But it will, in the end, be the single best way for the industry, and this country, to reach out to others on the planet, demonstrate leadership, protect health at home, and avoid health isolationist policies that are unworthy of a nation so rich in resources.

Chapter 10

Global Health Caring

Covenant in Innovation and Access to Medicines

Innovation in health care appears to be paradoxical: it provides simultaneously hope and fear. Hope to manage to tame at least temporarily disease and death; fear that innovation will raise the cost of health care up to a point where rationing becomes inevitable.[1]

Claude Le Pen, Director, Health Economics Laboratory,
University of Paris-Dauphine

Innovation has progressed beyond providing hope and fear: it now produces anger as well. It was bound to happen. As the investments in modern pharmaceutical discoveries and developments produced solutions for more conditions and as more people needed them, once-small and nearly-invisible drug budgets grew at a noticeable rate and to a notable size.

Lilliputian expenditures did not assume Gulliver's girth, but they received the attention of the giant come to town. Perhaps it was because the little pills came from companies that, by comparison, looked like giants alongside patients and other healers. In fact, some of the companies were giants and were bigger than some small nations. Perhaps, as in Gulliver's travels, the townspeople and the giant did not speak the same language or navigate the same waters, the giant having come from a land of research risk, competition and capital market demands. Speaking those words left the townspeople feeling adrift on lonely, unknown seas, fearing shipwrecks of disease and disability. Perhaps, like Gulliver, it was because the drug giant had traveled the world and had developed the wits to make his way in any country, while the Lilliputians were unaware of lands outside their own. Perhaps the people did not trust the giant's weapons—which it called prices and patents—fearing they'd be caught in the sights of an uncaring corporation, lacking in compassion for those who needed, but could not buy, the pills. Perhaps it was because . . . well, whatever the reason, the current relationship between the pharmaceutical industry and those it seeks to serve is no fairy tale.

Recounting the history of the industry and its relationships with governments and patients is unlikely to be of much value and is not my purpose here. Unraveling the mysteries of proprietary information and marketing strategy might be of some investigative interest, but it won't solve today's conflicts. Nor will progress be made by engaging in more finger-pointing, blame-assigning, or witch-hunting, either here or abroad. If the children's tale is instructive, however, then there might well be a brighter future ahead in the relationship between the pharmaceutical industry and those it serves, after all. Gulliver, you will recall, learns the language of Lilliput. He comes to be of great benefit to the people, prevents an invasion and saves the palace.

We should all hope that the giants of industry follow in the footsteps of Gulliver and provide us with the benefits we need today in health care. Never before in the history of mankind have so many people, suffering from so many diseases and disabilities, needed so many innovative solutions. As we hope for a future in which we have those innovative solutions on our pharmacy shelves and household medicine cabinets, we need to face the facts: finding and providing these solutions will certainly cost more than today's drug bills. But the price we will pay in early deaths, substantial disabilities and lost productivity if we choose to stop the search for new treatments and cures will certainly be higher.

Will we find those cures? Without a doubt. Never in history have we been more poised to reap the benefits of decades of research investments nor to grasp the discoveries of the scientific revolution at the frontiers of genomics and biotechnology. Decades of public and private investment in research are paying off. How we should reap the benefits of that research and how much more we can absorb into our health care systems will be among the most pressing questions of this decade. Will we endorse—not only with our voices, but also with our funds—the economics of discovery? Will we continue to support a public-private partnership in innovation? Will we continue to support a for-profit sector within health? Or will we erode the capacity of this nation to be innovative in the same ways that we have eroded our public health systems and crippled physician, nursing and hospital care—that is, by starving operating programs and ignoring investments that will bring improvements? How will we keep the pipelines flowing with new discoveries, healers and drugs and assure that those who need the cures get them? Will we, as Americans, come to see the needs of the developing world and recognize the imperative to support the search for solutions there, as well as here? Will other developed nations follow our lead in doing so?

Elsewhere in this book, I have addressed a number of global issues that drive back to the nature of the public policy climate in the U.S. today. I have argued that we practice "health isolationism" and urged against it. We act all too often as if health care in the U.S., including its economics, can be addressed solely within our borders. I have shown how in several ways—the need for subjects for clinical trials, the presence of infectious diseases, the likelihood of pandemics and the nature of bioterrorism—the U.S. is inextricably linked to other nations. Our fate hangs very much in delicate balance with theirs. In no sector is this truer than in biomedical solutions to today's global challenges. At precisely the time we need the medical innovation industry most, it is under renewed fire.

Shooting the Healer

This is not the first time in history that public ire has been leveled at healers. Healers have always been held accountable within their communities. Dating back to the earliest records, it is clear that they were punished for their misdeeds, not just rewarded for their skills.[2] Misstep, and the healer was held accountable. This is true in contemporary society as well. In the past several decades, healers in the U.S. have suffered one policy-directed retribution after another. Hospitals and physicians faced this in the 1980s and managed care suffered through hostilities as the millennium clock ticked through midnight. In our dissatisfaction with health care and our attempts to reform it, we selected one healer after another and laid the blame for our discontent at their feet. Spending too much on hospital care? Then certainly the cause must be super-charged fee structures, and the cure would be prospective payment systems that place hospitals at-risk financially in the care-giving process. Implementing those changes brought the industry to its knees and into the red, closing facilities and threatening community care in many locations. Spending too much on physician-driven care? Then certainly the cause was the indiscriminate overuse of resources by clinicians, and the cure would be tighter reign on spending by managed care and its controls. Too difficult to get treatments in managed care? Then certainly managed care was greedy and the cure would be litigation and patients' rights laws. Expenditures still growing? If all else failed, then surely every provider was committing fraud and could be threatened with fines and even jail time and led to see the wisdom of plea-bargaining for lower penalties.

It appears that the next of our healers in line to be demonized is the pharmaceutical industry. Compared to all the others, it is an easier target. It is a visible and, seemingly, the most reprehensible of the players in health care today. Some critics direct their ire at the profitability of the companies; others at the promotional tactics of marketing to physicians; many at the interference of healer-patient relationships in direct-to-consumer advertising; and several at the salaries of executives as a basis of contempt. Global public health activists cite the dearth of research and product development for diseases of the developing world, saying that the commercial returns to industry are out of balance with the gains that should be made against the needs of the poor around the world.

Aiming at the Wrong Target

Sadly, however, industry adversaries have not set their sights on drug companies alone. Unwittingly, they have targeted the broader, public-private alliance that produces innovations overall and brings them to us with stunning regularity and predictability. This innovation sector of health care is composed of three interrelated components—first, our biomedical research enterprise; second, our medical education institutions; and third, our pharmaceutical industry. Each depends on the other—and on public and private sector funds and favorable policy—to do an elegant dance of information, financing and human effort. This interdependent relationship optimizes the contribution they make, through innovation, to our personal and collective health and economy. This is an arena in which the interplay of these players results in a whole that is much greater than the sum of its parts. Cripple any part of this triad and the whole of the innovative machine will grind to a halt—not immediately, for certain, but surely over time. Yet pressures here and abroad threaten to do just that. The consequences will be felt here, and around the world. Consequences that we—and the rest of the world—should not take lightly.

The development of new knowledge is wasted effort unless it is used to develop products that will treat disease, and it is without value unless it is integrated into medical school teaching programs and results in clinicians that are better-prepared to address the diseases of their patients.

The training of new clinicians is incomplete unless they also participate in the development of new knowledge and learn the inquiry skills of research. Pharmaceutical solutions are fueled by these basic research discoveries, and the costliest part of the whole venture—clinical trials—is conducted mainly in medical schools. Medications are hollow promises without an educational system that prepares clinicians for the appropriate selection and use of the therapies. Ample evidence indicates that when these players within our innovative sector cooperate, the results are increased productivity.[3] Collaboration is not the fantasy of rhetoric; it is the reality and backbone of innovation in the U.S. today.

The Paradox of Value

The innovation segment of the American health care industry is on the firing line because of a somewhat unique position, I believe. Not just because of its weaknesses, but because of its strengths. Not just because of its liabilities, but because of its assets. Not because it is potentially a drain on national coffers, but because it is potentially such a boon to those coffers, as well. It has proven itself to be of such value that its discoveries dare not be denied to those in need. It has attracted so many stakeholders, with such keen interests, that the challenge of satisfying all of them may well be impossible unless we rise above our current crises and examine them from new perspectives. As in other areas of health care, the old covenant of grant has outlived its usefulness and is now in danger of destroying a principal engine of health and economic prosperity.

It is a paradox that something so valuable has become so vulnerable in today's health care and economic climate. I'll predict, and frankly without taking much risk in doing so, that the value of medicines will continue to increase and the vulnerability of medical innovation will as well. In fact, the controversies surrounding medical innovation are likely to get much worse before they get better. If these controversies stem the flow of resources into research, the result will be fewer discoveries. If these controversies stem the flow of resources into purchasing these products, the result will be fewer people treated efficiently, and more human suffering and economic loss.

The tragedy is unthinkable for patients in this country, and even more so for those around the world. Alzheimer's disease and congestive heart failure are the scourges of our own society, but the developing world suffers even more from diseases and from the economic consequences they cause. The ink is barely dry on a WHO report on the relationship between health and disease, but it should be required reading for everyone involved in crafting health or economic policy today. It demonstrates how defeating AIDS, malaria, and tuberculosis must be a key strategy in building the economies of developing world countries.[4] WHO proposes that investing an additional $27 billion—or .1% of GDP of the U.S., Europe and Japan—in health programs would save eight million lives and create economic gains of $186 billion. Our innovators have succeeded in developing some pharmaceutical products and public health strategies to combat these three diseases, but none is optimal and more research is needed to reach a more ideal therapy. What is true for these devastating diseases overseas is also true for conditions here. Will we continue to support ventures to find real, simple, tolerable medicines that will be total cures? Current medicines are the best that early innovation can offer, but they still involve side effects, complicated regimens and costly public health interventions. Will we ever develop something better for the millions who need help?

If we do succeed, it will be because the healers in biomedical research, medical education and pharmaceuticals who discover, develop and integrate innovations in health care have the support of the patients they treat and the communities—in this case the nations—within which they work. This calls for robust funding of biomedical research, adequate use of medicines, supportive pricing policies and protection of the intellectual property associated with the discovery.

Shining Some Light in the Black Box

Few people today understand the medical innovation sector in the U.S., which is the largest and most productive of all the world's nations. Even those who are a part of it have not grappled well with the interconnectedness of the enterprise. Its ownership is public and private. Its purpose is for-profit and not-for-profit. Its financing comes from private investment capital, philanthropy and government dollars. Its existence is enabled by the "tangibles" of funds and the "ethereals" of policies. Its organizations are highly decentralized and very complex. In those ways, it is like many of the innovation sectors in other parts of the world. In one way, however, it is fundamentally different. Its method of innovation allows the talent, peer review and creativity of scientists to pursue new knowledge and develop products, and the marketplace judgment of products to determine their value and willingness to use them. In other countries, research targets are pre-specified and governments set prices that keep product prices down and business investors away. Which is better? The prevailing opinion—and the scorecard of research results—says that, hands down, our model results in more prolific progress. Of the major drugs treating people today and responsible for stunning improvements in health, most were discovered and developed here in the U.S.

This system of discovery and development has been evolving for several hundred years and is reaching its maturity precisely during this time when it is coming under attack. To understand how and to see what is at risk, it is necessary to pull back the curtain and examine the nature of the research enterprise. This will be a simple review, to be sure, but one that is intended to demonstrate what is at stake in the public policies we must forge in this new century.

Federal research capacity is housed in many centers within the health, agriculture and national defense agencies of the government. The National Institutes of Health (NIH) is the largest of these agencies, with 15,600 employees and an annual budget that has grown from $300 at its founding in 1887 to over $20 billion today. The CDC is best known for its contribution to public health, but a number of its 8,500 employees and part of its $4.3 billion budget are devoted to research as well. The Veteran's Administration, the National Science Foundation, the U.S. Food and Nutrition Service, the Agency for Health Research and Quality, and Department of Defense operations at sites such as Walter Reed Army Hospital are also players.[5] Even regulatory and payment agencies, such as the Food and Drug Administration, the Center for Medicare and Medicaid Services, the Environmental Protection Agency and the Nuclear Regulatory Commission, support biomedical innovation. The work of these agencies is supported by the appropriation of federal funds for research, but direct Congressional funding is not the only way. Regulatory and tax policies also encourage research within the private sector, making the government and taxpayer indirect supporters of that research.

Each government research agency works in partnership with academic medicine. The structure of these biomedical research experts was articulated by Abraham Flexner[6], whose now-famous report detailed the faculty and facilities necessary to develop a profession of highly-skilled clinicians. His proposals have been refined and expanded and today, medical research—along with teaching and clinical care—forms the tripartite mission of medical education at the 125 medical schools, 400 major teaching hospitals and health systems and nearly 8,000 residency training programs in the nation. More than 100,000 faculty, 66,000 medical students and 98,000 medical residents participate in the training of our next generations of clinical healers. They receive research funding in the range of $12 billion each year—68% from government, 14% from the pharma-ceutical industry and 9% from philanthropic groups. While this is no longer true today, historically, with the tacit approval of those who paid for the health care delivered in medical schools, some patient-care dollars were also used to pay for research. Occasionally extra tests were done to collect data to enrich our understanding of illness, and higher costs for medical center hospitalization provided a funding stream to research at university medical centers.

Government agencies and educational institutions, in turn, work cooperatively with the private research-intensive industry. About 50 pharmaceutical companies in this coun-try contribute another $24 billion in research funding in the U.S. and nearly 250,000 jobs. The 1,300 biotechnology companies spend $14 billion and employ 174,000 people. Nearly 90 private research institutions, such as the Coriell Institute for Medical Research, also conduct research, and add another $3 billion.

If the U.S. is a hotbed of innovation, then regions with-in this nation are the places where the coals burn brightest. The concentration of funding and talent creates synergies in discovery. Companies tend to locate near academic institu-tions, and near each other. As a result, for example, Philadelphia, home of the nation's first hospital, is now home to more than 350 life sciences companies, employ-ing more than 50,000 workers. It ranks second nationally in pharmaceutical employment, third in biotechnology employment and fourth in medical device employment. Its universities attract $775 million annually in research, and private investment capital has followed—over $1.1 billion in venture funds since 1995. Support came not only from private and federal government sources, but from the state of Pennsylvania as well. The state invests $65 million per year in its universities, provides $100 million to create Life-Science Greenhouses and has passed favorable tax and business policy legislation to reduce the costs of doing busi-ness and create favorable business climates.[7] Philadelphia is only the entry, however, to a corridor of medical innovation that begins there and stretches to Boston.

Aside from today's benefits of being co-located on the eastern seaboard with other innovators, there are historical reasons why the industry is so concentrated there. The innovation sector began a slow, but steady, growth over the past century as the foundational building blocks that support discovery were laid. Philanthropy supported academic researchers until the mid-1900s, when federal funding began and the great medical research universities developed. Gradually, the small, family-owned—principally European—drug development and manufacturing companies, seeking better opportunities, moved to where the best scientific resources could be found. They came to the U.S., disembarking and settling in New York and Philadelphia, where they could recruit scientists trained in those university programs and work in a climate that rewarded discovery with patents and provided a large market in need of products. World wars required that some of those companies separate from their European parents, particularly if they were German, and demonstrate their loyalty to America as best they could or suffer confiscation of their assets. Loyal they became. They embarked on joint research programs with government to develop and produce penicillin for the fighting forces, and they offered deep discounts to veterans' health care programs after the war as further proof of citizenship and American spirit. For years after the war, they continued their research and development on diseases that were most common—or predicted to be most common—in this country.

Alongside other healers and taken in total, these innovation-sector research investments might appear to be large, but in reality they are quite small alongside other expenditures we make to manage our health and healing enterprise. Compare the total national public and private sector investment in biomedical innovation—$45 billion—to what we, as Americans, spend annually on health care:

$1.3 trillion. Or, from another perspective, medical research accounts for less than a nickel of every health care dollar and less than a penny of every federal dollar. That's less than 56 cents per American per day spent on medical research overall in the U.S., with well under half of that amount—19 cents—coming from federal sources.[8] Better yet, compare our research investments to non-health care, and some would say less essential, expenses. We spend more than twice the research investment—$100 billion— on fast food, $24 billion on accessories for our cars and trucks, $20 billion playing golf and $1 billion on Valentine's Day chocolate. The $45 billion for research pales by comparison to the costs of the disease challenges it seeks to address. The annual cost of uncured heart disease is $128 billion; of uncured cancer, $104 billion; of uncured Alzheimer's, $100 billion; of uncured diabetes, $92 billion; of uncured arthritis, $65; of uncured depression, $44 billion. Victor Fuchs has said that each nation chooses its own death rate by its choice of health as compared to other goals.[9] I would agree with him, and add that those choices involve not only what we decide to spend on health care services, but on biomedical research.

Even the cost of uncured disease here in the U.S., however, pales by comparison to the worldwide impact of disease and disability on health and the economy. In the last 40 years, life span in the developed world rose by 22 years, largely because of medicines. The developing world has seen improvements as well. In 1950, 15% of children died before their fifth birthday; today only 4% do. Nonetheless, the poorest nations face continuing devastation from several diseases—HIV/AIDS, malaria, tuberculosis, childhood diseases, tobacco-related illnesses and malnutrition— which alone are responsible for 8 million preventable deaths each year. By 2020, that picture will change. Death rates from these communicable diseases, which are either unknown or largely controlled in our country, will give way to conditions more like ours. Tobacco use will exceed every other disease, including HIV/AIDS. Heart disease, depression, cerebrovascular disease and lung conditions, such as chronic obstructive pulmonary disease and tuberculosis, will be the key health global concerns. Depression will cause the greatest burden, worldwide, on quality of life and disability, clearly affecting the productivity of the workforce in every nation.[10]

It is undeniable that health has value for its own sake, and we should care for others for that reason alone. But there are also compelling economic reasons to stem the tide of disease from these conditions. Health provides a workforce with the ability to be productive, and that productivity, in turn, creates better health. The impact would show up not only in annual returns, but would be cumulative as well, of course. For instance, a 20% reduction in deaths from cancer would be worth $10 trillion—double the national debt.[11] Among the working population, for every rise along the rung of the socioeconomic ladder, an individual experiences a corresponding improvement in health and reduction in mortality.[12] Economic development and the reduction of poverty throughout the world are dependent on a healthy population, capable of participating in the growth of an increasingly interdependent world economy.[13] Failure to improve the pace of economic development places us all at risk. Poverty is a growing cause of unrest, leading to threats of increasing violence throughout the world. It affects children disproportionately. As a result, they are malnourished and leave school to work. How can this not have life-long, multigenerational and global consequences?

Is this the concern of the American medical innovation sector? Yes. Why? This nation is a stakeholder—and a key player—in the future of the globe. That is why. As a result, its innovators—who are truly global themselves—are key players and may now be the most beneficial of the assets that the U.S. can offer its global neighbors. The work of the innovation segment of our health care system transcends any national boundary because disease transcends every national border. In my view, the innovation segment of the health care industry is the only true worldwide healer. No other component of health care crosses so many time zones, addresses so many global diseases and national needs, and adjusts to so many regulatory schemes and governmental systems. Interest groups agree, and as a result, a number of them from around the world currently demand the resources of our innovators to solve problems that lie outside our borders, laws, tax systems and funding. As such, our innovators confront a more complex set of cultural, legal, regulatory, research, marketing, pricing, and disease issues than any other healer can imagine. It is for that reason that the players within the innovation segment of health care—the biomedical research enterprise, the medical education system and the pharmaceutical industry—should now forge closer ties, recognize the interdependence, and invite those who want their healing into a covenant. It should come as no surprise that the covenant I would envision is a covenant of obligation, replacing the current covenant of grant. As in the case of all other covenants, this covenant must be a conscious, deliberate act of those healers who are the leadership engines of innovation.

Crafting an Innovation Covenant

If we, as Americans, are to do what I suggest and contribute our resources to world health in order to sustain economic development, and even to promote world peace, then we will need to support the ability of our innovators to deliver the solutions to today's disease problems. How might that happen? What would our innovator-healers ask of us in terms of support, and how would we perform within an interdependent relationship with them? What would be the terms and conditions that each would ask of the other now, given that the covenant was formed long ago and in ways that were not as mature as today's healing and

---

world climates demand?

The innovators are the superior party in this covenant and, as I have argued, the superior parties are the ones who initiate the covenant relationship. Our innovators have articulated what they need in order to continue to heal. Specifically, they have told us that their requirements are resources for research, appropriate product access and use in the marketplace, and protection of the innovative ideas themselves from piracy committed by others.

Resources for Research Ventures

Highest on the list of what innovators say they require for their ventures are resources, both financial and human. On the financial side, innovators need more funds. Recently, Congress decided to meet their request for more financial resources by appropriating higher levels of funding for the NIH. In addition to the increased dollars, Congress and disease interest groups also acted on another request: to allow science to drive research projects and limit the "earmarking" of funds for particular projects. Our innovators have argued that following scientific leads is the best way to achieve disease solutions. New knowledge, they have successfully argued, rarely proceeds along a course plotted by politics; earmarks were getting in the way of progress. This, it seems, qualifies as a request within the spirit of a covenant by our healers, and it seems that we, as parties to that covenant, heard them and responded appropriately.

Other financial resources have been provided by partnerships with industry and by capitalizing on the fruits of academic work. These resources for research ventures have come from the collaborative efforts of academic investigators, federal funding sources and the pharmaceutical industry. Though highly successful, these relationships are currently at risk and the covenant demands that innovators better define and defend collaboration. Collaborative relationships are now suspect, and concerns about conflicts of interest threaten the reputations of scientists and cooperative efforts overall. This is not the first time that researchers have been criticized or have voiced concerns themselves about the challenges of working with new partners.

The alarm sounded by critics today—that industry may have undue influence—is similar to the one made concerning federal government funding of research in the 1950s. In that era, government was beginning to replace private philanthropy as a major source of money for research efforts, raising fears that these funds would distort the research mission. What we take for granted today—that government does and should fund research—was a controversial idea just a few decades ago. Scientists feared that their research ventures would be "directed" by government and that they would no longer be free to pursue their scientific leads as they believed best. As was the case then, and as should be the case now, any threat—real or perceived—should be balanced by the opportunities for a research enterprise that is ever more vibrant and productive, and by mechanisms to ensure that the scientific process proceeds as society would expect it should to develop important innovations. Doing so should not weaken the joint efforts. In fact, collaboration among various parties—interdependent as they are—should be strengthened, not weakened. Knowledge flows both ways between the bench and the bedside, and only through widespread cooperation among the players will we realize the real value of innovation. Further, though federal support for biomedical research has grown tremendously in the past several decades, it represents a declining share of biomedical research overall. The private sectors of industry and philanthropy—and, in particular, industry—contribute an ever-growing share of the research resources. To ignore that and separate these dynamic forces in discovery from one other is to weaken all the partners.

Those who fear that the universities and government laboratories, and their federal research counterparts, will be at the mercy of powerful companies have only to review the national policies that have encouraged innovators in government and academia to capitalize on their work. These create a balance among the partners and result in additional funding streams for research. Stevenson-Wydler Technology Transfer Act of 1980 accelerated the translation of research results from federal laboratories into commercial products; and the Federal Technology Transfer Act of 1986 provided incentives for federal-industry research. The Bayh-Dole Act of 1980 provides incentives for universities to patent their findings, and income. University licensing income increased from $186 million to $725 million between 1991 and 1997.[14] The Small Business Innovation Development Act of 1982 facilitated the growth of small companies created by scientists dedicated to transferring their discoveries to the market. Some will be critical, regardless of Congressional oversight and pubic accountability, but their arguments, while passionate, do not address the bigger questions of how we, in this nation, will support innovation to solve our own, and the world's, disease problems. The more worrisome issue today is not the occasional conflict in research partnerships; instead, it is the availability of talented scientists able to join in those research ventures in the future. Science—the discovery of the unknown—is no longer attractive to many students, and fewer of them are choosing the difficult and expensive educational path that science requires.

Besides scientists, the other human resource that our innovators require is clinical trial subjects. Traditionally, patient care settings in academic health centers were ideal sources for investigators. The advent of managed care and, in fact, all cost-controlled care changed that. Managed care, while a seemingly natural organizational structure for conducting research, has not embraced any but the most directly cost-relevant studies of health economics and outcomes. Clinical trials have not been a part of the managed care contribution to innovation, even when managed care patients are cared for in the academic health centers that formerly were the clinical trial powerhouses of the world. Though it has never been documented, it is assumed that research-related care is more expensive than other care, and so managed care has shied away. In fact, until recently, and under public pressure and state legislation, some managed care plans refused to pay for any care when the patient was included in clinical research, even if some of the care would have been deemed medically necessary. Further, managed care has not reached out to its members to encourage their participation in research, as numerous clinical trials go begging for subjects. As a result, new organizations—including Physician Based Research Networks (PBRNs) and Contract Research Organizations (CROs)—have emerged to conduct clinical trials and new methods of recruitment—including the internet—have been used. Despite this, many clinical trials go begging for subjects. Over 41,000 clinical trials are being conducted today, and of those underway, 80% are not meeting their enrollment deadlines, spending an estimated $1 billion just to recruit patients.[15] Since pharmaceutical companies sponsor more than 80% of the approved clinical trials in the U.S.,[16] the sheer volume of the effort makes the collaboration among these innovators necessary. This, in turn creates yet another target for criticism about the partnership. As a result, the academic health centers that are the mainstay of medical education and clinical research are faced with a double-barreled threat: they lack the financial resources necessary to conduct clinical trials, and they face additional scrutiny and continued oversight because of their relationships with their collaborative partners. Because they are dangerously underfunded, these centers—and the translational research and medical education they provide—are a disadvantaged and threatened partner in the innovation triad.

Protecting the Ideas

Plant a rice field, tend it, grow it, harvest it and sell it. If you're the farmer, the rice you hold in your hands is tangible evidence that you own it. Plant an idea, tend it, grow it, harvest it, sell it. If you're the inventor, there is no real, tangible "stuff" to hold in your hand. Is it yours? Should it be yours? For how long and under what circumstances should you have the rights to it? When might someone else have the rights? Are there ever circumstances when those rights can, or should, be taken from you?

If you are the innovator, your "stuff" is intellectual property and you have a legal right to call it yours. This is true not only in health care innovation, but also in the industrial, scientific, literary and artistic fields.[17] According to the World Intellectual Property Organization (WIPO), those rights are extended to literary, artistic and scientific works, performances of performing artists, phonograms and broadcasts, inventions in all fields of human endeavor, scientific discoveries, industrial designs and trademarks, service marks, commercial names, and designations.[18] Intellectual property, unlike rice, bricks and mortar, inventory, and other corporate assets, is intangible; it does not have physical characteristics. Our innovators tell us that this ownership is critical to maintaining a pipeline of new discoveries. Is intellectual property important? Yes, it is. One study calculated that, on average, 62% of a company's value lies in intangible assets[19], which are patents, copyrights or trademarks. In the health care industry, specifically the innovation sector, it is clear why patents are important. It is not the pills in the warehouse that have value, but the knowledge created when they were discovered and developed. Patent protection ensures that innovators have protection against intellectual pirates, similar to the protections farmers enjoy from the theft of crops from their fields.

The U.S. Constitution underscores the importance of patents[20], and subsequent laws reinforce their value.[21] Internationally, as well, countries agreed to certain obligations regarding Intellectual Property Rights in 1967 with the creation of the WIPO, an agency of the United Nations. Prior to WIPO, many countries excluded pharmaceuticals, considering drugs to be of such great importance to the national welfare that patents should not create barriers to access.[22] Over time, other nations came to recognize that innovation was important and, further, that without protections piracy would plague the vulnerable industries of informatics, entertainment, specialty chemicals, and pharmaceuticals, and so patent protections were provided to the innovators. Recognizing the value of patents is one matter; protecting them as the world changes is quite another. With the increasing globalization of the world economy, IP rights have emerged as an item of major political conflict among nations and across sectors. Harmonization of IP laws is a key component and central controversy of international trade negotiations, and pharmaceuticals are at issue because they are not considered ordinary goods or products—they are essential goods. As such, they are integral to securing access to health care, a major objective of the WHO.[23]

Research and development for most industries is grounded in IP protection, and the value has been documented in numerous sources.[24] In the case of medical innovation, the discovery enterprise is robust, and the U.S. and its firms lead the way. Over 40% of innovative drugs in the last three decades were discovered in this country,[25] and most of them—94%—by the pharmaceutical sector. Academia and government accounted for only 3.6% and 1%, respectively, of new discoveries.[26] The policies that, in part, fuel this productivity are not without critics. Both here and abroad, the greatest concern is that patent protection increases drug costs by allowing powerful companies to have a monopoly over the idea. As a result of high prices, many who might truly benefit from the therapy are unable to afford it.

The results of patent studies will likely always be considered biased toward industry. But the fact is, a number of these studies have found that improving intellectual property protection does not have a measurable impact on prices of existing drugs and that patent-protected products face therapeutic competition. They also found large, powerful customers who bargained well for better prices and, eventually, generic competition.[27] More indicative of the value of patents is the degree to which protection drives investment in risky research[28] and the reality that regions and countries without such protection—including Latin America, South America, Eastern Europe, and India—do not become the incubators for new scientific inquiry and helpful medicines.[29] This is the case even when patent protections are not eliminated, but only "weakened." Canada, for instance, used to apply compulsory licensing to pharmaceuticals. That is, it compelled the patent holder to license rights to a third party to produce and sell a product, with royalties paid back to the innovator as determined by the government. The U.S. International Trade Commission reports that those compulsory licensing requirements had a significant, negative impact on investment levels in the Canadian pharmaceutical industry, particularly investment by research-based companies. Fewer new products were introduced until after 1987, when compulsory licensing was phased out.

Will the U.S.-based innovators—both companies and scientists—convince us that patent protection is the mainstay for future innovation, discovery and economic growth? The stakes are high, but the outcome is uncertain. Intellectual property is high on the list of concerns for the pharmaceutical and biotechnology industries, but it should be equally important for all those in the innovation sector, and for all of us who will depend on the discoveries they produce for our future health. Patents are not about reaping returns for today's products as much as they are a method to assure funding for tomorrow's products. Society has critical needs that may only be addressed if patent issues are addressed. What can we expect of our innovators in caring for the world? How should national emergencies, which can result in compulsory licensing, be defined and declared? Will patent-free zones be declared? How would they be defined: by disease, by geography, by community? How can our covenant with innovators sustain their work to provide cures to less-developed countries? Do American innovators or Americans in general have a covenant obligation to countries that do not recognize our patents?

Using the Discoveries

Supporting research ventures with funds and talent and providing for the ownership of the discoveries, however, is only halfway to success unless the technologies that result are used. Medicines are of no value in company warehouses or on pharmacy shelves. We have to use them. When we do, they cost; and increasingly, as so many headlines declare, they are costing us more. We spend more on medicines today. That's undeniable. With more people aging and taking the increasing number of new drugs available,[31] there could be no other outcome. Whether branded prescription drugs or generics, whether over-the-counter drugs or herbals, our interest in and need for a pharmaceutical solution is greater than ever. In 2001, the nation's prescription drug budget was $117 billion, or 9% of every health care dollar we spent. The average drug expenditure per person per day in this country is about $1.19. That is a bit higher than the average $1.15 we spend on telephone service, and shy of the $1.57 spent on auto repairs, $3.75 on clothes, and $8.69 on food. The share of spending was split nearly evenly between generic and patented drugs. The increase in the rate of our spending was driven by several factors: better diagnosis and treatment of diseases, an aging population (the elderly generally consume more drugs), the availability of new drugs, an increase in the number of drugs that patients take, new drugs recently introduced onto the market, and price inflation.[32] We feed our hunger for longer and more pleasant lives with more products, and they are doing better things for our health and economy.[33] Death rates from childhood diseases, sexually transmitted diseases, rheumatic fever and rheumatic heart disease, atherosclerosis, ulcer, ischemic heart disease, and hypertension are down by remarkable levels, all attributable to vaccines and pharmaceuticals.[34]

That drugs are blamed for spending increases is no surprise; they are the most visible of the fruits of research. A researcher who discovers the underlying cause of Alzheimer's disease can bank the cash from medical prizes. A company that develops a drug that reverses the process of Alzheimer's dementia can bankrupt the pharmacy. The spending increase has become so visible and volatile, however, that innovation overall is sometimes blamed for the increasing cost of health care today. It is not the first time that this criticism has been leveled, but it has been a serious enough concern that some policy experts warn, privately, that perhaps Congress should not increase NIH funding as promised because the country can ill afford the cost of the discoveries that will result. These criticisms ignore the fact that the nation and the world cannot afford to stop the progress that biomedical innovation can bring, especially at a time when too many helpful treatments seem so close to reality. Perhaps, as some analysts believe, the root of this spending controversy is the fact that not all patients in the U.S. and overseas today who need access to medicines have reimbursement systems to fund their purchase—as is so often the case with other forms of health care. While the drug budget may be small overall nationally, it can represent a burdensome expenditure for some patients—the 25% of elderly, for example, who lack drug coverage; or the obese person whose drug bills are typically 80% greater than non-obese persons with similar conditions. If access to financing to help those who need it is necessary, then by all means, it should be pursued. Demonizing the innovators, however, is no solution to the problems of financing.

Companies have not only been demonized for drug spending, however. As drugs are used in the marketplace, they are also criticized for conflicts of interest in their collaborations within the innovation sector. In the flow of new knowledge between the researcher, the clinician and the pharmaceutical industry, the use of a product, once it reaches the bedside, creates even more new insights. Unproven drugs are tested in isolation, in tightly controlled situations, against a placebo. They are not used that way in real patient care. As new products are introduced, research continues and cooperation among the collaborators must continue as well. These studies—sometimes required by regulators, but often pursued by the innovators—help develop better understanding and new uses for the drugs; so much so that the secondary indications of drugs can eventually exceed 40% of revenues.[35] These collaborations, when they involve industry education, are even more suspect. Industry support of education is substantial, reaching over $1 billion each year and accounting for more than 40% of the continuing medical education provided by medical schools. As the number of new drugs increases, so does the level of industry support for continuing medical education, growing 71% since 1996.[36] This happens on the heels of increased industry support of academic research: from 4% in the 1960s to 14% by 1997.

As the distance between academia and industry narrowed, some critics believed that the relationship was so close as to contaminate not only the agenda, but the objectivity, of investigators, educators, and prescribers. A number of articles have detailed the risks of conflicts of interest[37] and others have posed solutions to safeguarding objectivity, both for the investigator and the university involved.[38] It would now be wise to determine if the organizational changes suggested by some, including the development of new structures and layers of accountability, are necessary. One proposal calls for the creation of separate new entities to do research and to hold equity and receive royalties. While this might seem useful, it may also only succeed in attracting the best and the brightest away for the teaching and service roles of academic medicine. Other proposals call for industry to cease physician education altogether, claiming that for a company to educate about its product is, *a priori*, a conflict of interest.

Is this really necessary? Has biomedical research and physician education truly been compromised because of the relationship among the parties? Or is compromise assumed because the private, for-profit sector is involved, and even the prescriber, the academic and his institution stand to gain financially from discoveries? Is there really an ethical matter at hand, or is it our pervasive discomfort with profit in the healing enterprise? Might this also be just a phase of coming to grips with the costs of new discoveries, and might we all be getting cold feet as the bills of innovation come due?

Enabling Our Innovators to Become Global Healers

We, here in the U.S., might well put our innovation giant to work solving the disease problems of the world, for the needs are great and the giant's talent is immense. As we do, however, we must be thoughtful and strategic. We should sort out where the giant can help and where its girth, regardless of how generous, may not be enough to create the healthy world we would like to enjoy. To begin, we should consider what we—and the giant—are up against. We should address questions such as these:

- How can we better address poverty? Branko Milanovic, a senior World Bank economist, recently assessed world poverty and confirmed what is apparent on the evening news: income disparities are worsening within and between countries.[39] Slower growth in rural areas, generally, and particularly in rural areas of China, India and Bangladesh, is a major cause. These regions cannot keep up with the more rapid economic development of urban areas and the OECD nations. World inequality is a tension, therefore, between the wealth of the U.S., Japan, France, Germany and the United Kingdom and the poverty of China and India. The richest one percent—50 million—of the world's people hold wealth equal to the poorest 57 percent—2.7 billion people. It would seem to be self-evident that the poor of the world would have greater health needs and the nations within which they live have fewer resources with which to provide care. Our intuition should be supplemented, however, with the insights into the distribution of goods and services in relation to health. The work of Norman Daniels is instructive here.[40] Daniels describes how the distribution of income, education, political participation and control of life and work affect health, how inequalities reduce health, and how fair distribution would improve health. He and his colleagues have documented how health correlates with income and other measures of status at the individual level. In other words, it is not just access to care that produces health. Even when a person has access to care, some health conditions have progressed too far for health services to make up for years of physical stress.

The implications for this should be clear: simply sending medical teams and donating drugs to poor nations will not, alone, solve the problems of poverty and income disparity. Elsewhere in this book, in the discussion of drug donations, I noted the challenges of delivering drug therapies in countries without adequate transportation systems or public education, or in countries where civil disputes, war and corruption are the norm. Beyond those challenges are those related to economic, educational and social development that must keep pace with the improving health of the people. Simply providing improved health care will not change the economy of a poor nation, and while our innovation giant may provide solutions to some of the health challenges, it should not be expected to solve the fundamental problems that caused the sicknesses at the outset. We might prevail upon our innovators to provide anti-retroviral medicines for the young women who have been sold by their families into slavery to brothels in the Far East and who now have AIDS as a result, but that will not address the poverty that caused them to become slaves. We might prevail upon other innovators to provide anti-depressant medicines to farmers in the Punjab to stem the rising tide of suicides there, but medicines alone will not alleviate the farmers' poverty by restoring their lands, promoting agricultural diversity, and improving market conditions. Our foreign policy and international aid programs, and the domestic agricultural, educational and development programs must be engaged to address those issues as well.

- How can we better engage our wealth, and that of potential partners, in healing the world? As Americans we should—and we do—decry the poverty of some in our nation, but the work of Milanovic demonstrates how little we comprehend the devastation of poverty worldwide. An American in the bottom 10% of income in this country has greater wealth than two-thirds of the world's population, and those of us in the top 10% (25 million) of income hold wealth equal to the poorest 43% (2 billion) of others in the world. How will we engage our assets to help others who need it? Will we do this through tax-supported ventures, through philanthropy, through public service, by supporting products in our markets so that our innovators have resources available to research developing-world diseases? Our wealth can be put to work in many ways.

- How can we engage other developed-world commercial markets? American philanthropy and government funding of research are important forms of wealth sharing, but together they cannot sustain the research and development efforts necessary to solve the disease problems of the developing world. Support from the European and Japanese commercial markets is also necessary. Within each of our wealthier markets, we support innovation in what we choose to purchase and how much we are willing to pay for those goods. The choice to purchase care is a choice to support the capital structure of the innovation sector. It infuses capital back into innovation. Doing that encourages investors to likewise infuse their capital—and assume some risk—in the research and development ventures that lie ahead. We need individuals willing to risk nearly a decade of advanced education and six-figure educational debts to become clinicians and researchers. We need individual and institutional investors to risk losing their money on biotechnology and pharmaceutical companies involved in $800 million-per-product discoveries.

- Can we come to peace with profit in health care? In order to convince investors to spend their lives and their dollars—or Euros or Yen—on innovations, an even more fundamental shift is required. We must come to terms with a for-profit sector within health care, including a for-profit sector that works in collaboration with government, academia and not-for-profits. If we can do this, then we can end many of the unproductive debates of the current day and stem the tide of incursions into intellectual property ownership. The choice, it seems to me, is simple: do we, as Americans, want to encourage private investors to risk their assets in pursuit of more innovation, or do we not? Do we, as Americans, want to encourage other nations to do likewise? Would we, as Americans, prefer to fund the full cost of education for individuals and take the risks of drug research failure with tax dollars?

- How can we pursue stronger innovation partnerships within this nation? Neither the public nor the private sectors can address the problems of global health alone. Legislated funds for research and public health will never be sufficient to tackle the world's disease problems, and legislated anti-innovation and commercial market policies will only cripple a giant poised to contribute its talent to healing the world needs. Partnership implies more than "doing no harm," however. It implies that the partners will work collaboratively at every stage of the venture. Within the sphere of global caring, this will involve setting an agenda for research, clinical training and product development and pursuing the critical targets of opportunity and need. It will involve detailing the public and private policies that will support progress, and enumerating the public and private assets that should be engaged to address the needs of the globe, not just our own nation. True, there should be oversight to assure that the public trust is not violated, but that oversight should not impede progress on the road to disease solutions.

- How can we pursue stronger partnerships with other developed nations? Our cross-national efforts should entail engaging other developed nations in health care innovation and economic development to assure that Americans, alone, do not unfairly shoulder the world's burdens. These discussions will be difficult, particularly as they relate to the support of products in the marketplaces of Europe and Japan. Many developed nations have created unfavorable climates for health care and innovation which have, in part, driven the innovators to the U.S. Some have set product prices that require companies to charge higher prices in the U.S. in order to recoup investment costs and conduct research on new drugs. While there are some hopeful signs that other developed nations—particularly Germany and Ireland—may be willing to reconsider national policies concerning innovation, creating those changes in both the public policies and the prices in commercial markets will not be easy.

- How can we invite partnerships with developing nations? Dependence and independence are aspects of covenant that are immature and unworthy of the healing ventures to which we should aspire. Recognizing and acting within interdependence should be the goal as we deal with any nation, no matter how poor or distressed, just as it is with any patient, no matter how poor or distressed.

- How can we engage our innovators to address the problems of developing world diseases? Some of our most respected scientists, Dr. Anthony Fauci among them, believe that progress made so far in research to combat HIV/AIDS demonstrates that, if applied well, financial and human resources can solve the seemingly unsolvable problems of disease. Yet only 1% of drugs approved in the last 25 years are directed at solving the infectious tropical diseases that comprise so much of the disease burden of the developing world. In a recent study, major pharmaceutical companies indicated they spent less than 1% of their research resources on these diseases, and the public sector is estimated to be spending less than $75 million.[41] Some advocates have advanced proposals to require companies to invest in developing-world diseases[42], and the government funds an

International Center for Tropical Disease Research that issues challenge grants to those who commit their own resources to this arena. The Gates Foundation has emerged as a major funder of developing-world disease innovation, and at a recent meeting of government, industry and academia, our innovators met to assess and correct barriers to research.[43] All these are hopeful signs. Are they enough to address the needs of poor nations for our help, and the needs of this nation to lend it?

The current hostility and mistrust that confront our innovation sector as it attempts to solve our disease riddles are an unfortunate distraction from the task at hand to heal the world. It is my hope that new dialogues can begin. Creating the relationships will require change on the part of all who are involved. For their part, the innovators must become more engaged in telling their story and participating in solving not just the disease, but the health care financing problems. For our part as patients, we must become more involved in appropriately using their discoveries—and being willing to pay for them when we can. As a nation, we must be prepared to fund care for those who cannot afford to pay for it themselves. Most of all, however, we must recognize the consequences of abandoning a century-long tradition of being the most innovative nation in the world. Neither we, nor the world, can afford a kink in the innovation pipeline.

Part 4

HEALING HEALTH CARE

In some ways healing has changed substantially since healers first created their covenant oaths. Healers today have greater capabilities to influence the course of our health and disease. They are better educated and have highly evolved diagnostic and healing tools in their arsenal. The number and types of healers—at least in the way I define them—have changed as well. The healing arts are not just a clinical skill. Today they comprise business, organizational, and project skills as well. Today, healers are not just the traditional physicians, surgeons, and pharmacists of ancient times, nor are they the allied health professionals who readily come to mind. Healers are all those who touch the health care enterprise. This includes those who manage health information on the worldwide web, develop and market health care products, and most important, control the access and reimbursement streams that fuel patient care.

In at least one significant way, however, nothing has changed. Although the relationships between patients and their healers are in tremendous flux, patients still expect today's healers to act within the covenant to which they have ascribed for thousands of years. Many healers are willing to do so and hold dearly to their obligations despite mounting pressures within health care today. For these healers, their patients, and communities, steps to reinvigorate existing covenants and create new covenants of obligation may well be the most productive steps to take in assuring a healing enterprise for the future.

If health care is healed, it will be because healers continue to embrace covenants. If health care is healed, it will be because healers call today's patients and communities into new covenants of caring. If health care is healed, it will be because patients and communities responded. If health care is healed, new covenants of obligation will serve as the foundation of the healing enterprise for generations to come.

Chapter 11

Emerging Models

Healing and Living Within Covenants

Noisy, curious healers who make house calls will have the time of their lives![1]

Patch Adams, M.D.

I met Patch Adams. I was his patient and so I feel qualified to talk on his behalf. Patch Adams describes his approach in *Gesundheit! Bringing Good Health to You, the Medical System, and Society Through Physician Service, Complementary Therapies, Humor and Joy*, and I know it's for real.

It wasn't a house call. I met Dr. Patch Adams at National Airport in Washington, D.C. in the fall of 1992. It was an early Friday evening and I was waiting to board a flight for home after a long week's work on the road: tired from travel, stressed from meetings, and very much in need of a vacation. I was seated at the boarding gate waiting for the flight, when I glanced over my shoulder and saw a very tall, strange character coming through the metal detector. He was dressed more outrageously than any portrayal Robin Williams ever managed in the film version of Dr. Adams' life—a rubber chicken, immense floppy shoes, ballooned pantaloons, and a huge nose stand out most clearly in my memory. He was accompanied by a tall woman who was also dressed to draw attention—a cross between Olive Oyl, Raggedy Ann, and Minnie Pearl. He must have sensed the tension in my executive life from across the room. He headed straight for the seat next to me. For nearly 45 minutes as we awaited the flight's departure for Newark, he teased, he played, he offered a lollipop. He made whistle and hum sounds, but he never spoke. He answered none of my questions, but he engaged me in his brand of healing, delightfully. Having no idea who he was or what this was about, I was polite, but also afraid, amused, and curious. Mostly, I laughed—apparently the medicine he was prescribing, and I have since come to learn, good for the immune system. I noticed others in the gate area: they kept their distance, but they watched all the while. They also laughed. Perhaps this was Dr. Adams' view of public health. Not only did he cure me of the fatigue of the moment, but he helped the whole group. I took the lollipop to be polite, but never ate it, for the obvious reason that I suspected it contained a substance that precipitated his unusual behavior. Until the movie "trailers" for Patch Adams arrived in theaters, it did not occur to me that he was a physician, acting as a healer within the covenant he defines, healing everywhere he goes.

Covenant does not require healers to make house calls or to "act-up" in airports, but I'd like to think that more healers can have fun, fulfilling, and satisfying practices. I'd like to think that this will contribute to the effectiveness of their healing and that not only their patients, but they themselves, will thrive and enjoy longevity. Unfortunately, as the years pass, I see fewer and fewer healers with the kind of enthusiasm that drives Patch Adams. The stress they face in their work is draining the soul from their healing. Many want to reconnect with the spirit that first led them into health care, and for them, there are models of healing covenants that can re-inspire visions and reinvigorate their energies. This chapter is dedicated to those healers, and to those of us as patients and communities who will venture out to support them as they work to heal us.

Not all of the extraordinary healers I know have articulated their missions or expressed them as outrageously or as well as Dr. Patch Adams, but some of them have. Few of them have published their views, and even fewer are known by the public-at-large. None of them is likely to appear on the silver screen, so they are largely unsung heroes except within the spheres of health care where only close colleagues and friends know their work. Although those healers have not embraced a formal covenant, they have acted within one. Although they might not choose to portray their life's work as having been lived within the covenants of obligation that I propose, I believe they would see themselves in the stories I tell about them and others who work within covenant. Although they have never specifically mentioned covenant in their work, their writings, or their talks, they act as if notions of covenant were central to their own personal, organizing principles.

These healers share a number of characteristics in common with Patch Adams, and since his life and views are the best known of those contemporary covenant healers, it tells the story of the others. Like Dr. Adams, these healers look beyond the mechanics of the physical body into a wider array of needs the people they serve have—be they a patient ill with some malady or a healthy person avoiding sickness or improving their fitness. Like Patch Adams, they prefer preventing illness and supporting health over crisis management of illness and disability. They have a passion for what they do in caring for others and they are always striving to do it better. They don't dress in red rubber noses, but they have taken risks to engage the resources they needed to create successful practices, as Dr. Adams did. They haven't all defied the institutions of health care and its bureaucracies, but most of them have, and all of them have been willing to engage in nontraditional ventures to accomplish their mission. Like Dr. Adams, they are scholars in their own fields, but they never shied from the opportunity to learn from others or to integrate learned approaches from other fields. They work in teams, and they inspire leadership. Acting as leaders, they have invited others into the covenant, whether as patients, as customers, as employees, or as colleagues. They took fewer vacations than they needed, and they were certainly tired at times, but none of them burned out. They have worked long past retirement age or "retired" into other healing ventures. And like Patch Adams, Dr. Gesundheit himself, they are strong personalities and a pleasure to be with.

Healers and Their Emerging Covenants

Covenant pioneers in contemporary healing go beyond good customer service. Patients, after all are not just "consumers." They have some of the same needs and wants as consumers—courtesy, timely service, and affordability, for example—but they have needs that go beyond those of mere consumers. A customer can be inconvenienced. A patient can also suffer the fear, vulnerability, guilt, and change in social and economic status that come with being out of control because of their illness. The intention of these healers, then, is not to grow market share or to limit health care utilization, though those outcomes are frequently the result of their efforts. Their intention is to relieve the suffering that accompanies disease and disability. It is unlikely that they are known to each other, as there is no trade association or professional society that embraces those who feel the pull of covenant to guide their endeavors. Their stories are largely anecdotal, as few studies have been undertaken to develop a comprehensive picture of what their practices contribute to health and healing. Nonetheless, their contributions are real and important for sharing. Their covenants are implicit, because few explicit covenants have been written. Today's health policy climate is conflict-ridden and anger is frequently directed at healers. Leaders in health care are too often criticized for lacking easy answers to tough questions. In an attempt to heal health care, those innovators who are striving to be healers of patients, communities, and other healers deserve some recognition and continued encouragement for their efforts.

Some of these healers are professionals we do not traditionally view as being within the healing enterprise. One that comes to mind is an advertising executive, Gil Bashe.[2]

His early life experience as a medic in the Israeli army gave him an appreciation for the needs of patients and the importance of nurturing them that translates into a passion for communicating health issues in a way that improves patient knowledge and thus their health. He tells stories about how soldiers in the Israeli army, tough as they come, would need caring when they were ill with relatively simple conditions. He tells an even more compelling story about how he, with the help of others in his unit, cared for a young enemy Syrian soldier in battle, dragging him off the field under cover and treating him for what was already a partial amputation of his leg. Gil says, "There are many ways to communicate, and even in the presence of an enemy unit and unable to understand the language, we could see the spark in this soldier's eye that he understood we would care for him. Providing care for him was life-giving for us as well as for him." Gil's mission is to make communications as much a part of life-giving care as the other therapies that healers employ. He wants information, itself, to be healing. Gil should be applauded for this, as should others who strive for quality communications with patients.

It is reassuring to know, in the information age, that others are following in Bashe's footsteps. Brother-and-sister team Julie and Paul Lerner developed and published a guide to health care services in New York, in response to problems Julie encountered during her experience with non-Hodgkin's lymphoma. They work with other patient groups, encouraging them to demand more information, compassionate care, and less bureaucratic relationships with payers. They use information as tools of empowerment into the hands of other patients.

Michael O'Neil's own experience as a patient in a hospital led him to understand the importance, not only of information, but also of connecting with others during the isolation that illness causes. He created GetWellNetwork to assure that hospitalized patients can not only get information about their condition, but support from those who care for them through interactive distance communications.

On the creative side of communications, physician-brothers John and Mathew Clarke have written, arranged, produced, and performed rap music health education campaigns on such critical teen-health concerns as HIV/AIDS prevention, smoking, substance abuse, and asthma under the name "Health-Rap." Their research has indicated that teens will be more receptive to health messages in rap-music formats.

Similar ventures are underway through the Internet and are now too numerous to mention. Unfortunately, though many sites would claim to be covenantal, not all of these ventures are. Some contain inaccurate and biased information and masquerade as legitimate sources of valid clinical information. Few sites are monitored for quality, and only recently have e-health commerce groups met to form standards of performance that characterize a covenant with patients and communities. One notable exception is DiabetesWell, designed by Dr. Joe Prendergast.[3] This web-based site provides information on diabetes that includes quarterly patient assessments, counseling, and recommendations for diet, medication, and exercise. Patient test data are collected and monitored by the site, which is staffed by Prendergast and a staff of physicians and nurse specialists. New research and information are provided to patients through daily e-mails designed to be read in one minute. True to the nature of monitoring quality in the covenant, Dr. Prendergast tracks the impact of his e-care on patients. Rates of hospital admissions and deaths from diabetes are substantially reduced in his subscribers.

Other covenant pioneers are business executives. Matt Emmens had such passion for healing potential that he left the comfort of a good, secure job to risk it all in a start-up company. That company became the platform for one of the largest pharmaceutical research companies in the world today. Des Cummings created a new health care system, based on new paradigms, in a new town. Des and

Matt worked together to fund and launch the search for innovative solutions in health care. They called it the Center for Health Futures, and its work is to link traditional healers with other healers and communities. Rich Rakowski took disease management to a new level, integrating communication technology with highly skilled nurses who kept in touch with patients by phone.

Business executive Pat Charmel was profiled in Inc. magazine as a hands-on hospital CEO.[4] Griffin Hospital, which he heads, embarked on a multiyear project to satisfy its customers. In the midst of reimbursement rate slashes, revenue declines, and competitive consolidation, this community hospital challenged the impossible—to "just say yes" to whatever would satisfy their patients. What the hospital team did was characteristic of covenant relationships: they listened. Sometimes this meant listening to each other as they detailed the bad experiences they or family members had in hospitals. They posed as patients to see what patient care was like at other institutions thought to be "better." It also meant listening to their own patients. Then it meant changing their directions, their procedures, even their bathtubs, if that would satisfy patients. It meant creating community access to the Internet for research, visits by therapy dogs, and places to bake cookies in the oncology unit. It also meant forcing changes, changes that were not always well received at first. But eventually staff turnover slowed, staff designed even more responsive programs, occupancy is up, and 400 community volunteers provide any service patients need at the moment—including, for one patient, seeing that income tax forms left in the car got mailed on time.

Entrepreneur Brian Crawford has initiated a number of projects, but his most recent is also the most innovative. Brian was concerned that social isolation took too great a toll on the health of older people and saw a way to link frail, elderly, homebound patients with other, usually elderly, people who were still active in their communities. These active elderly were trained to act as community-based healer-visitors, agreeing to visit as "care companions" those frail elderly to coach, engage, and monitor their health status. The care companions are volunteers, but their time translates into tax-free "time dollars" they may "spend" later if they require a similar service. In this way, people are caring for each other in ways that no traditional clinical healer could and no current financing system could afford. The satisfaction of all those involved is very high. In fact, many care companions have created such strong relationships with their patients that they visit daily, not weekly as the program requires.

Some new covenant healers have personal experience with disease or with special patient needs. If they do, they tend to become organizers. Charles (Charlie) B. Inlander and Abbey Meyers created separate venues for patients to act collectively and have a voice in their personal care. In each of their organizations, they have created mutually supportive covenants with patients, and together they challenge healers. Myrl Weinberg took her passion for patients overseas, creating links between patient groups in the U.S., Europe, and Japan to facilitate an international dialogue that would improve patient care and empowerment.

Corporations are also healers. CVS, the largest pharmacy in the nation, has invited customers into a covenant regarding medication safety.[5] The company encourages its patients to provide complete information to its pharmacists about their prescriptions, over-the-counter drugs, vitamins, minerals, nutraceuticals, and herbal medicines they are taking. In an atmosphere of assured confidentiality, CVS pharmacists can caution against the negative effects that some combinations are known to cause.

Other healers support the health policy process. Judy Miller Jones has nurtured the nation's national policy wonks since the Carter era, creating a cadre of reciprocal relationships with them and enabling those relationships, all for the benefit of improving the quality of health policy analysis and decision making. Dr. Art Sprenkle, a physician who held positions in the Washington State legislature and was medical director of a health plan, has used his insights to bring together physicians, Washington State government offices, pharmaceutical companies, and the press to improve clinical care in the state.

Researchers like Dr. P. Roy Vagelos are covenant healers. His passion for patients and the mechanisms of disease led him to ground-breaking ideas in drug development and stirred him to challenge other physicians in the way they managed disease. Roy was unusual as a researcher in the days when he explored the healing potential of research. First, he worked as a researcher for a pharmaceutical company at a time when researchers shunned the industry, fearing that working for a company would damage their careers. Roy put those fears aside. Then, he developed the business and management skills needed to turn the labs and clinics into highly successful discovery centers, beating the odds in discovering and developing more drugs than other companies in the industry. Finally, he translated all of those skills into not only managing the internal vision of the company, but communicating that vision through tough times weathered by the industry when the capital markets were losing confidence and investors were leaving biomedicine in droves. He held prices at or below the Consumer Price Index long before other companies followed suit, and he made a valuable parasitic medicine available at no cost to the people of the developing world who could not afford it. He retired to devote his experience to education, new research ventures, and philanthropy.

Maurice R. Hilleman, Ph.D., broke through barriers, plunged into a field that was highly controversial—vaccines—and brought prevention to the world's children. He pioneered vaccine research in children and was one of the first to address the ethical issues of informed parent consent and community concurrence with studies of vaccines. Visiting local neighborhoods, community leaders, and churches in the Philadelphia area, Dr. Hilleman worked through the concerns about vaccine research and produced some of the most valuable vaccine products available today. One vaccine alone, the Measles-Mumps-Rubella vaccine—which he developed, in part, through throat cultures from his own daughter Jeryl Lynn's illness—is estimated to save the nation $5 billion in direct and indirect medical costs for each birth cohort that is vaccinated. He might have retired long ago, but he has not. Instead, he has continued his research and to advise others in his field of expertise.

Two individuals are unique in their ability to walk both the trenches and the hallowed halls of public health. They have cared for patients individually and have mastered the politics of caring for them as populations. Dr. Bill Foege is one of the most notable of this group for his role in eradicating smallpox from the globe. Medicine and peace are inherent to Dr. Foege's inimitable style in all of his work. He traveled in West Africa in the midst of a smallpox outbreak without enough vaccine to immunize everyone at risk. He developed new strategies to contain the disease in Africa and other parts of the world and convinced government health officials to try his radical approaches. He worked in war-torn zones to do it and was held at gunpoint by rebels and in detention twice.

When he returned to the United States, Dr. Foege was appointed to head the Centers for Disease Control and Prevention at a time when it was reeling from the ill-effects of the Swine Flu Immunization campaign and reports of Guillain-Barre Syndrome supposedly caused by the vaccine. He repaired the image of the agency and restored the trust of the nation in its programs and policies, in time to confront a growing number of public health crises: toxic shock syndrome, vaccine safety, Reye's syndrome, and HIV/AIDS. His considerable skill is now applied as an advisor to The Gates Foundation, as it addresses the needs of the developing world for disease solutions.

Dr. Foege's experiences and skills are similar to those of the soft-spoken medical missionary, Sister Maura O'Donohue, M.D., a physician and surgeon who practiced for fourteen years in Ethiopia during the wars and for nine years on HIV/AIDS in the developing world. Like Bill Foege, Sister Maura walks the halls of power where she articulates the needs of her patients well. Some healers practicing in war-torn, famine-struck regions are more at home in their field clinics than in policy and political settings. Sister Maura, a rare breed among them, is facile in both. Her political skills promote the true changes that global institutions must make to save lives. Like Bill Foege, her efforts have resulted in negotiated solutions to global problems of death from disease and malnutrition.

A few pioneers in healing today have crafted the reciprocal relationships central to a covenant of obligation; they are teaching this way of healing to other healers and evaluating and publishing the results of these ventures. As healers, they have proposed new relationships to their patients and their patients have accepted the offer. And now, the healers and the patients are in a reciprocal endeavor participating in and generating the outcomes of covanental healing approaches.

The list of all those who have engaged covenant, though not specifically saying so, could fill a book. Knowing more about these and others who have approached healing with such respect could create models for others who follow them into much more demanding territory to address many more challenging problems today. Since these relationships are being explored in greater depth in a project on Relationship-Centered Care sponsored by the Pew Foundation and the Fetzer Foundation, the future may well yield greater insights and more models of covenant caring.

Over time, these relationships have evolved and are still evolving—neither healer nor patient at this point can say where the relationship will lead. As a result, a significant challenge awaits these healers, the systems within which they work, and the health care payers and policymakers who shape them all. The challenge will be to assure that, over time, the regulatory and payment environments don't get in the way. Today's regulated health care is so constrained that the sacredness of these relationships is endangered. New regulatory and payment environments must keep pace with these changes to allow for the growing covenant-style care and not "lock in" noncovenant systems of management. The complexity of the regulations that guide the practice and the reimbursement of healing, as Uwe Reinhardt has said, can make "a crook" of anyone in health care.[6] It would be a tragedy if those involved in returning to the roots of caring were prevented from doing so. It is critical, then, that those regulators and legislators who frame the legal structure for payment examine their own role in healing and enter into the covenant accordingly.

Cooperative Health Care Clinics:
A Covenant Between Patients and Healers

The Cooperative Health Care Clinic (CHCC)[7] is one of the programs worthy of protecting against rigid systems of payment and regulation. It is an innovative model in which care is provided to older patients by a team composed of a physician, nurse, pharmacist, and other healers in a group setting. It was developed by John Scott, M.D. and colleagues with funding from Kaiser Permanente and first piloted within the Kaiser plan. Based on findings from research conducted to date, the CHCC is a cost-effective delivery style that helps physicians and health care plan administrators improve the quality of care provided to older adults with multiple disease conditions.

The CHCC model addresses one of the major challenges of health care today—that physicians' time spent on direct patient care has been seriously eroded by various mandates of managed care. In the CHCC model, groups of fifteen to twenty patients meet monthly in an "expanded doctor's office visit" that includes care delivery, education, social time, and a question-and-answer session. Patients or their physicians have the option to request time for private visits following the group session, if either should feel the need. In the traditional way that we speak about health care today, we would say that the CHCC model encourages patients to be active participants in the management of their health care rather than dependent recipients of care. In the language of covenants, the CHCC model moves beyond the usual covenant of grant and encourages several types of covenants of obligation between the healers and the patients: first, between the patients within the group; second, between the healers in the group; and third, between the patients and healers together. By all accounts, both the healers and the patients who participate in this form of care are living up to their obligations. They attend the meetings regularly and provide continuing support to each other and their families, including when their conditions cause hospitalizations or death. No study has yet been completed to capture the richness of the relationships, but they are clear from observing the groups in action, from the anecdotes provided by all the participants—patients as well as healers—and from the outcomes measured in the participants in the project.

The initial CHCC program was a one-year, randomized, controlled study funded by Kaiser Permanente and included about three hundred patients. The promising findings of the first study attracted the attention of the Robert Wood Johnson Foundation, which subsequently funded a larger study of eight hundred patients. In both of these studies, the experimental groups attended CHCC sessions and control groups received traditional primary care. The results were favorable. The participating patients showed improvement in their ability to manage activities of daily living, improvement in patient satisfaction, 20%-30% decrease in hospitalization, more than 20% decrease in emergency room use, and a decrease in nursing home referrals. Patients liked this care model so much that they stayed with the health plan. Even physician satisfaction was improved, so much so that some of them said they would never again want to practice any other way.

The economic analyses conducted by the CHCC are preliminary, but it appears that among these very old and frail patients, savings have been approximately $3 per member per month. Economists are in the process of applying these findings to a broader spectrum of patients, as defined by diagnosis, health status, and utilization. Savings for a broader and largely healthier group of patients are anticipated to be in the range of $50 per member per month. Currently, there are great expectations and significant planning efforts associated with the future of the CHCC. Kaiser Permanente has a goal to establish 100 CHCC groups of 20 individuals for 2,000 of its most needy enrollees.

Covenants with the Uninsured

There is no more challenging issue in health care politics today than how to deal with the growing problem of the uninsured. Those who lack insurance because small business employers cannot obtain or afford coverage for their employees, those who earn too much to qualify for low-income programs and those who are too young for Medicare are a growing segment of those who need care and the funds to finance it. Providing insurance to the uninsured was only partially resolved in programs of the last few decades. Policymakers and politicians have yet to resolve the issue by crafting a final solution that will have sufficient support for enactment into law. Burdened by other patient rights proposals, including proposals to give patients the right to sue for denials of care, some employers predict that their continuing coverage of health benefits is in jeopardy. The number of uninsured may be destined to grow.

A number of communities, in meeting their part of the covenant have designed programs to provide managed care for the uninsured. The Center for Studying Health System Change is tracking 12 communities intensively.[8] In each case, the community is attempting to provide for primary and preventive care, while avoiding the expensive inpatient and emergency care that sometimes results from a failure to prevent and treat conditions early. These communities use existing charity care funding, Disproportionate Share Hospital (DSH) funding, and local tax revenues to provide access to managed care for those who are not eligible for other publicly funded programs like Medicare and Medicaid. They do not provide the identical benefit package as entitlement programs, but they actively monitor and transfer the patients to public programs when they become eligible. They use a variety of strategies to control costs, including physician primary care managers, provider networks, 24-hour help lines to divert patients from unnecessary emergency room visits, social services, language translators, and low-cost transportation to health care facilities.

A project funded by the Robert Wood Johnson Foundation called "Reach Out, Physicians' Initiative to Expand Care to Underserved Americans" has modeled the provision of care for the uninsured through networks of volunteer physicians.[9] Medical societies, group practices, not-for-profit groups, and religious organizations sponsored projects to increase access to care, under the leadership of physicians in local communities who recruited and organized participation. Development grants from the Foundation supported the organization of the care, which was provided in freestanding clinics, referral networks, primary care networks, and public-private partnerships for primary and surgical care. Approximately 11,000 physicians provided care to nearly 200,000 patients during the four years of the program and, because the projects have demonstrated their value, more than three-quarters are expected to receive local support to continue now that the grant funding period has ended.

Nursing Center concepts have developed out of advanced nursing practices that originated in 1965 and provided general primary care, as well as special care in schools and in nurse-midwifery, in areas where physician care was unavailable and insurance unaffordable. Of patients in nurse practices, 20%-50% are uninsured. They tend to see their nurse practitioners somewhat more often, but they use hospital and emergency care less frequently. In some cases these practice arrangements are collaborative with physicians, in others they are independent practices that are fully managed and supervised by nurses, and in half of the states today, nurses can provide primary care and prescribe medications without the supervision of physicians or without collaborative agreements with them.[10]

In an effort to use information technology, the Greater New York Hospital Association (GNYHA) is in the process of developing a system, called the Health Insurance Training and Education (HITE) Network, to inform New York's nearly 3 million uninsured about the resources available for their care.[11] In this project, these people will be linked with a variety of resources that are already available, but underutilized. Concerned for the growing number of uninsured, as well as for the number who are eligible for services but not accessing those services, HITE assumes that these individuals are unaware of the resources and simply need to be linked with them. Services such as health insurance subsidies, breast cancer screening, HIV testing, flu shots, free medications, and low-cost care will be made known through outreach and information using a web site containing state-specific resources and trained personnel to help uninsured individuals access the information.

In a radically different model, and one that addresses the affordability problems of the uninsured and the underinsured, the American Association of Patients and Providers (AAPP) has established SimpleCare.[12] The program is built on the vision of both traditional healers such as doctors of medicine and osteopathy, chiropractors, podiatrists, and others considered alternative or complementary healers, such as massage therapists, acupuncturists, nurses, and physician assistants working together with patients. The AAPP recognizes that each of these healers offers a unique perspective and can help the patient in need, and that they can coexist when patients are allowed to choose their healers. Its goal is to return to a simple system of health care, avoiding the administrative expense and paperwork burdens that have so confused patients and drained the resources of healers. In the SimpleCare program, patients pay for services at the time of the visit in cash, by check, or by charge card at a rate reduced from most third-party visits, usually 35%-50% less. The healer does not bill the insurance company, nor does it provide information to allow the patient to file claims. For uninsured patients who cannot afford the care, some communities have bartering options in which patients can "pay back" their health care costs by providing services to others in the community. The AAPP is not the only such discount program. North American Care operates a similar program, with discounts of 20%-70% for cash up front.

Celebration Health: A Covenant Between Healers and Communities

Healers and their communities are also pioneering covenants as communities are becoming increasingly receptive to new relationships with healers,[13] and as community leaders become aware of how they can support health and healing within their official roles. In one recent study of community attitudes, it was clear that community views of health and healing are ready for new, broader definitions of health and covenants of obligation. Definitions of health are moving away from the avoidance of disease and toward the active pursuit of wellness and an appreciation for the non-medical quality of life factors in communities. People are discouraged with the health of their own communities, lack confidence in their leaders and institutions, and are ready to play a more active role to improve health. Health care reform is viewed as an individual as well as a national responsibility, and most people now believe that they can help by becoming more focused on prevention and on cost-conscious buying of health care services. Declining moral values and selfishness are viewed as barriers to improvements in health, and the definitions of a healthy community have become more comprehensive. Communities perceive themselves as healthy when the crime rate is low; when they can raise their children in a good place; when children's needs are addressed, including child abuse, child care, and education; and where strong family life, positive race relations, and affordable housing is predominant. The usual measures that health care has come to be concerned about—access, quality, and affordability—were considered critical determinants of health for only slightly more than half of the people surveyed. Communities are looking beyond the clinical offices and institutions that deliver care.[14]

It was into that community reality that Disney and its fantasy-world designers stepped when building the twenty-first-century town of Celebration in central Florida. These visionaries did not neglect the health care needs of the community. They collaborated with the Florida Hospital Health System, part of the Adventist Health System, and Celebration Health was conceived. Florida Hospital Health System was a logical choice for several reasons: It has over 90 years of medical leadership serving central Florida; it is central Florida's largest health care provider; it is the largest integrated health system in the nation; and it is part of the Adventist Health System, a unique system founded on healthy lifestyle principles. These healthy lifestyle principles have been examined in a study of 50,000 people who have lived the lifestyle advocated by the Adventist Health System for 25 years. They were found to be among the healthiest people in the world.[15]

The Florida Hospital Health System was asked to address the needs of the community in creative and interactive ways, and the Celebration Health facility became the anchor of the innovation in health and healing services. It is a unique setting that delivers hospital care, but its primary focus is on community care, wellness, and disease prevention. The facility provides a location for physician offices and includes a major fitness center, rehabilitation center, community pharmacy, and food service. In addition, it houses patient education and risk management programs that go beyond the usual reduction of risk behaviors to encompass elements of life and health that create not only disease reduction or health promotion, but also optimum health. In its approach to treating the whole person, Celebration Health has incorporated eight guiding principles for individuals who are seeking a healthy life: Choice, Rest, Environment, Activities, Trust in God, Interpersonal Relationships, Outlook, and Nutrition.[16]

Patients, known as "guests," play a central, directive, and interactive role in their care and health improvement plans. The facility offers a mix of conventional customs and futuristic concepts where old-fashioned, individualized, personal attention is combined with the power of new technology and paradigms for caring. The setting is Disney-like in its quality, thoughtful planning, and characterization as a center for creating and maintaining healthy lifestyles. The Celebration Health experience is consistent with the anticipated future of health care and certainly the direction in which today's empowered patient is moving. This model emphasizes holistic health and healing, and the health system provides individuals with facilities, staff, and opportunities to experience optimum health at whatever their age and health status. The goal is for all people in the community, not only those who are ill and are the inpatient "guests," to achieve the best possible health outcomes from their encounters with healers.

The centerpiece of Celebration Health is a change from traditional models of care based on acute encounters with medicine to a focus on a healthy lifestyle integrated with the traditional health care competencies of primary, acute, surgical, and emergency care. In this transition, Celebration Health recognizes the challenges facing health care today, in which most health problems stem from diseases individuals bring on themselves from lifestyle choices and personal mismanagement of chronic conditions. The hallmark of Celebration Health care, however, is the recognition of the mutuality of the relationships between each of the players—the patient, the hospital, and the community. In this shift, although the hospital may be the anchor for healing within the community, it is not the center of the care. It is but one player in a continuum of healing services that helps individuals change the way they live in order to successfully prevent and manage disease. Every component of the design and management of Celebration Health promotes this paradigm shift in the creation of healing for the community.

Engaging Other Healers in the Community Covenant
To promote the transformation of American health care, Celebration Health's leadership enlisted the support and collaboration of approximately 35 partners, all of whom are working cooperatively to integrate innovations in healing that support the goals of the community. These partnerships support Celebration Health with a wide range of activities, programs, and equipment to promote health. In return, these companies use this community setting to further develop and test the latest in technology, information services, and patient support strategies. As a result, new methods are developed and then the center is used for training and demonstrations to other parts of the country.

Through the work of one of the partners, the Center for Health Futures, Celebration Health is a party to identifying, developing, and assessing the effectiveness of new models of care. Wyeth-Ayerst works with Celebration Health to develop and maintain a Center for Women's Health Services. Women who receive obstetric and gynecologic services at physicians' offices on site have access to extensive web-based information services and are encouraged to research their questions and conditions prior to physician visits. GlaxoWellcome works with Celebration Health to pioneer innovative disease management programs and outcomes research. One disease management initiative is a pilot program to better manage chronic headaches. This program identifies chronic headache sufferers, educates them to better understand their symptoms and the mechanisms that trigger pain, and telephones them later to assess the success of the education in controlling their chronic headaches.

GlaxoWellcome also worked with Celebration Health on a smoking cessation project. Celebration Health staff noticed that when patients were in the hospital, surrounded by concerned family, they were more receptive to education about smoking and quitting than at other times. This led to inpatient counseling for patient and family coupled with pharmaceutical care and resulted in quit rates twice those of other model programs. The AGFA Medical Division of Bayer developed the radiology department to meet the health care demands of the future and showcase a state-of-the-art Picture Archival Communications System (PACS) that creates the highest quality diagnostic images and simultaneously streamlines the diagnostic process. Celebration Health serves as a demonstration center for training other radiology departments now making the transition to digital technology. Ethicon Endo-Surgery, Inc., a Johnson & Johnson Company, showcases its surgical tools in the operating room and uses it as a test site for new minimally invasive tools and services to advance surgical outcomes. Celebration Health will oversee educational programs on the Ethicon Endo-Surgery Mammotome Breast Biopsy System, demonstrated to be three times more accurate than a core needle biopsy. General Electric Medical Systems was involved in early strategic discussions about Celebration Health's design and now is a center for GE Medical's state-of-the-art diagnostic imaging equipment. Approximately a dozen types of GE Medical's diagnostic imaging equipment can be found at Celebration Health, including the Stenoscope mobile digital imaging systems, the AMX-4+ mobile X-ray system, the Millennium MG multigeometry nuclear imaging system, the Advantx DRS integrated digital radiology system, and the Signa Conquest MR system.

Reaching Out to the Surrounding Community

These Celebration Health project partners are impressive, the facility is beautiful, well equipped, and well staffed. It is a center for health that reaches out to the central Florida area and to the nation—and eventually to the world. An example is a project with AstraZeneca, which partnered with Celebration Health to develop a Digestive Health Center in central Florida. The center is developing comprehensive best practice models in the care management of patients with gastrointestinal (GI) disorders, including outreach to the community to identify and treat patients with GI disease. This model will be replicated throughout the Florida Hospital Health System and Adventist Health System.

Another example of reaching out, this time to the Florida Governor's Office, was the formation of the Community Health Improvement Council (CHIC). The CHIC provides a committed infrastructure for addressing health and disease issues within the state and will invest $8 million over eight years into central Florida health improvements. As a result of working with the Governor's Office, new resources for health care, most recently for congestive heart failure, have received support in the state's budget. Since the CHIC membership also includes the Central Florida Health Care Coalition, a group composed of over

200 employers in the region and involving the largest employers in the nation, projects with employers are being planned.

Celebration Health has its critics. They argue that the facility and its service components are only possible because of the extensive partnerships with Disney and other corporations drawn to Orlando because of its tourist potential and Disney association. As a matter of fact, those elements have facilitated some of the interactions. The Orlando site is a preferred location for medical conventions, and Celebration Health can easily originate satellite-beamed surgeries and educational sessions into the Orlando Convention Center, where large numbers of clinicians are meeting. But in truth, it is the attitude of the leadership, not the location of the building, that makes Celebration Health what it is. It is the nature of the healer-patient and healer-community relationships that creates the "green field" for the experimentation and success that the organization clearly appears to be enjoying. Furthermore, no one at Celebration Health will claim that their relationships are truly unique, as they have learned in their work with other communities.

Reaching Out to Other Communities

Celebration Health and a number of other communities are charter members of the Accelerating Community Transformation (ACT) Project.[17] ACT is a multidimensional, five-year applied research project guided by the broad and ambitious vision of building healthier communities, first in the United States and, ultimately, throughout the world. ACT builds community partnerships and civic infrastructures to achieve and demonstrate measurable improvements in community health and quality of life. The ACT Project has ambitious goals:

- To establish and refine community visions of healthy and sustainable futures

- To develop clear statements of desired outcomes and

how to achieve them

- To develop a software tool to measure outcomes of community health in a standardized and efficient way and to link outcomes to performance

- To measure and track indicators of community improvement

- To identify, create and document collaborative approaches and interventions "that work," creating a repertoire of "best practices" to increase health and quality of life that can be shared with other communities.

To date there are nearly thirty operative ACT sites in various stages of implementation in seventeen states. By design, the locations, social and economic characteristics, and demographics of the ACT Project site communities are diverse and represent a cross section of America. They have a track record in applying the principles and values of healthier communities, and they want to further build capacity to improve health and quality of life. For example, two of the program sites illustrate the vast difference between the sites in the area of geography. One is a small, old, southern town with a population of approximately 25,000 that began as a health resort many years ago. All of the organizations and agencies involved in this project are located in a small vicinity; they are all familiar with one another, have established contacts, and have worked together for many years. In contrast, another ACT site covers an area of approximately 10,000 square miles over 15 counties in 4 states.

In the course of their work, ACT communities are addressing pressing public and community health issues. One community ranked 50th in the United States in its rate of infant mortality when it began its healthy community initiative. Another community had lost 40% of its population in years immediately prior to the implementation of ACT due to unemployment when major employers pulled out of the area. In their projects, various communities are addressing low immunization rates among vulnerable populations; substance abuse; domestic and community violence; identification of, and treatment for, diseases such as asthma, cardiovascular conditions, diabetes and depression; and achieving Healthy People 2000 Objectives. The community goals, however, are not all health related, as other factors clearly influence health status. Some communities are focusing on improving regional economic health; increasing high school completion and GED attainment; developing workforces, job retraining, and adapting to changes in community jobs; decreasing homelessness and increasing affordable housing; improving racial and ethnic harmony; developing urban and community neighborhoods; improving cooperation and collaboration among community agencies; and improving transitions from school to work.

Like the other projects that represent emerging covenant, this one is new, but there are notable examples of progress in the ACT communities. The sense of leadership on the part of healers and reciprocity and responsibility on the part of communities defy the current wisdom about what change is possible in this country today. One community trained over 150 volunteers who are currently providing respite care to caregivers throughout the community. In another community, the ACT program instituted "community forums" to convene representatives from five or six towns in a single county to identify and collaborate on problem issues. In one of these forums, between 30% and 40% of the participants are high school teenagers. Student participation has given them a sense of their own leadership ability and provided the impetus to take responsibility for, and ownership of, their community.

ACT Community Outcomes Toolkit
The Outcomes Toolkit is a new software-supported methodology to design, organize, and monitor measurable

---

indicators of community health and quality of life.[18] It is a performance-based planning tool that incorporates the many stages of community development through a fully integrated software package. The Toolkit provides step-by-step guidance to its users to: create a shared vision, develop action plans, identify and define outcomes and indicators, set measurable targets, identify data sources and data collection methodologies, analyze results, and generate reports. The Outcomes Toolkit grew from questions regarding what factors in a community affect the quality of life and health of individuals and which of those factors are amenable to change. Because of the pioneering nature of the Toolkit, its development involved qualitative research by a team of professionals who visited multiple ACT sites. The team included a cultural anthropologist, an ethnographer, public health and community development experts, and others. The development process involved iterative steps in which the team designed, built, and tested the software.

The Toolkit fosters collaboration between public and private sectors, and organizations and agencies by linking the continuum of community development activities through common goals, objectives, standards, and data collection methods. The software is installed on multiple computers in organizations throughout a community to enhance data collection, organization, and information sharing. The various sites using the Toolkit in a community are networked via the Internet to enable information sharing, data entry from multiple locations, the creation of outcome measures, and a database incorporating data from the multiple sites. Participating ACT program organizations can use predefined outcome measures and/or establish their own indicators and, in doing so, use data from any number of primary or secondary sources. For example, a community might incorporate data from the local health department, hospital, and coroner's office and compare it to national standards to measure and assess infant mortality rates.

The Outcomes Toolkit is an important project emerging from the partnership between Celebration Health and the Center for Health Futures because it allows for outreach to so many other communities throughout the nation and, perhaps eventually, throughout the world. It not only measures the traditional inputs, processes, and outcomes that support health care, but also addresses the measurement of outcomes related to education, criminal justice, and the local economy, each of which contributes to the health of individuals and the community. In contrast to patient level outcome measures, the use of outcome measurement at the community level is much less advanced, yet, increasingly, that is where health care decisions are being made. Thus, the development and implementation of the Outcomes Toolkit is a tangible contribution to measurement of outcomes in community health, well-being, and quality of life in a standardized way. This has been recognized by a number of organizations that are now in the process of exploring the use of the Outcomes Toolkit, including the Centers for Disease Control, United Way, local Chambers of Commerce, and a number of community foundations.

Covenant and the Pressing Needs of the Future

Every one of the examples mentioned here—whether individuals, organizations, companies, or communities—takes a step in the direction of covenants and, in most cases, covenants of obligation with the partners they engage for the benefit of healing. The success of these covenants should be celebrated and the new challenges ahead examined. It is important to find ways to support them, as the needs for the future are so great.

Beyond the efforts of healers, however, are the important gestures of patients and communities who "reach back" when the covenant hand of healing is extended. Sally Jeffcoat, CEO of St. Joseph's Hospital, describes the outpouring of community assistance during the 2001 Houston floods. People and businesses arrived with food, refrigeration, and cooking trailers. They also helped to relocate patients when all the power systems—including the backups—were taken out of commission by the high waters caused by torrential rains. Physicians tell me of patients who send letters or cards to them and their office staff, bring cookies, and send flowers. Are these trivial gestures? Not in the eyes of those who receive them.

As we confront the growth of consumer-driven and empowered health care demands, the growing number of therapeutic alternatives arising from research, the pace of faster e-commerce lifestyles, and the aging of the population, the models of care we have traditionally known will be less viable. The foundations of the values and the ethics will not, however. As I've noted in other sections of this book, what we have gained in information in our modern era has been more than offset by what we have lost in wisdom. It is in the wisdom of the covenant healer that we may well find the answers to the complexity we fear will overwhelm us in this new millennium. These healers and the relationships they are crafting with patients and communities are well worth preserving, enabling, and modeling.

Chapter 12

Healing Health Care

Crafting Covenants for Today

> *Health policies are rarely derived from explicit and systematic analysis of the moral values that shape them. Much of the art of national and international politics consists in structuring decision-making in such a way that value issues are not confronted. The aim is to keep peace between, and within, divergent belief systems. However, once framed, a health policy unerringly reveals the values that drive a society; and these cannot escape examination retrospectively.*[1]

Edmund Pellegrino

Coming Full Circle

This book ends where it began, back in Greece in 1984, where ethicists and academics, government representatives from many nations, theologians from the world's religions, and experts from the clinical and scientific disciplines of medicine and public health engaged in a dialogue about health policy and human values. The group explored how ethical and religious values affected the health policy decisions of the world's nations. Dr. Pellegrino was one of the medical ethicists whose observations shaped the discussions. It was at that meeting that he made the comment quoted above. His reflection was true to the exploration of national health policy at that time, and it remains true in health care practices and national health care policy today. The policies that have shaped the nation's care over the important and fast-moving decades of the last half-century did not explicitly address the covenant relationships among those who were a party to them—or should have been. As a nation and within our clinical relationships, we did not confront the values that framed the foundation of the healer-patient relationship. We did not examine the responsibilities that patients and communities had towards themselves and each other for the quality of their own health and healing. Yet, it is possible, now, to look back and retrospectively assess what happened to the covenants that were the basis for the health and aspects of personal and community life. It is possible to determine how and when the covenant in health care was lost and how policies and practices might have been enriched if covenants had been engaged. Had we engaged in covenant-building, we might not have left so many of our dying in intractable pain and hounded so many of our healers for treating them. We might not have neglected the perspectives of the animal rights activists so long that some would resort to extreme positions and strategies, threatening researchers and leaving potentially solvable disease problems suspended in damaged labs and destroyed data. Had we felt the reciprocity in the healer patient relationship, we might never have transformed our insurance systems into no-fault financing systems, removing much of the incentives for patient self-care and prevention. Had we acknowledged the obligations of communities, we would not have allowed our public health infrastructure to crumble or become so eager to assume that healers, captive to capitation payment systems, would absorb the increasing costs associated with social problems. If we recognized the importance of the covenantal trust between patient and healer, we might not sell and resell encounter data without the knowledge of either, or for a purpose to which neither had explicitly agreed. If we and others were globally in an international covenant of caring, we might have approached the problems in pharmaceutical donations differently—not as a rationale for pummeling the donors, but as an opportunity to save lives and improve health systems. Had we as Americans been willing to participate in clinical trials, people in developing nations might never have been pressed into service as research subjects. Had we come to peace with profit-making ventures and private investment in health care, we might now have more venture capital available to develop the new drugs and technologies the world needs for healing.

If covenants of obligation become more explicit in our relationships, we might more satisfactorily resolve the problems we face in health care today:

- If traditional healers—allopathic physicians—felt more "in covenant" with other healers, would they be more willing to embrace nontraditional healers and methods and bring them into their practices, and would clinical practice become more integrated? Would they be more accepting of direct-to-consumer advertising as an educational and compliance strategy with an appropriate place in health care? Would they be more open to nurse practitioners and other nonphysicians who provide care to the uninsured who lack access to care?

- If alternative healers felt more "in covenant" with patients, would they more carefully limit the claims associated with their practices to those truly demonstrated as valid, avoiding the potentially ineffective and potentially harmful approaches that may be philosophically attractive, but not genuinely beneficial to health?

- If the news media felt more "in covenant" with patients and communities, would they improve the quality of information dissemination and reporting and develop methods to ensure accuracy in reporting on the health care arena?

- If communities felt more "in covenant," would they comprehensively address the social problems of racial, ethnic, and gender bias that drives violence and higher utilization of health care? Would they protect the young and the old with safer streets? Would they work toward cleaner air and living conditions to prevent asthma disability? Would they address the problems of unemployment and poverty that create health risks?

- If citizens of the nation felt "in covenant" with each other and our healers, would we be more inclined to contribute to tax-supported or other health care financing pools to pay for care for those who cannot afford it? Would we be more willing to adhere to lifestyle and health care practices that control costs? Would we be willing to require that each of us do so? Would we require that, much like children who receive immunizations for school entry, the elderly be likewise immunized against preventable adult diseases to be eligible for Medicare coverage?

- If patients and communities felt "in covenant" with our healers, would we be more willing to see our own role in shaping the status of health? Would we recognize that our own behaviors and the health of the communities we live in also play a role in the quality of our lives, the status of our health, and the cost of our care?

- If citizens of the world felt more "in covenant" with each other, would we more actively address the risks of disease transmission in travel and immigration? Would those in developed nations reach out to those in poorer countries with health and economic aid, recognizing that when one nation is at risk, the world shares in the consequences?

Whatever the problems in the headlines today, in the years to come the challenges for health care will become greater. The public may focus on the immediate concerns of cost, quality, and access to care, but those in the healing enterprises know that there are a number of fundamental questions that have only begun to emerge:

- How will we support the academic health centers that train new healers and research disease without full funding of biomedical research projects or the patient care dollars to support the effort?

- How will bioethical and biogenetic decisions be made as the science and technology of health care outstrip the capacity of this nation to address its values and craft legislation accordingly?

- How will the healing and health care financing needs of an aging baby-boomer society be met?

- To what degree will alternative therapies be legitimized, not through research but due to patient demand and willingness to self-pay? Will the impact of these therapies be positive on healing, health care costs, and mainstream clinical care?

- What is the likelihood that the nation will be confronted with emerging infections, increasing antibiotic resistance, and bio-terrorism? To what degree will those factors change the safety of cities and threaten the public's health?

- How will the growing number of clinical and pharmaceutical solutions to lifestyle desires, choices, and problems be financed?

- How will those sectors outside health care, particularly those in the financial and electronic commerce industries, affect the course of healing?

These issues are all the more complex as the nation faces the realities of post-terrorism planning and health preparedness funding. Now, more than ever, the nature of the relationships we have with each other—and with those throughout the world—are critical to our health and healing. Now, more than ever, we should commit to the development of the covenants that were the roots of the healing enterprise from its formation.

Only One Step Along The Way
The meeting in Athens was the beginning of this exploration into the roots of healing within cultures and the importance of covenants in healing relationships. This last chapter will

not be the end of either; it is merely a step along the way. It is my intention that this review of our collective healing history will result in a dialogue about covenants, and that new covenants will emerge in today's healing enterprise, thus shaping our healing future. It appears to me that there are principles in ancient covenants relevant to health care today that will help us craft a covenant-centered future.

Principle Number One: Covenants Flow from the Senior Party and Are Preceded by Gifts

Before inviting someone into a covenant, gifts are given. We in this country cannot deny that we are among the most gifted and privileged of all the people in the world. We enjoy the freedom that democracy and capitalism ensures. Our healing enterprise grew from that democracy and the risks taken by healers—and other investors—who willingly invested in building our collective healing capacity. Because of them, the resources have been plentiful and gifts have flowed abundantly. The nation has developed extraordinary scientific and healing resources and possesses the talent and the technology to shape a better health future for all people—not just for the "insured" patients or for those living in our country, but also for people lacking the resources for care here and overseas. It has crafted the sciences and the systems that make a difference in our own lives and the lives of others.

For all the complaints about the state of health care today, we should not ignore the reality of the gifts we have received from our healers and should acknowledge that we have asked for and have received the most well endowed health care system on the globe. For all the problems in health services, there remain more opportunities than there are obstacles. Our healers have given gifts to us as individual patients, as well. They have studied hard, worked long hours, taken personal risks, contributed their talents, and produced many of the miracles that were asked of them.

These gifts, given and received, form the basis of the early covenants that were established here and that should evolve into the basis of new covenants of obligation. It was healers, through their oaths, who invited us into covenants and, by virtue of their expertise, remain the senior parties today. It is the healers who should now take the lead in proposing the new covenant. There are some who may believe that healers are no longer the senior parties or, by virtue of the current patient-empowered climate, should not retain the rights of such expert positioning within the proposal of covenants. For all the faults of healing in health care today, however, our healers remain the most skilled of all the parties at living within the covenants of the oaths they have taken. Unlike the rest of us, they understand covenants in a way that patients and communities do not. They are, therefore, the best teachers and leaders into a covenant lifestyle that the future demands.

Principle Number Two: Covenants Do Not End
If covenants are embraced, neither this nor any other effort to explore them can be the end of the story. The beginning of a covenant can be dated; the ending cannot. Covenants are established and they evolve. They should not wither. They do not die. There is no "stepping outside" of the covenant for a vacation or a "break." Covenants, established by our forbears in healing, have framed relationships between healers and patients for generations. Healers passed down their healing ethic to subsequent generations of healers, sharing even the specific oaths to serve patients. As oaths are revitalized today, healers are signaling to the patients and communities that the covenant created thousands of years ago is still the basis of the healing relationships by which healers themselves wish to live.

There are no exit clauses in covenants. There are no buy-out provisions in covenants. To paraphrase Professor May, once a person abides in a covenant, he does not step outside of it. Do it well or do it poorly, do it awake or do it in sleep, the covenant role endures. Just as healers practice their skills and are available to patients at all times, so, too, should patients and communities practice their roles continually. Healthy behaviors are no less a concern when buying groceries, driving a car, or watching television than they are during office visits to the physician. Once engaged in a covenant of obligation, healing should be "top-of-mind" for patients and communities, not just for the healers who serve them.

Principle Number Three: Covenants Change Over Time

At the beginning of a covenant, it is impossible to know where the relationship will lead and what the covenant relationship will require of its parties. It is this element of evolution that distinguishes covenants from contracts. Contracts spell out every step and, even at the beginning, define the end. Covenants, by definition, cannot do this. It is impossible to say how each party will influence the other and how the needs and demands upon those involved will change.

At present, many of the parties to healing are re-examining the nature of the healing enterprise and the relationships involved. It would be wise for all concerned that this examination results in new covenant of obligation relationships among the many healers in health care today, between healers and patients, and between healers and communities. When the newly defined healers I have enumerated accept their responsibilities to the covenant, they will be more likely to shape positive health care climates. When patients and communities accept responsibilities and obligations, they will help carry the load that has been shouldered so predominately by healers. The relationships that create healing and quality health care outcomes will become the shared responsibility of everyone. Currently, some of the players central to the healing enterprises are able to ignore their roles as healers. In the future, having accepted a covenant of obligation, none of the parties will be able to shift their responsibilities to others and expect that healing will simply be "granted."

Coming into Covenants of Obligation

Covenants of obligation address the challenges of this new era. The existing covenants of grant should be replaced with the more mature covenants of obligation. We as a nation are not satisfied with the health care services we receive. We want more and better care. We demand new advances in research, and we are worried about how we will pay for it. The old covenants of grant that existed between healers and patients have run their course and are no longer sufficient for our health care challenges. The old covenants of grant did not effectively engage all those involved in healing. They did not engage the patients and the communities that are such an important determinant of health today. In order to satisfy the nation's wants, we must acknowledge that all those who "practice" within the healing enterprise—healers, patients, and communities—achieve health and healing within mutually supportive relationships.

Each party must feel obligated to the other. Each party to the covenant must be willing to reciprocate with the other in the healing process. Each must be willing to do his part in finding the best solution to the important lifestyle, policy, political and business decisions that are pending at the beginning of the new millennium. These solutions will shape the future of our health and that of other nations, as well. None of us—healer, patient, or community—can expect that health care will be healed unless we all participate.

None of us can expect that the world will be healed unless we reach out to make it happen. In the case of global health, we are the superior parties. We have the wealth; we own the technology. We have the talent, the incentives, and the resources to invite the world into a covenant of obligation for the healing of all. In this way, we can contribute our assets and elicit from them the mature response of interdependence to create the healing climate for their nations, and thereby, for the world. None of us can expect to be insulated from the consequences of our behavior—whether that behavior is our personal health practices or our policy positions on helping the needy nations of the world. Whether we are patients, healers, or communities, whether we are rich nations or poor ones, we cannot shun the opportunity that a covenant of obligation in healing can create. Mutual obligations will benefit us all.

If covenants, particularly covenants of obligation, are to be the order of the future, how will this be accomplished? Who will be party to these covenants? What processes and documents will frame them? How will those who wish to engage in covenants prepare for them and execute them? Will everyone embrace covenants? Can they be required to do so? What about those who may reject the invitation to join in covenant, and what are our responsibilities to them?

Creating covenants of obligation will require six essential conditions. Some of these are obvious and will be familiar to those who have tackled any new program and or project. Some are well-honed skills of healers, patient advocates, and community leaders. These skills draw upon the leadership development, strategic planning, policymaking and other processes already used by those in the health care community.

First, there must be an intention to develop and enter into a covenant of obligation. Being in a covenant is no accident. It will not occur because one "just happens" to be in a particular job or position in the health care arena, because one has made an appointment to visit a healer, or because one is a resident of a community. Compare it to a wedding and a marriage. A marriage does not "happen" because a man and a woman show up in church at the appointed hour. The marriage covenant is struck because both parties have committed to going forward in their relationship over time. Particularly on the part of the party who first proposes the marriage, or covenant, the intention must be clear—it must be intentional. As the expert party who makes the proposal, healers must have the intention to form covenants with each other, with their patients, and with communities. Without that intention, the next steps cannot and will not be taken.

The second essential condition calls for a purging of the immediate past, a clearance, or "letting go" of any biases that might interfere with new styles of relating. This includes releasing the prejudice, ideas, likes and dislikes about the past relationship. Emptying out will free the mind and the heart to consider new ways of relating to the covenant in general and relating to the parties who will become part of the covenant specifically. This will not be easy. Large numbers of interlocking contracts are in place in health care today. These contracts are layered over old, dysfunctional covenants of grant. Biases among patients, healers, and communities are strong, and many of them are negative. It will not be possible to engage in covenants if we continue to believe that patients are irresponsible and ignorant, healers are greedy and unethical, and communities are disengaged and disinterested. New covenants require new ideas and a past that is purged, resolved, and left behind. New covenants require a fresh start and a clean slate.

A third essential condition prescribes that covenants must be rooted. The best roots for grasping covenants of obligation are those from the ancient past. Today's health care ground is, frankly, not sacred enough for a covenant of obligation to be proposed, root, and grow again. Our ground has been eroded and is no longer fertile soil in which to plant a practice as paradigm-shifting and potentially radical as a covenant of obligation. As the modern scientific era and the wealth of the nation produced its fruits, the old covenants of grant could have matured into covenants of obligation. They did not. Instead, the existing covenants of grant began to break down, burdened by new, complex, and interlocking contractual arrangements that characterized changes in health financing over the past 50 years. New players in health care, policy, politics, insurance, advertising, media, and electronic communications did not recognize themselves as healers, did not embrace the healer's covenant or adopt healing roles. Patients and communities did not mature into accepting responsibilities for the state of their own health. The confluence of these factors in this modern era limits our ability to mature our healing covenants toward those of obligation to one another. Perhaps by returning to the sacredness of healing and the interdependence of the relationships, the roots of healing can take hold again in fertile soil.

New covenants must be connected for the fourth essential condition. Interconnections with those in the covenant of obligation are essential to maintaining it. Hippocrates was wise in holding physicians accountable to one another in a covenant of obligation. Those relationships of obligation supported the difficult demands of research, learning, and practice. The obligation to one another ensured that no physician was left without peers in the demanding arenas of science and skill that were called for in healing. This should stand as a lesson for those developing and engaging in covenants of obligation today, whether patients, healers, or communities. Maintaining and restoring health, and treating and healing disease cannot be accomplished without the connections to other patients, healers, and communities. Each party to the covenant will perform better within a covenant and will meet his obligations more completely if he reciprocates with others in peer relationships. Much as healers gain support for the demands of their roles by connecting with other healers, so, too, will patients gain support by connecting with other patients and communities. Each party will do well within covenants if he contributes something to the healing of others, for it is frequently in giving that we receive the most.

The fifth essential condition demands that those who

develop and work within covenants must pause from time to time to reconsider the relationship. The work of health care is demanding, and recreating covenants will make the tasks of healing even more so. This call for covenants is intended to ease the crises we will most certainly face without them, but covenants are hard work. They require near constant attention to the ebbs and flows of human relations. Covenants are not intellectual constructs, but heart-focused, soul-driven lifestyles. Covenants are not only for the good of the patient, but for the good of the healer as well. Overworked, stressed-out, and unhealthy healers cannot give what they do not have. Patients whose lives have been altered by disease or who face critical disease crises need the pause to sort out what changes they want and are willing to seek from their healers. Communities and nations, too, will change as economic circumstances, employment, immigration, and disasters take hold. Covenants are destined to change. It is, therefore, important that, from time to time, the parties to the covenants reconsider and recommit to them. This takes an occasional pause to reassess their workings to determine if changes are needed. Some couples do this within marriage. They reassess their relationship to determine if changes should be made. Not a bad idea for covenants in health care, either.

The sixth, and final, essential condition asks that covenants cause the parties to stretch into and beyond their capabilities in creating, sustaining, and healing their health and the health of others. If we are to embrace an idea as fundamental and radical as covenant, we should set our sights high. We should call out the best in ourselves as patients, healers, and communities. We should seek the best within the relationships we have.

Too often in health care we have limited the capacity to do better, believing that we cannot, or that others around us cannot, successfully perform to the goal. Yet, the history of health care is one of remarkable progress on all fronts.

New funds have appeared from private, public and commercial sources to build the infrastructures wanted, healers have adapted their practices to what the nation wanted, and new medicines have spilled out of pipelines with increasing regularity. Today, there is tremendous wealth and diversity in personnel and resources. The health workforce is one of the best-educated groups of all the sectors of the economy. It is already bound by covenant. These resources are not some albatross around the neck of the nation, but the wings that will enable us to soar to new heights of healing. Covenant may well be one of the flight paths towards the change we so desire today. As we work toward creating these new covenants within this country, we should stretch all the more, to reach beyond our borders. It matters little for us to enjoy health here if we will fear our global neighbors for the pathogens they may harbor in a handshake. Global covenants of healing are one signpost on the path to world peace.

Who Should Create New Covenants of Obligation?
Donald Berwick, of the Institute for Health Care Improvement, says that all those who "shape the experience of patients and the social investment in care" should be party to the ethical ideals of healers.[2] I agree. Even though he is referring to "ethics" and I to "covenant," our perspectives are so similar as to be indistinguishable. I'll be more specific. Everyone who works in a professional or volunteer position in a healing enterprise should define him- or herself as a healer, should be a party to a covenant, and should adopt a covenant of obligation in relation to the patients they serve. This is independent of the education or position of those healers. It is independent of whether the healer serves one patient or a million patients. It is independent of whether the service is clerical or clinical. It is independent of whether the patient served is a single individual or the collective whole. As a result, I include physicians and policymakers, surgeons and clerks,[3] legislators

and litigators, advertisers, marketers, and e-commerce entrepreneurs. I also include newscasters, insurance company clerks, and pharmaceutical sales representatives. These individuals form the initial covenants of obligation—those that exist among healers and are at the foundation of all the other covenants. They are the senior parties who will invite each other and others—the patients and the communities—into the reciprocal relationships that will create the new covenants of obligation that I propose.

The creation of these covenants will not happen by myth or by magic. The identity as a healer, the intention to create covenants and act within them, will not ensure that these covenants arise full-grown like some goddess of old from the head of her father. The creation of these new covenants of obligation will emerge from a new generation of leaders in health care who may now be appearing on the scene. These are leaders worthy of being nurtured by the rest of us. These are leaders whose intentions will span beyond the limits of the sitting president and congressional majority. They are not leaders who will deliver solutions, but the leaders who will facilitate the processes to find solutions. They will be able, at all times, to see the viewpoint of others, to believe in the value of collaboration and synergy, to resolve conflicts, and to park their egos at the door. They will articulate the necessity of making sacrifices for the good of the whole nation, for those served and for those who serve.

Health care today is on the verge of change from external forces, particularly from the information technology and e-commerce sectors. The leadership required to manage the challenges will come from the most covenant-centered individuals if it emerges from inside of health care. This leadership will have communication and peace-building skills that will enable us to come together long enough to get beyond the cynicism in our attitudes today. These leaders will be, at their core, healers. They will understand that healing—especially healing a chronically ill patient like today's health care system—does not happen overnight They will understand that they must be cautious and, most important, do no further harm.

These leaders will, first of all, heal health care. They will help create the sanctuaries of tolerance for bringing today's healers together to search for their commitment to covenant. Once they are united in trust, they will use that emotional glue to approach patients and communities. Since patients carry with them the vestiges of the covenants established throughout history, they will be inclined to welcome the invitation to participate.

What Will a Covenant of Obligation Look Like?

A covenant of obligation will be an explicit statement of relationship. It will be reciprocal. I have only been able to locate one healer with a clear statement of such a covenant. It was developed by the staff and patients of Indiana Health Centers, Inc.[4] This healer is a Community Health Center (CHC) composed of clinical sites and satellites. It is a safety-net provider established to care for the uninsured, the underinsured, and those lacking access to care. As such, it is dedicated to serving those too often at the margins of our communities. If healers can create covenants of obligation within these settings and amidst the resource constraints of caring for the poor and the disadvantaged, we all can.

Their covenant of obligation addresses access, affordability, quality convenience, prevention and dignity. It says:

Each Indiana Health Centers person promises . . .	Your responsibility is . . .
. . . to provide quality to keep you healthy	. . . to schedule and keep your services, appointments for immunizations, annual exams, WIC and cancer, and other screenings

. . . to provide quality nutrition and WIC services, as well as quality medical care when you are ill, and to have a medical provider you can reach by telephone when we are closed

. . . to call us when you have a health problem or nutritional concern

. . . to be open at times that work for you, including evenings and weekends

. . . to let us know if our evening and weekend hours work for you

. . . to make every attempt to honor appointment times

. . . to make appointments whenever possible, to make appointments at convenient time, to make every effort to be on time for an appointment, and to call if you can't keep your appointment

. . . to take a personal interest in your health and keep all personal information private

. . . to give us accurate information about you and your health, and to make sure we can always contact you if necessary

. . . to treat you with respect and courtesy

. . . to treat us and other clients with respect and courtesy

. . . to ask for and consider your input

. . . to complete the client satisfaction survey

. . . to keep the cost as low as possible

. . . to pay your fees for medical services when due, to tell us if you have any insurance coverage, to take advantage of any health insurance program you might qualify for, to provide us with accurate financial information

. . . to refer you to other services that would be helpful

. . . to consider using the referral and let us know if it works for you

. . . to offer many services that help you stay well

. . . to use as many of our services at each visit as possible

Other covenants may be stated in different terms because they will be uniquely structured to fit the nature of those within the relationship. The covenant of caring that emergency personnel have with their communities will differ from those that primary care physicians have with patients and families. The covenant that health care trade associations have with their members will differ from those that their members have with the patients and communities they serve. The covenant of state public health officials will be different in times of crises than in times of quiescence.

Some covenants may be totally personal—as between a healer and a patient. Some may be organizational—as between a hospital and a community. Since oaths have been used to structure and define covenants, most parties will choose to state their covenants in that way. Covenants won't be the answer to every dilemma, but they will be the starting point for resolving many. These covenants will probably be short, so that they are easily remembered. It is not the document, after all, that will be important, but the degree to which the reciprocal promises live in the hearts and inform the heads of those who are party to it. These covenants will also provide for some sort of reconciliation process, as everyone is fallible and will fail to live up to the spirit of the covenant on occasion. Building back the trust and reentering the relationship will require the parties to restore their standing in the covenant when it breaks down.

Covenants in Action

Do covenants work? Do they make a difference in practice? For true covenants of obligation, it is not yet clear. So few can be identified, and none is sufficiently longstanding to be measured at this point. Many hospitals and health care institutions now post patient rights and, less often, patient responsibility statements, but the statement of the Indiana Health Centers, Inc. stands alone as a true, reciprocal covenant of obligation developed between healers and patients.

In addition to the covenant of grant established in the Hippocratic Oath, which has been measured and found to have a positive impact on practice,[5] there are three others worthy of note and discussion. One is from a corporation, one is from an association and the other is from an individual.

The first is the Johnson & Johnson Credo. This credo is typical of a covenant of grant, but it is notable because its impact has been measured.[6] It reads:

Our Credo

We believe our first responsibility is to the doctors, nurses, and patients, to mothers and all others who use our products and services. In meeting their needs everything we do must be of high quality. We must constantly strive to reduce our costs in order to maintain reasonable prices. Customers' orders must be serviced promptly and accurately. Our suppliers and distributors must have an opportunity to make a fair profit.

We are responsible to our employees, the men and women who work with us throughout the world. Everyone must be considered as an individual. We must respect their dignity and recognize their merit. They must have a sense of security in their jobs. Compensation must be fair and adequate, and working conditions clean, orderly, and safe. Employees must feel free to make suggestions and complaints. There must be equal opportunity for employment development and advancement for those qualified. We must provide competent management, and their actions must be just and ethical.

We are responsible to the communities in which we live and work and to the world community as well. We must be good citizens—support good works and charities and bear our fair share of taxes. We must encourage civic improvements and better health and education. We must maintain in good order the property we are privileged to use, protecting the environment and natural resources.

Our final responsibility is to our stockholders. Business must make a sound profit. We must experiment with new ideas. Research must be carried on, innovative programs developed, and mistakes paid for. New equipment must be purchased, new facilities provided and new products launched. Reserves must be created to provide for adverse times. When we operate according to these principals, the stockholder should realize a fair return.

In this credo, Johnson & Johnson, as a corporation, holds itself accountable to patients, family members, employees, communities, and stockholders. It grants them quality products, working opportunities, good neighbor relations, and returns on investment. The credo was written in the mid-1940s by the late Robert Wood Johnson, the company's leader, and was the guiding principal of his own management of the company. In 1972, it was the theme of the company's annual report and the basis of a series of meetings for company employees, led by the new chairman, Philip B. Hoffman. The credo formed a number of important corporate decisions, including the decision to maintain the company's headquarters in an urban area and support the redevelopment of the city rather than flee to more desirable settings in the country.

The credo was tested most severely in 1982 when a criminal poisoning of Tylenol® resulted in a number of deaths. The company encountered a crisis of unprecedented proportions. No crisis management plan could have anticipated the turn of events and the demands on the company to cooperate with so many government officials, press contacts, consumers and customers. The company and a number of knowledgeable observers credit the credo with guiding corporate actions through the hour-by-hour responses that, within five months, led to its re-launch of Tylenol® into the marketplace, the repackaging of consumer goods to prevent similar tampering, and the recapturing of 70% of the market it had previously held.

In another example, the National Health Council, an association of over 100 health groups, developed concepts of patient rights and responsibilities. The Council is composed of both patient and healer organizations, and these rights and responsibilities were developed through extensive research with patients across the country. This statement, like the one developed by Indiana Health Centers, Inc., moves in the direction of reciprocity between healers and their patients:

All patients have the right to:

1. Informed consent in treatment decisions, timely access to specialty care, and confidentiality protections.

2. Concise and easily understood information about their coverage.

3. Know how coverage payment decisions are made and how they can be fairly and openly appealed.

4. Complete and easily understood information about the costs of their coverage and care.

5. A reasonable choice of providers and useful information about provider options.

6. Know what provider incentives or restrictions might influence practice patterns.

All patients, to the extent capable, have the responsibility to:

7. Pursue healthy lifestyles.

8. Become knowledgeable about their health plans.

9. Actively participate in decisions about their health care.

10. Cooperate fully on mutually accepted courses of treatment.[7]

In the final example, an individual, Martin Wasserman, M.D., J.D., at his swearing-in as Secretary of the Maryland Department of Health and Mental Hygiene, crafted a "Health Pledge to the People:"

- To protect and promote the health of the public by

creating healthy people in healthy communities

- To strengthen partnerships between the state and local government, the business community, and all of the health care providers in Maryland

- To build a world class and professional organization grounded in the principles of quality, accountability, cultural sensitivity, and efficiency.

This pledge, particularly the second item, established an explicit covenant of obligation among a broader group of healers and others within the state. The state's Department of Health and Mental Hygiene reached out to form a relationship between community health departments, healers, and communities through businesses. The pledge not only guided the efforts of the state's Department of Health; it was also signed by 24 local health officers and 7 facilities, and it was supported by over 200 quality teams. As a result, the Department of Health and Mental Hygiene was the only department-wide winner of the Governor's Gold Quality Award in 1997, which was based on the Baldridge quality award criteria. No other department in Maryland has won that award since. In addition, the pledge formed the basis for extensive outreach to communities. When the Health Care Financing Administration approved a Medicaid waiver for the State of Maryland in record time, it commented that the state had secured the highest involvement of the public in any state up to that point. The state continues to involve the public, respecting citizen time by scheduling meetings in multiple locations so that no individual must travel more than one hour to participate.[8]

Evolution of Covenants Over Time
Those who engage each other in covenant terms are changed by the nature of their relationships. Much like young couples who marry with ideal expectations and later face difficult realities, each party to a covenant is challenged in ways that would not have been possible had they

not entered into the covenant in the first place.

In healer-patient covenants in clinical settings neither party knows, at the outset, how the relationship will unfold. What diseases will befall the patient? What diagnostics or therapeutics will the healer be called upon to use? How rapidly will health care technology develop? How will the interaction between the two parties change each one as they work together over the years for the benefit of the patient's health—and perhaps for the healer's health as well? What will each party teach the other?

In a healer-community relationship neither party knows how the other will be required to change perspective in order to advance the covenant. How will communities respond to a healer's call for better education and social issue management to address, for example, problems of drug abuse, teen pregnancy, smoking, and obesity that drive health care costs? How will healers respond to the problems of violence that lead to increased health care utilization? How will the cost of caring for the uninsured be distributed among the community and its healers during economic recessions and periods of high unemployment?

In the case of the patient-community relationship the evolution is even more uncertain. How will communities be defined? To which community does a patient belong: the one in which they are employed, where they live, or where they worship? To what degree are local employers a part of the community that should be engaged in solutions to health problems? Who will act as the voice of the community and have the "standing" to bring various groups within the community together to improve health? What are the limits of community control in cases where the community also feels responsible for health care? Are there limits to the degree that a community and its healers should feel responsible for individual patients, including those who may not be inclined to practice healthy behaviors or respond within the covenant themselves?

No Easy Answers

By now, some readers are hoping for some final answers, and perhaps some easy answers, at that. However, this book was not intended as a scholarly analysis of the history of medicine, the ethics of medical care, or the theology of covenants. It was not intended to describe each of the health care or global issues of the day and present an analysis complete with prescriptive solutions. In fact, discussing such a scholarly analysis of even one of the dilemmas mentioned here would require several volumes, as the field of global political and health care publications readily demonstrates.

This book was intended to be a practical exploration of selected pivotal issues for healers, patients, and communities interested in understanding and influencing the important decisions in the public policies of tomorrow's health care. It was intended to raise the questions that could frame discussions for those who are parties to the covenant that may be the better way to create the future. Each of the issues we face in health care today is a long-term work in progress. Each one is complex enough that none is likely to be resolved in the near future. Pausing now to consider how covenants may lead to solutions is the next important step along the path of healing health care. I believe that pausing to develop covenants where they are most needed is the best prescription for the maladies that ail our failing health care system and that plague too many parts of the world. Covenants created by those in health care will help to resolve the conflicts that seem so intractable to us now.

This book was not intended to tinker at the margins of new health care financing proposals. There are very talented and dedicated people in the policy arena and health care enterprise who are crafting the incremental changes that will make health care accessible and affordable for decades to come. I cannot contribute to those efforts except by raising issues of covenant and suggesting that mutual obligations among all the players within health care will help. This book is, instead, intended to radically challenge the nature of the relationships that are the foundations of health care today. On a new footing in relationships, the payment and financing issues can be more productively and easily addressed.

Furthermore, this book was not intended to tinker with the margins of health care companies. To do so would not help the future, it would harm it. Investors have long recognized that the health sector contributes to the economy in a number of ways. Health care has produced a growing number of jobs for an expanding workforce and kept the nation in the forefront of development as well. Health care was founded on solid science and increasingly productive, exportable technology. Demand-driven care has been good for health care. New technologies replaced old ones with greater effectiveness and, over time, efficiency. Health care contributed not only to national pride, but to a favorable balance of trade.

This book was not intended to shoot at a single, clear target with magic bullets. The targets in health care and on the globe are too numerous, too fast moving, and there are no magic bullets. This book was not intended to offer specific solutions or to propose changes to "fix" health care—save one. It is my contention that if health care and the world is to be healed, everyone involved in the healing enterprises of the day—the healers themselves, patients, and communities—must enter into new and reinvigorated covenant relationships, and we in the U.S. must reach out to the world. Any reader who has made it through the entire text has encountered nearly four hundred questions in its various chapters. Yes, there have been precious few answers. But there are ways to reach toward those answers and find the right ones. The best way, I believe, is to reach back into the roots of healing and covenants—specifically covenants of obligation. What better time than now?

Epilogue

Questions About Covenants in Health Care Today

Writing this book has been an examination of the health care enterprise with its ancient roots from a new perspective. I enjoyed exploring the role that covenants can play in recreating the relationships necessary for healing ventures in the future. Along the way, I've had numerous discussions with others about this project. Most of the discussions were with healers, whether they were members of the audience at presentations on this topic or reviewers of drafts of this text. These individuals have been generous with their time and willingness to imagine health care with covenants of obligation as a core principle. Their willingness was not surprising to me, as so many healers already ascribe to an oath to guide their practices.

Some of the discussions have been with patients. Their reactions have been ultimately positive, as well, and that has surprised me. After venting their anger over the state of health care today, they readily accepted the notion that they, too, are responsible for their health, and that they have been less than faithful to the self-care and lifestyle choices that would improve their health and reduce the costs of care. Both groups—physicians and patients—were equally frustrated and looking for a solution. Both feel vulnerable. Neither wants health care wars to escalate.

Some of the discussions have been with communities, and in particular, employer or workplace communities. Privately, their reactions have also been positive, though concerned. In our conversations, they worry about the reactions of their employees, and in particular their unions, if they embrace covenant notions. They, too, are looking for solutions and feel more trapped than ever in the current paradigm of payment and contracting.

All of these discussions challenged my thinking about covenants and this manuscript. Each discussion raised questions that are best addressed at the end, because they frame the future of a covenant-focused dialogue so well.

Why invite controversy by discussing the animal research debate?

I'll deal with the toughest question first. It was the most difficult to resolve and involved the most soul searching. One reviewer suggested removing the chapter on animal research altogether, advising that the issue was contentious enough to create distractions that would interrupt the other messages on the central premises of the book.

It was a tough call to decide to keep that chapter. I have high regard for the views of this advisor. He is right: The issues involved in subjecting animals to research procedures for the benefit of humans (and other animals) may create controversy. However, I feel a responsibility to the health policy community, to researchers, to patients in need of research-driven cures, and even to my friends in the animal welfare community, to attempt to bring some peace to this issue by including their concerns in the context of covenant. To do less is to ignore my responsibility to each of them as a health policy analyst, observer, and negotiator. I hope they will likewise feel a responsibility—I am inviting a covenant here—to engage in a discussion of the issues and not in the politics of personal destruction. I hope all the stakeholders involved will consider dealing with each other and their constituencies within a covenant that respects the views and obligations of each. I hope they will value my intention to assist with a resolution to this important arena of ethics, research, and respect for all concerned. As in all the issues, it should be clear that there is much at stake, and in the years since publication of the first edition, the issues have become even more contentious. As a result, I've allowed this chapter to remain, and I feel even more clearly that we must find new ways to address the conflicts we face in this aspect of healing.

Why address international issues? Aren't our own issues compelling enough?
This question was raised in the first edition, which contained only one chapter on healing the globe. It was related to the donation of pharmaceuticals to the developing world. Our national consciousness changed radically when the World Trade Center towers fell to the ground, but perhaps not permanently. As this second edition goes to press, we Americans face a change in some aspects of our daily lives, but we have returned to an essentially peaceful and uninterrupted American "way of living."

In this edition, I've chosen to deal with the global issues and problems of the developing world in a more expended way for two reasons. The first, as in the previous edition, is to continue to place our own problems, opportunities, and assets in a broader perspective. The second, which is even more significant, is to drive home an important point—that we, here in the U.S., may live in privilege, but we do not live in isolation. The writing about infectious diseases makes that point most clearly. The chapter on drug donations calls for an evaluation of the values we hold as human beings and as Americans, whose wealth relative to the rest of the world gives us the ability to help others. The chapter on clinical trials is intended to alert us to the problems of victimizing research subjects—too often for our benefit. The chapter on global caring addresses the assets we have developed that we must now continue to support and to share. Helping others in dire need allows us to reconnect with our humanity and the importance of compassion. Helping those around the world sensitizes us to the needs of the poor at home.

Lending our assistance and donating our technologies to those abroad satisfies the needs I believe we all have to view healing as a gift to be shared, not a commodity to be bargained. In our sharing, we will realize our prosperity. It is an inroad to creating global health, peace, and prosperity. To help is not just good will, it is good health, good business, good policy, and good politics. It is good for world peace. It is good for global prosperity.

Finally, I fear that health policy in the U.S. today is in danger of devolving into tactical elements of program operations, PMPMs,[1] "cap" rates, and budget requirements. The health care enterprise is much more complex, multi-faceted, demanding, and global than the current and most pressing concerns of today's budget battles. Unless we address these longer-term and more global issues today, the problems brewing outside our borders will become domestic crises, and we will be unprepared to address them.

Why aren't there more prescriptions and specific directions?
By definition, only the parties to the covenant can work out the specifics. I've been about as specific as I can be in the examples and policy issues I've included and other suggestions I've made. I've outlined who the parties to various covenants might be and have pointed them in a direction. Only they can determine if they want to walk the path. Once underway, they'll decide how fast to progress and whether to detour from the route. Taking the first steps will not be easy, but the next steps will be even harder and no observer can second-guess the results.

It is along the way in the covenant relationship that the toughest questions must be addressed. These are the questions that we have avoided so well in the past several decades. They are questions of reciprocity and responsibility: If a patient can sue a managed care provider for failure to provide care (e.g., experimental therapies not covered by contract), can managed care sue patients for failure to follow medical advice? If patients do not take their medicines or change their lifestyles, should managed care be responsible for covering the cost of the more expensive diseases that will result? If employers cover the cost of a flu shot, can they deny sick leave to employees who choose not to be immunized but then get the flu? If the nation allows its citizens to carry guns, can insurers levy a surcharge for the likelihood of higher emergency room costs in areas of high gun ownership? In other areas of our lives we pay—financially—for the consequences of our choices. If we change an airline ticket, arrive late to get our children from daycare, check-out of hotels early, or fail to show up for restaurant reservations, we incur financial penalties. Should it be any different in health care?

Talking about covenant is easy. Living covenant is not. As the first edition was reviewed, I was cautioned that even proposing covenants was likely to be controversial, including among physicians, who fare best in the analysis here. I did not begin to write with a bias toward any group, but over the course of my research and this examination, I became sympathetic to physicians and managed care providers. It strikes me that public policy has presented them an impossible task: provide, in some parental fashion, for all the desires of patients and communities who are insulated from the payment for care and the consequences of decisions. Nonetheless, I was warned that the relationships within health care today in some parts of the country were so contentious that there is "no turning back" from the politics of destruction that lay ahead. If the concept of covenants is controversial for physicians, who have long held them, then they may be all the more challenging for patients and communities. That being the case, I'll choose to start slowly, introducing the concept and its rationale. Later, perhaps, will come a time for more prescriptive directions.

At this point, if all I can do is to define the shape of the table at which all the relevant parties to a covenant can sit, and propose a paradigm and a vocabulary for the first discussion, it may be enough for now. To do more at this time would be to prematurely suppose an outcome that only a covenant can determine. Worse, it might even frighten some people away.

Why so many questions and so few answers?
Few health care problems and policy issues today have clear answers or easy resolutions, and I can't imagine that the next several decades will be any easier for any of us—healers, patients, or communities. Today's health policy, which is so dominated by the economics of care, could benefit from an infusion of new ideas to frame our analyses. This is an offering of that type. I wanted to bring a new perspective, some structure for analysis, a vocabulary for negotiations, and some tools to help.

Health care today could also benefit from an infusion of new questions. It is not only the answers to questions that are important, but the questions themselves. Some say, in fact, that the right question is more important than the right answer. Ancient wisdom says we can afford to be inefficient if we are working on the right question. Stephen Covey's work on effectiveness is built, in part, on a similar notion: that it is of little value to focus on how fast one can climb a ladder, if that ladder is leaning against the wrong tree.[2]

I applaud everyone in health care, e-commerce, and telecommunications working to create efficiencies. Their work deserves support, encouragement, and reward. Squeezing the cents from the dollars is a good thing. Squeezing the soul from the system of care is not. I'll continue to pose the questions that get to the soul of healing.

Will health care in the future be consumer-centric? Is covenant-centric going against the tide?
First of all, I'd like to get past calling patients "consumers."

Doing so might well help us improve the "friendliness" of our services, but patients are not just consumers, they are more than that, since healing relationships are covenantal and therefore sacred. The terms are problematic here, and I struggled with what to call patients in this new edition because "patient" did not seem right either. "Patient" does not account for the healthy person before their illness struck, before their encounter with our health care system, caring for themselves. People? Individuals? Persons? Consumers? I gave up and returned to "patient."

That being said, yes, I believe health care of the near future will be consumer-centric, but I hope it does not end there. Consumer-centrism is most likely a phase of our development as a society as a whole, and it may be a healthy transition away from "any-color-as-long-as-it's-black" delivery of health care. I hope that it will only be a phase and that we transition beyond it. Health care will benefit from consumers with the incentive to care for their health and the personal skills to do so. Healers and communities can and should help them do that, and doing so may be the most important covenant-focused activity that healers and communities can fulfill in the near future. Healers and communities should avoid strengthening the dependencies that have been created over the past 50 years in this country, however. A consumer-centric attitude should transition towards interdependence among consumers, communities, and healers. If health care of the future is only consumer centered, lacking in covenants of obligation among the parties involved, the many challenges we face now will become serious problems, and the many opportunities before us today to solve problems won't be realized.

Why all the emphasis on spirituality? Are you advocating more of it within health care? Isn't there a role for today's practice of medicine?
This book did not start out to be a discussion of spirituality in health care. Those issues were included as the research

path led in that direction. I was quite surprised to see the wealth of information available and the ties between healing and spirituality—right down to the root of the words that we use. After some thought, I had to admit it: health and disease are still mysteries, still fraught with powerful and unknown forces that we, as patients, want to be controlled for our benefit. Being modern, scientific people has not changed that. Even modern genomics and high-science medicine has not eliminated the mystery of disease and death. If anything, it is all the more mysterious and frightening, and hence, all the more a subject we should discuss openly.

I am not at all opposed to today's standard medical practices and have been the beneficiary of some of the best this nation has to offer. It is not this book that is out of balance in addressing spiritual issues in a policy context, however. In my view, the current practice of medicine is out of balance with what patients expect. After thousands of generations of linking healing and spirituality, I am convinced that it is so in-bred that we take it for granted. We may not ask for it, but it is something we want. Deny it to us and we'll feel it missing.

The fundamental underpinning of a covenant is a sacred relationship. As patients and as healers we want it within our healing enterprises. I hope that this work will encourage us to reinvigorate the language and the practice of covenants. I also hope that we'll decide it's worth paying for—which, in my opinion, it is.

How can you expect that we can do what you advocate when all of our policy discussions are political debates? How can we get Congress involved?
We should talk to each other, not to Congress, about what ails us in health care. It is my observation that we turn to Congress reluctantly, and in anger, when the relationship between us breaks down, and we want the Congress to impose controls to fix the "other guy." I was in the audience at one of the farewell addresses of Congressman Barber

Conable, at his departure to head the World Bank. "Do not expect us to lead," he announced. "We were elected to represent, not to lead. In that regard, we will have to be dragged kicking and screaming into any issue we deal with." Reluctant congressmen, dragged into issues after years of local constituent anger and hostility, are not in the best frame of mind for crafting a health care future. Perhaps if we talked to each other, we could sort out our needs, our wants, and our differences of opinion. This means that every encounter, every phone call, and every e-mail becomes an opportunity to deal with someone else in the covenant. Take those opportunities. In those instances where Congress is already involved, let's at least advise them to avoid rash solutions and eleventh-hour compromises that please no one. Doing the first will take our time; doing the latter will require our restraint. Doing both is absolutely essential.

Everyone else is addressing trends from another perspective. They say the reason we are in crisis is demographics, costs, or greed. Why are you taking such a different tack?
Yes, my approach is different, and it focuses on the nature of the relationships we have with each other as we approach health and healing. I think we've made several mistakes. First, we forgot that our patients were also citizens and had recourse to their governments for relief when they did not like the care they received. We let them approach government for solutions, while we in health care paid too little attention to government as it emerged as a potent force in national health care planning, management, and payment. With government investment came government micromanagement. Second, we allowed contracts to replace the traditional covenants. Doing so, we not only abandoned democracy, we abandoned covenants. Third, we allowed the nation to develop an antipathy to profit within the health care sector. This was very foolish. We are an otherwise capitalist culture and we need investors willing to risk their capital to improve health care knowledge and

systems—and young people willing to incur hefty six-figure debt to complete medical and post-doctoral training. Fourth, we failed to understand the inter-relatedness of health and disease across national borders. We did not recognize that diseases from other parts of the world—intentionally or accidentally—could arrive in our land, and that the resources we had developed to safeguard our own health should be used to protect ourselves by protecting others as well.

Focusing on covenants dos not minimize the contributions of other health policy analysts, I just see our problems, and the roadmap to their solutions, in a slightly different way. We need their perspectives and analyses to address the dilemmas we face today. Neither of these approaches—the traditional or the covenant—is sufficient; both are necessary.

How can covenants help the uninsured in this country? Aren't doctors and managed care just shirking their responsibilities to make care available to them?
This is my favorite question. It may be my next book. It is such an immense topic that it deserves a book, or several! Some of the best minds in the country are struggling with this issue, and they have my respect. I hope they are prepared to fail, because, in my view, the current paradigm of health care financing provides them with few opportunities for success. Today, these policy and political leaders—along with healers, employers, and health plans—are confronting the challenge of retrofitting new, escalating, unrelenting demands into old laws, regulations, and systems. It's a tight fit for a swelling foot in a worn-out shoe. The employer-based and tax-funded insurance systems have matured into no-fault financing systems precisely at the time when employment patterns changed, science produced cures, and consumers aged and emerged as politically savvy, demanding change agents. My friends in the health care financing battles will make incremental changes, but they will not have the wherewithal for true

reform unless the underlying relationships among the parties to the covenant engage each other first in the ways I have proposed.

In the meantime, it is my view that the healers in this country are already doing their part by providing a substantial amount of care to the uninsured. Whether they are physicians, nurses, institutions, or pharmaceutical companies, their products and services are available for free and at reduced charges for those who cannot afford them. Even those healers who work in medical advertising provide free services. They develop and air public health service messages. Providing care for those who cannot afford it is within the covenants that shape healing practices and, in my view, healers have done their part within the covenant.

It is time now to address similar covenant-focused questions to patients and communities. Should patients who can afford coverage but decline to get it be required to do so? Automobile insurance is required in most states; should health care be required as well? Can patients who engage in high-risk lifestyles that drive up costs be required to change their behaviors? For example, should high-calorie, high-fat processed foods be taxed like cigarettes are taxed and for the same purpose—to reduce consumption, to fund health messages, and perhaps to fund health care that treats diseases associated with obesity? Should those who demand cost-increasing health care mandates be required to find funding sources in some other pocket than their own? Legislating that our healers provide care to Medicare and Medicaid patients at lower rates and without patient subsidies is driving some healers away from treating government-funded patients altogether. Is this what we want? All-or-nothing care? Should every new mandate that increases the cost of coverage be matched with a patient— or community-focused responsibility that will create savings in some other part of the employer or managed care budget?

It seems to me that the uninsured challenge us with

questions about what we value in this country, how health care stacks up in that value equation, and what kind of responsibility we feel to ourselves and to others as a result. It is clear to me that we value health and health care, and well we should. I have seen health care systems on five other continents, and this one (even at its worst) is by far the best. We value health and health care above many other things in our lives, and we want everyone to enjoy its benefits as well. We value it so highly that we believe cost should never be a barrier to receiving care. When cost is a barrier, we believe that health care should be free—a gift, if you will. This is not a new idea. Health and healing have always been a gift, from the deity, as the early chapters in this book describe. Our attitudes are no different than those of our ancestors; our behaviors, however, are different. Inherent in the gift-giving of a covenant tradition is the proscription to be a giver as well as a receiver. In the ancient tradition, the Israelites received gifts as a part of their covenant and were then enjoined to preserve their own health, protect the health of others, and give to others in recognition of what they had received. Therein lies a message for all of us today.

I may sound like a broken record here, but caring for the uninsured is a responsibility of the patient, the healer, and the community. Patients do their part through healthy lifestyles, practicing prevention, and securing coverage when it is offered to them. Healers do their part in providing free and reduced-price care. Communities do their part by supporting free and reduced-price clinics, whether through tax dollars or philanthropy.

What I fear most today, in our political climate, is that communities will band together and use legislation or regulation to set prices, require free care, and shift the patient's and community's responsibility for financing even more of the care to the healers. If the community wants all of its members to receive care, the community should be willing to step forward and pay for it, not legislate healers to do it for them. Medi-Cal, on behalf of taxpayers, pays a physician $43.25 to fix a broken arm, while veterinarians in the state get $500–$800 for repairing a dog's broken leg. It seems to me that's a misplacement of payment priorities.

Isn't "concierge" or "boutique" medicine a clear violation of the healing covenant?

"Concierge" or "boutique" medicine is a term used to describe an emerging clinical practice model. In these physician practices, patients pay much higher fees—ranging from $4,000 to $20,000—to physicians, who care for far fewer patients and are therefore able to provide a higher level of service. Patients get access to cell phone numbers, have home visits and examinations, are accompanied on visits to specialists, and are offered other amenities. In other segments of the economy, there is nothing usual about paying more for a higher quality of service or for more personal care. In health care, however, this type of service has been criticized as contributing to two-tier medicine in a nation that abhors class distinction. The phenomenon has been described variously as a response to market forces, as physician greed, and as the natural outgrowth of clinician dissatisfaction with the constraints of practicing under managed care and government-restricted payment schemes.

Concierge, or boutique, medicine is not a violation of the healing covenant. Covenants, after all, are created by the parties involved. In typical style, the "senior" party—the physician—is offering this relationship to the "junior" party—the patient, specifying the nature of the care and the cost of that care. It is not clear from press reports of these practices if the covenant reflects a true obligation on the part of patients at all, or if it is merely additional services of the grant—type of covenants I have outlined in this book. For example, if the physician uses the additional fees as an excuse to create even greater dependencies, then neither

---

the patient nor the healing relationship will mature. If, on the other hand, the physician educates and empowers patients to make better decisions on a day-to-day basis and creates interdependencies, then a truly mature healing relationship can evolve. That will be good for the healer as well as for the patient. Healthier patients will be more productive employees. It's hard to argue against something that is so good for so many people, including those who are not funding the higher level of care. The real objection, it seems to me, stems from those who want similar service but are unwilling to pay for it. Their objections are not persuasive to me.

Do people have a right to health care?
I get this question after nearly every presentation, probably because the notion of "rights" is promoted in health care reform proposals today. To begin, I'll distinguish between "healing" and "health care" because those terms are often used interchangeably when this question is posed. "Healing" is what we seek when we see a physician, take a drug, or enter a surgical suite. Will we get "healing?" Perhaps. Is it our right to have it? No. That's a strong statement, but I can find no historical or covenant rationale for saying "yes." In fact, "healing" is a gift and, as such, must be freely given by the giver; it cannot be legislated as a "right." The giver cannot be forced into giving, and particularly in the case of healing, with its tradition of emanation from the divine. Physicians, surgeons, and pharmaceutical companies in a covenant model are aligned with healing forces beyond themselves and are frequently operating within the many mysteries of life—in fact, within the greatest mysteries of life and death. To assume that even with modern science they can vanquish still-unknown sources with regularity is naïve. When we do not secure the healing we want, we sometimes believe that it is because our healers have withheld their technology or skill from us, and we claim our right to more. We believe so strongly that heal-

ing is our right, we will go to a great extent to get more access to health care in order to get it, including through litigation.

What about "health care?" Is "health care" a right? Is receiving any or all of the health care that we want—or even need—a right? Again, I can find no justification for that. Historically, it was the king or the employer who recognized that a healthy workforce was a productive workforce, and so provided health care for the economic benefits that would result. In today's health care system, with large and growing numbers of uninsured and underinsured this is an increasingly important question, particularly as we shift the responsibility for funding care to providers. In my view the best way to answer a question is with a statement and another question: Whether health care is a right is a question we can all answer. For me, yes, it is a right. In order to secure it, as an employer, I provide insurance for my employees; as an individual, I manage the insurance benefit wisely; as a taxpayer, I contribute to the federal and state programs that fund care; and as a philanthropist, I provide additional funds for programs that care for the needy. Are you willing to do the same? If so, then by your own actions you, too, demonstrate in the best possible ways that health care is a right.

Notes

Preface

[1]Charles Inlander, National Public Radio, "Marketplace," September 21, 2001.
[2]John H. Bryant and Zbigniew Bankowski, "Health Policy: Ethics and Human Values-An International Dialogue," XVIIIth Council for International Organizations of Medical Sciences (CIOMS), Switzerland: CIOMS, 1984.

Introduction

[1]Guenter Risse, *Mending Bodies, Saving Souls: A History of Hospitals*, New York: Oxford University Press, 1999, pp. 577–578.
[2]National Health Statistics Group, Office of the Actuary, "National health expenditures, 1996," *Health Care Financing Review*, 19(1) Health Care Financing Administration (HCFA) pub. No. 03400, Washington D.C.: U.S. Government Printing Office, Fall, 1997.
[3]Statistical Abstract of the United States: 1998 (118th edition), Washington, D.C.: U.S. Bureau of the Census, 1998, p. 129.
[4]Commonwealth Fund, *From Bench to Bedside: Preserving the Research Mission of Academic Health Centers: Findings and Recommendations of The Commonwealth Fund Task Force on Academic Health Centers*, New York: The Commonwealth Fund, April, 1999.
[5]Life expectancy at birth by race and sex: United States, 1940, 1950, 1960 and 1970–1995. U.S. National Center for Health Statistics, "Monthly Vital Statistics Report," *Vital Statistics of the United States*, Vol. 45, No. 11(S)2, June 12, 1997. Also at http://www.cdc.gov/nchswww/data/mv4511s2.pdf. Accessed July 1, 1999.
[6]"The gerontocrats," *Economist*, May 13, 1995, p. 32.
[7]http://www.aarp.org. Accessed February 15, 2000.
[8]National Health Statistics Group, Office of the Actuary, "National health expenditures, 1996," *Health Care Financing Review*, 19(1), Health Care Financing Administration (HCFA) pub. No. 03400, Washington, D.C.: U.S. Government Printing Office, Fall 1997.
[9]"Comparing health care," *Fortune*, July 27, 1992, p. 80.
[10]Institute for the Future, Robert Wood Johnson Foundation, "Health and Health Care 2010." Available at http://www.rwjf.org/iftf. Accessed February 25, 2000.
[11]Projections concerning health care expenditures are updated routinely by the Congressional Budget Office. Available at http://www.cbo.gov. Accessed November 17, 1999.
[12]David Emmons and Gregory Wozniak, "Physician contractual arrangements with managed care organizations," *Socioeconomic Characteristics of Medical Practice*, Chicago, IL: American Medical Association, 1997.
[13]"What the doctor ordered," *Time*, 1952, 60(7):38–44.
[14]R. Blendon, K. Scoles, C. Desoches, J. Yound, M. Herrmann, J. Schmidt, M.

Kim, "Americans' health priorities revisited after September 11," *Health Affairs Web Exclusive*, November 13, 2001, available at htpp://healthaffairs.org. Accessed November 20, 2001.

15R. Winslow, "U.S. hospitals may need $10 billion to be prepared for bioterror attack," *Wall Street Journal*, November 29, 2001, p. B-8, col. 5–6.

16Charles Morris, "The health-care economy is nothing to fear," *Atlantic Monthly*, December, 1999, pp. 86–96.

17D. Wessel, "Rising medical costs can be a good thing," *Wall Street Journal*, July 26, 2001, p. A1, col. 5.

18D. Leonhardt, "Health care as main engine: Is that so bad?," *New York Times*, November 11, 2001, Section 3, p. 1, col. 1–5, p. 12, col. 1–5.

Chapter 1

1W.F. Buckley, Jr., "Mr. Goodwin's great society," *National Review*, 1965, 17(36):760.

2For an examination of the gift related to the law, see Alan M. Dershowitz, *The Genesis of Justice*, Warner Books, New York, 2000.

3David B. Morris, *The Culture of Pain*, Berkeley: University of California Press, 1991, p. 44.

4Lakshmi Raman and Gerald A. Winer, "Evidence of Immanent Justice Reasoning in Adults." Paper presented at the 107th Annual American Psychological Association Convention, Boston, 1999.

5H. Koenig, M. McCullough, D. Larson, *Handbook of Religion and Health*, New York, Oxford University Press, 2000.

6H.G. Koenig, J. Hays, D. Larson, "Does religious attendance prolong survival?" *J Gerontol A Biol Sci Med Sci*, 1999, 54:M370–M377.

7R. Hummer, R. Rogers, C. Nam, C. Ellison, "Religious involvement and U.S. adult mortality," *Demography*, 1999, 63:273–285.

8Lynn Lamberg, "Native American physician incorporates tradition into mainstream medical care," *JAMA*, September 20, 2000, 284(11):1370.

Chapter 2

1S. Rushworth, Sam Woods, *American Healing*, Barrytown, NY: Station Hill Press, 1992, p. 35.

2Steven H. Gifis, *Barron's Law Dictionary*, Woodbury, NY: Barron's Educational, 1975, p. 49.

3William F. May, *The Physician's Covenant: Images of the Healer in Medical Ethics*, Philadelphia, PA: Westminster Press, 1983, p. 119.

4May, p. 108.

5Charles G. Cumston, *An Introduction to the History of Medicine*, London: Dawsons of Pall Mall, 1968, pp. 86–87.

6Irving I. Edgar, *The Origins of the Healing Art: A Psycho-Evolutionary Approach to the History of Medicine*, New York: Philosophical Library, 1978, p. 138.

7Edgar, pp. 135–138.

8Indiana University School of Medicine, 1997–1998 Student Manual. Available at http://www.medlib.iupui.edu/osca/smoath.htm. Accessed April 3, 2000.

9"Islamic Code of Medical Ethics, Declaration of Kuwait," adopted by the International Conference on Islamic Medicine, 1981. Available at http://www.phrusa.org/research/medicsoath.htm. Accessed October 31, 1999.

10J.A. Benson, "Contemporary Use of Oaths and Covenants." Paper presented at the Institute of Medicine, Washington, D.C., October 13, 1998.

[11]Information on White Coat Ceremonies and the work of the Arnold P. Gold Foundation can be accessed at http://humanism-in-medicine.org. Accessed November 21, 2001.

[12]R. Lowes, "Swearing off the oath," *New Physician*, April, 1995.

[13]K.D. Clouser, "A covenant between physician and patient: An innovation by a graduating class," *Annals of Internal Medicine*, 1985, 10(6):941–943.

[14]Gifis, p. 44.

[15]Gifis, p. 45.

[16]Gifis, p. 45.

[17]Donald Berwick, P. Janeway, P. Hiatt and R. Smith, "An ethical code for everybody in health care," *Brit Med J*, 1997, 15:1633–1634.

[18]Frank J. Molnar et al., "Assess the quality of newspaper medical advice columns for elderly readers," *California Medical Association Journal*, 1999, 161:393–395.

[19]This is true in public health as well as individual clinical healing encounters. See J. Katz, "Patient preferences and health disparities," *JAMA*, September 26, 2001, 286(12):1506–1509. This study noted that even patients who tended to avoid care received higher immunization rates when they were cared for within managed care settings. The authors concluded that individual resistance could be overcome with the right (healer) interventions. This, it seems to me, represents the continuing trend of healers to accept responsibility that is better left to patients.

[20]Eli Ginzberg, "Ten encounters with the U.S. health sector, 1930–1999," *JAMA*, 1999, 282:1665–1668.

[21]S. Fox, L. Rainie, *The Online Health Care Revolution: How the Web Helps Americans Take Better Care of Themselves*. Washington D.C., The Pew Charitable Trust, 2000.

[22]M. McFarlane, S. Bull, C. Raitjeijer, "The internet as a newly emerging risk environment for sexually transmitted diseases," *JAMA*, July 26, 2000, 284(4):443–449.

[23]Elia Kacapyr, "What's wrong with this picture?," *American Demographics*, September, 1998, pp. 18–19.

[24]In *The Physician's Covenant: Images of the Healer in Medical Ethics*, Philadelphia, PA: Westminster Press, 1983. William May describes the model of the physician-patient relationship in parent-child terms.

Chapter 3

[1]A. Etzioni, "The Responsive Community: A Communitarian Perspective" (Presidential Address, American Sociological Association, August 20, 1995), *Amer Sociological Rev*, February, 1996, pp. 1–11.

[2]A.D. Speigel, "Hammurabi's managed health care: Circa 1700 BC," *Managed Care*, May, 1997. Available at http://www.managedcaremag.com/archiveMC/9705/9705.hammurabi.shtml. Accessed November 29, 1998.

[3]Institute of Medicine, Committee on Quality of Health in America, *To Err Is Human: Building a Safer Health System*, National Academy Press, Washington, D.C., 2000.

[4]George Lundberg, *Severed Trust: Why American Medicine Hasn't Been Fixed*, New York: Basic Books, 2000.

[5]Rates of noncompliance for epilepsy range from 30%–50% [I.E. Leppik, "How to get patients with epilepsy to take their medication: The problem of noncompliance," *Postgrad Med*, 1990, 88:253–256]; for arthritis from 55%–71% [W. van Elmeren and B. Horisberger, eds., *Socioeconomic Evaluation of Drug Therapy*,

New York: Springer-Verlag, 1998]; for hypertension to 40% [L.T. Clark, "Improving compliance and increasing control of hypertension: Needs of special hypertensive population," *Amer Heart J*, 1991:664–669]; and for diabetes from 40%–50% [M. Nagasawa, M.C. Smith and J.H. Barnes, "Meta-analysis of correlates of diabetes patients' compliance with prescribed medications," *The Diabetes Educator*, 1989, 16(3):192–200]. Even organ transplant patients, for whom medications prevent organ rejection and death, have noncompliance rates of near 20% [M. Rovelli, D. Palmeri, F. Vossler, S. Bartus, D. Hull and R. Schweitzer, "Noncompliance in organ transplant recipients," *Transplantation Proceedings*, 1989; 21:833–834]. The cost in terms of additional doctor visits is high. Excess hospital admissions are placed at $25 billion per year, nursing home admissions at $5 billion and lost productivity in the workplace at $50 billion [Task Force for Compliance, "Noncompliance with Medications: An Economic Tragedy with Important Implications for Health Care Reform," November, 1993, revised April, 1994. For further information, contact John Hawks, Task Force Executive Director, 2300 N. Charles Street, Suite 200, Baltimore, MD 21218, phone: 410-467-1100]. Even in an aggressive intervention program using pharmacists to improve compliance for lipid-lowering agents, the compliance rates rose only to 84%. That increase is better than most programs, but it is still not good enough if we are to achieve the cost-management goals that the public and payers have set for health care [B.M. Blum, J.M. McKenney, M.J. Cziraky and R.K. Elswick "Interim report for Project ImPACT: Hyperlipidemia," *J Amer Pharm Assoc*, 38(5):529–534].

[6]J.M. McGinnis and W.H. Foege, "Actual causes of death in the United States," *JAMA*, 1993, 270(18):2207–2212.

[7]C.L. Murray and A.D. Lopes, "Alternative projections of mortality and disability by cause 1990–2020: Global burden of disease study," *Lancet*, 1997, 349:1498–1504.

[8]N. Pronk, M. Goodman, R. O'Connor and B. Martinson, "Relationship between modifiable health risks and short-term health care charges." *JAMA*, 1999, 282(23):2235–2239.

[9]Centers for Disease Control and Prevention, "Tobacco Use—United States, 1900–1999," *JAMA*, 282(23):2202–2204.

[10]Lewin Group, "Costs of Obesity," for the American Obesity Association, Obesity Conference, Washington, D.C., September 15, 1999.

[11]Centers for Disease Control and Prevention, Healthy People 2000 Progress Review, last updated on December 15, 1999. Available at http:/www.odphp. pdophs.dhhs.gov/pubs/hp2000. Accessed February 4, 2000.

[12]An entire issue of the Journal of the American Medical Association was devoted to obesity, edited by Richard M. Glass, M.D. and Phil B. Fontararosa, M.D., *JAMA*, 1999, 282(16):1493–1588.

[13]"Inside the industry—Obesity drugs: Drugmakers vie for market share," *American Health Line*, November 5, 1998.

[14]H. Taylor, The Harris Poll #60, *Public Health*, October 20, 1999.

[15]P.S. Mead, L. Slutskey, V. Dietz, L. McCaid, J. Bresee, C. Shapiro, P. Griffin and R. Tauxe, "Food-related illness and death in the United States," *Emerging Infectious Diseases*, 1999, 5(5). Available at http://www.edc.gov/mcidod /EID/vol5no5/mead.htm. Accessed September 18, 1999.

[16]Centers for Disease Control and Prevention, "Current trends in childhood lead poisoning—United States: Report to the Congress by the Agency for Toxic Substances and Disease Registry," *MMWR*, 1988, 37(32):481–485. See also, "About Lead Poisoning," Alliance to End Childhood Lead Poisoning. Available at http://www.aeclp.org.

[17]J. Steinhauer, "Plan to fight West Nile Virus outlined," *New York Times*, December 17, 1999, p. 83.

[18]Personal communication with Robert Howard, Special Assistant for Media Relations, Center for Infectious Diseases, Centers for Disease Control and Prevention.

[19]National Center for Environmental Health, Centers for Disease Control and Prevention, "Air Pollution and Respiratory Health." Available at http://www.cdc.gov/nceh/publicatns/1994/cdc/brochures/airpollu.htm. Accessed February 21, 2000.

[20]National Center for Chronic Disease Prevention and Health Promotion, Centers for Disease Control and Prevention, "Teen Pregnancy." Available at http://www.cdc.gov/needphp/teen/html. Accessed August 16, 1999.

[21]Division of Child Development, Disability and Health, Centers for Disease Control and Prevention, "Fetal Alcohol Syndrome." Available at http://www.cdc.gov/nceh/programs/cddh/fashome.htm. Accessed August 20, 1999.

[22]D.R. Rice, E.J. MacKenzie, A.S. Jones, S.R. Kaufman, G.V. DeLissovoy, W. Max, E. McLaughlin, T.R. Miller, L.S. Robertson, D.S. Salkever and G.S. Smith, *Cost of Injury in the United States*, Baltimore, MD: The Johns Hopkins University Press, 1989.

[23]T.R. Miller, M.N. Pindus, J.B. Douglass and S.B. Rossman, *Databook on Nonfatal Injury: Incidence, Costs and Consequences*, Washington, D.C.: Urban Institute Press, 1995.

[24]National Highway Traffic Safety Administration (NHTSA), *Promoting Safe Passage into the 21st Century*, Washington, D.C.: NHTSA, 1999.

[25]NHTSA, *National occupant protection use survey—1996, Research Note*, Washington, D.C.: NHTSA, 1997.

[26]P.J. Cook, B.A. Lawrence, J. Ludwig and T.R. Miller, "The medical costs of gunshot injuries in the United States," *JAMA*, 1999, (282):447–454.

[27]National Center for Injury Prevention and Control, Centers for Disease Control and Prevention, "Unintentional Injury." Available at http://www.cdc.gov/ncipc. Accessed November 12, 1999.

Chapter 4

[1]Jayne Mackta, "The case for communication," *Lab Animal*, February 2000, 29(2):38–40.

[2]Purnell Chopin, "Report from the president," Howard Hughes Medical Institute Bulletin, December, 1998. Available at http://www.hhmi.org/annual98/report/index.html. Accessed December 23, 1999.

[3]Pharmaceutical Research and Manufacturers of America, *2001–2002 Annual Report: New Medicines*, New Hope, PhRMA, Washington, D.C., 2001, and Statement on the President's 2002 Budget Request, at www4.od.nhi.gov/office of budget/press2002/pdf. Accessed November 20, 2001.

[4]Lawrence Goldstein, "Investing in tomorrow's health care today," *Howard Hughes Medical Institute Bulletin*, February, 1996. Available at http://www.hhmi.org/communic/bulletin/Feb98/invest.htm. Accessed December 23, 1999.

[5]L. Goldstein, Available at http://www.hhmi.org/communic/bulletin/Feb98/invest.htm. Accessed December 23, 1999.

[6]Pharmaceutical Research and Manufacturers of America, *1999 Industry Profile*, Washington, D.C.: PhRMA, 1999, p. 13.

[7]Information available at http://www.AMProgress.org. Accessed February 11, 2000. Other activist activity at the University of Minnesota can be found in: Will Woodward, "On campus, animal rights vs. animal researchers: University of

---

Minnesota emerges as a focal point," *Washington Post*, November 5, 1999, p. A01.

[8]Meredith Wadman, "U.S. Senate gets tough on animal activists," *Nature*, June 3, 1999, p. 397.

[9]U.S. Department of Agriculture, Office of Communications, *Agriculture Fact Book*, Washington, D.C.: USDA, 1996.

[10]Katie McCabe, "Who will live and who will die?" *The Washingtonian*, August 1986, p. 114.

[11]Cited in Martin S. Pernick, *A Calculus of Suffering: Pain, Professionalism and Anesthesia in Nineteenth-Century America*, New York: Columbia University Press, 1985, p. 156.

[12]Vicki D. Thompson Wylder, *Judy Chicago: Trials and Tributes*, Tallahassee, Florida: Florida State University Museum of Fine Arts, 1999.

[13]John G. Hubbell, "The 'animal rights' war on medicine," *Reader's Digest*, June, 1990, pp. 70–76.

[14]Personal Communication, HSUS Office of Membership.

[15]Report of confidential interviews, cited in New Jersey Association for Biomedical Research, The HSUS 2020 Initiative and Animal Rights, Strategic Health Policy International, 1999.

[16]The total amount of funds dedicated to identifying alternatives to the use of animals in research has not been tallied, but is estimated to be well over $7 million annually. Funds are provided by both public and private sector sources, including the National Institutes of Health, the National Toxicology Program, the Johns Hopkins Center for Alternatives to Animals in Testing, Proctor & Gamble, and the Alternatives Research and Development Foundation. Personal communication with Joanne Zurlow, Ph.D., Associate Director, Center for Alternatives to Animals in Testing.

[17]Sam Howe Verhovek, "Radical Animal Rights Groups Step Up Protests," *New York Times*, November 11, 2001, p. A24, col. 1.

Chapter 5

[1]The National Center for Health Services Research Agency was created nearly 25 years ago. The agency has since been renamed. It is now known as the Agency for Healthcare Research and Quality (AHRQ) and had a fiscal year 2000 budget of $107.05 million. This is not the only federal agency that conducts or funds this type of research. The Health Care Financing Administration, the Centers for Disease Control and Prevention, the Department of Defense, the Veterans Administration, and the Health Resources and Services Administration also conduct research to understand the delivery of health care.

[2]California Health Care Association, "National Survey: Confidentiality of Medical Records," January 29, 1999. Available at http://www.chcf.org. Accessed October 12, 1999.

[3]Robert O'Harrow, Jr., "Prescription sales: Privacy fears," *Washington Post*, February 15, 1998, pp. A1, A18–19.

[4]The defendants in this case include CVS Pharmacy, Inc., Elensys Care Service, Inc., GlaxoWellcome, Inc., Warner-Lambert Company, Merck & Co., Inc., Biotech, Inc., Biogen, Inc., and Hoffman-LaRoche, Inc. Commonwealth of Massachusetts, Superior Court Department of the Trial Court, Civil Action No. 9800897-F.

[5]The first comment period ended on February 17, 2000 and resulted in more than 50,000 comments. A second comment period ended on March 30, 2001 and generated an additional 24,000 comments. The health care industry must

now be compliant with the regulation by April 14, 2003. Several parts of the rule are in serious debate and it is unclear if privacy regulation will be reconsidered because there are still differences of opinion on the best ways to preserve privacy. Many of those variations are at the state level. Of the five major bills introduced in the 105th Congress, the only major differences among these bills lie in how the federal standard would affect the flexibility of state laws. In the absence of federal law, the states have acted to set standards of their own. Prior to 1999, only seven states had set regulations concerning how insurers could use medical records. Twenty-eight states included in their legislation the duty for physicians, insurers, health care institutions, and other providers to maintain the confidentiality of computerized medical records. Concerning the penalties for unauthorized disclosure, seventeen states established civil penalties, nine states have criminal penalties, and five states have both types of penalties. The remaining nineteen states established neither criminal nor civil penalties for unauthorized disclosure of medical records.

[6]Charles Greene Cumston, *An Introduction to the History of Medicine*, London, Dawsons of Pall Mall, 1968, pp. 86–87.

[7]"Health Care Information Privacy," Louis Harris and Associates poll conducted for Equifax, 1993.

[8]Steven Jacobsen, Zhisen Xia, Mary Campion et al., "Potential effect of authorization bias on medical record research," *Mayo Clin Prac*, 1999, 74:330–338.

[9]Victor G. Freeman, Saif S. Rathore, Kevin P. Weinfurt, Kevin A. Schulman and Daniel P. Sulmasy, "Lying for patients: Physician deception of third-party payers," *Arch Intern Med*, 1999, 159:2263–2270.

[10]Max Frankel, "Snoops or germs?," *New York Times Magazine*, September 13, 1998, p. 44.

Chapter 6

[1]Oskar Kraus, *Albert Schweitzer: His Work and His Philosophy*, London: Adam & Charles Slack, 1944, p. 26.

[2]Stuart Grossman, et al., "Correlation of patient and caregiver ratings of cancer pain," *J Pain and Symptom Manage*, 1991, 6(2):53–57; Jamie H. Von Roenn et al., "Physician attitudes and practice in cancer pain management," *Ann Intern Med*, 1993, 119(2):121–126.

[3]National Pain Survey, Conducted for Ortho-McNeil Pharmaceutical, 1999; "Acute pain management: Operative or medical procedures and trauma," *Clinical Practice Guideline No. 1*, AHCPR Publication No. 92-0032, Rockville, MD: Agency for Health Care Policy and Research, Department of Health and Human Services, February, 1992.

[4]Clermont E. Dionne, "Low back pain," in Iain Crombie, Peter Croft, Steven Linton, Linda LeResche, and Michael Von Korff (eds.), *Epidemiology of Pain*, Seattle, WA: International Association for the Study of Pain, 1999, pp. 283–297.

[5]Reva C. Lawrence et al., "Estimates of the prevalence of arthritis and selected musculoskeletal disorders in the United States," *Arthritis and Rheum*, 1998, 41(5):778–799.

[6]Marilyn Marchione, "Headaches: Common, painful and expensive," *Scripps Howard News Service*, November 23, 1999.

[7]"Pain and Absenteeism in the Workplace," Study conducted for Ortho-McNeil Pharmaceutical, 1997; "International Pain Survey," conducted for Ortho-McNeil Pharmaceutical, 1999.

[8]*The NIH Guide: New Directions in Pain Research I*, Washington, D.C.: Government Printing Office, 1998.

9P. Wall and M. Jones, Defeating Pain, *The War Against a Silent Epidemic*, Plenum, New York, 1991.

10International Association for the Study of Pain, Subcommittee on Taxonomy, "Part II: Pain terms: A current list with definitions and notes on usage," *Pain*, 1979, 6:249–252.

11E.J. Cassell, *The Nature of Suffering and the Goals of Medicine*, New York: Oxford University Press, 1991, p. 36.

12National Hospice Organization (NHO), 1700 Diagonal Road, Suite 300, Alexandria, VA 22314. Available at http://www.nho.org. Accessed October 15, 1999.

13C.S. Hill, "The negative influence of licensing and disciplinary boards and drug enforcement agencies on pain treatment with opioid analgesics," *J Pharm Care, Pain and Symptom Control*, 1993, 1:43–62; R. Nowak, "Cops and doctors: Drug busts hamper pain therapy," *J NIH Res*, 1980, 4:27–28.

14National Hospice Organization (NHO), 1700 Diagonal Road, Suite 300, Alexandria, VA 22314. Available at http://www.nho.org. Accessed October 15, 1999.

15J. Porter, and H. Jick, "Addiction rate in patients treated with narcotics," *New Engl J Med*, 1980, 302:123; R.K. Portnoy, and K.M. Foley, "Chronic use of opioid analgesics in non-malignant pain: Report of 38 cases," *Pain*, 1986, 25:171–186; E.M. Marks, and E.J. Sashar, "Undertreatment of medical inpatients with narcotic analgesics," *Ann Intern Med*, 1973, 78:173–181.

16According to the joint statement of the American Academy of Pain Medicine and the American Pain Society, physicians need not fear respiratory depression and other side effects of pain medicines, which are rare and can be managed with diet and other medical supports. Sedation and nausea are early side effects that usually dissipate with continued use of the medication, 1998.

17E. Emanuel, "Euthanasia and physician-assisted suicide: Attitudes and experiences of oncology patients," *Lancet*, 1996, 347(9018):1805; K.M. Foley, "The relationship of pain and symptom management to patient request for physician-assisted suicide," *J Pain and Symptom Manage*, 1991, 6:289–297.

18Richard Schulz, and Scott R. Beach, "Caregiving as a risk factor for mortality: The caregiver health effects study," *JAMA*, 1999, 282(23):2215–2219.

19Family Caregivers Association, 10400 Connecticut Ave., Kensington, MD 20895-3994. Available at http://www.nfcacares.org. Accessed December 3, 1999.

20Committee on Psychosocial Aspects of Child and Family Health, American Academy of Pediatrics, and Task Force on Pain in Infants, Children, and Adolescents, "The Assessment and Management of Acute Pain in Infants, Children and Adolescents," *Pediatrics*, 108(3):793–797.

21Joint Statement of the American Pain Society and the American Academy of Pain Management, 1998.

22Alabama, Alaska, Arizona, Arkansas, California, Colorado, Florida, Georgia, Iowa, Kansas, Louisiana, Massachusetts, Maryland, Minnesota, Missouri, Montana, Nebraska, Nevada, New Jersey, New Mexico, North Dakota, Ohio, Oklahoma, Oregon, Pennsylvania, Rhode Island, Tennessee, Texas, Utah, Vermont, Virginia, Washington, West Virginia, Wisconsin, Wyoming.

23Iowa, Rhode Island, South Dakota, Virginia, Oklahoma, South Carolina, Virginia, West Virginia, Arkansas and Maryland.

24Alabama, Arkansas, Illinois, Kansas, Maryland, Missouri, Vermont (some of these measures strengthen the language of earlier legislation).

25The American Academy of Pain Medicine, The American Pain Society, The Federation of State Medical Boards of the U.S., The Medical Board of California,

The National Academy of Sciences, Institute of Medicine, The National Conference of Commissioners on Uniform State Laws, The National Conference of State Legislatures, The State Cancer Pain Initiatives.

[26]Joel B. Obermeyer, "Doctors urged to treat pain," *News and Observer* (Raleigh, NC), October 26, 1999.

[27]Jerome Groopman, "Separating Death from Agony," *New York Times*, November 9, 2001, p. A25, col. 1.

[28]Paul Tough, "The Alchemy of Oxycontin," *New York Times Magazine*, July 29, 2001, pp. 32–38, 52, 62–3. This article was one of many, including front-page stories recounting addiction and trafficking in Oxycontin®.

[29]The "Circle of Life Awards" is a program of the American Hospital Association, the American Medical Association, the American Association of Homes and Services for the Aging, and the National Hospice and Palliative Care Organization, with grant funds from the Robert Wood Johnson Foundation. This award is an annual program recognizing excellence in end-of-life care, including the management of pain.

[30]World Health Organization, *Cancer pain relief.* Geneva: WHO, 1986.

[31]William T. McGivney and Glenna M. Crooks, "The care of patients with severe chronic pain in terminal illness," *JAMA*, 1984, 251(9):1181–1188.

Chapter 7

[1]Kurt Vonnegut, Jr., *Breakfast of Champions.* New York: Dell Publishing, 1973, p. XX.

[2]Poll Data Booklet, Vol. 2, *Research!America*, p. 2. Also available at http://www.researchamerica.org/opinions/2000polls.generalversion_files/frame. htm. Accessed January 7, 2002.

[3]Merck & Co., Inc. established a relationship with the Instituto Nacional de Biodiversidad of Costa Rica to support the search for and cataloging of plants native to that nation's rain forests, in return for the rights to screen those products for bioactive compounds. Available at http://www.inbio.ac.cr/en/inbio/Inbio.htm. Accessed November 21, 2001. Shaman Pharmaceuticals is a company devoted to producing medicines from natural sources in the rain forests. Additional information can be found at: http://www.well.com/user/hlr/tomorrow/shaman.html. See also http://www.shamanbotanicals.com. Accessed November 21, 2001.

[4]Charles G. Cumston, *An Introduction to the History of Medicine.* London: Dawson's of Pall Mall, 1968, p. 86.

[5]Irving I. Edgar, *The Origins of the Healing Art: A Psycho-Evolutionary Approach to the History of Medicine.* New York: Philosophical Library, 1978, p. 137.

[6]"Islamic Code of Medical Ethics, Declaration of Kuwait," adopted by the International Conference on Islamic Medicine, 1981. Available at http://www.phrusa.org/research/medicsoath.htm. Accessed October 31, 1999.

[7]J.P. Bull, "The historical development of clinical therapeutic trials," *Journal Chronic Disease*, 1959, 10:218–248.

[8]L.M. Friedman, C.D. Furberg, and D.L. DeMets, *Fundamentals of Clinical Trials*, 3rd ed. New York: Springer Publishing, 1998.

[9]F.L. Iber, W.A. Riley and P.J. Murray, *Conducting Clinical Trials.* New York: Plenum, 1987.

[10]*NIH inventory of clinical trials: Fiscal Year 1979, Vol. I.* National Institutes of Health, Division of Research Grants, Research Analysis and Evaluation Branch, Bethesda, MD.

[11]Friedman, et al., *Fundamentals of Clinical Trials.*

12The archive of NIH Clinical trials can be searched at http://clinicaltrials.gov. Accessed November 21, 2001.

13Kathleen Drennan, "Have the ultimate benefits of clinical trials been maligned beyond repair?," *Drug Discovery Today*, 6 (12): 597–599.

14*The Globalization of Clinical Trials: A Growing Challenge in Protecting Human Subjects*, Department of Health and Human Services, Office of the Inspector General, December 2001, OEI-01-00-00190. Available at http://oig.hhs.gov/oei. Accessed January 13, 2002.

15The group of founding members includes Public Responsibility in Medicine and Research, the Association of American Universities, the Association of American Medical Colleges, the National Health Council, the Consortium of Social Science Association, the Federation of American Societies for Experimental Biology and the National Association of State University and Land-Grant Colleges. Representatives of the public will join the board of the group and institutions will apply for accreditation, which can be granted following site-visits to the institution and adherence to guidelines and principles of the group.

16R.B. Standler, "Nonconsensual Medical Experiments on Human Beings," May 1999. Available at http://www.rbs2.com.

17Katz, *Experimentation with Human Beings*, 1972, pp. 9–65.

18The Willowbrook Hepatitis study was carried out from 1963 to 1966 at the Willowbrook State School, an institution for "mentally defective persons." Some children were deliberately injected with the hepatitis virus, others were fed extracts of stools from infected individuals, and still others received injections of purified virus. Information is available at http://hstraining.orda.ucsb.edu/training/willowbrook.htm. Accessed July 5, 2001.

19James H. Jones, *Bad Blood: The Tuskegee Syphilis Experiment*. New York: Free Press, 1993.

20Vickie L. Shavers, Charles F. Lynch, and Leon F. Burmeister, "Knowledge of the Tuskegee Study and its impact on the willingness to participate in medical research studies," *Journal of the National Medical Association*, December 2000, 92 (12), pp. 563–572.

21An article by Henry Beecher reviews 22 studies, conducted in prestigious medical institutions and published in prestigious journals, where human subjects encountered risks without their knowledge or consent. Henry Beecher, "Ethics and clinical research," *New England Journal of Medicine (NEJM)*, 274 (1966): 1354–60.

22P.M. McNeill, "Experimentation in human beings," In H. Kuhse and P. Singer (eds.) *Companion to Bioethics*. Oxford: Blackwell, 1998, pp. 369–378.

23G.J. Annas, L.H. Glantz, and B.F. Katz, *Informed Consent to Human Experimentation*. Cambridge, MA: Ballinger, 1977.

24Cited in Martin S. Pernick, *A Calculus of Suffering: Pain, Professionalism and Anesthesia in Nineteenth-Century America*. New York: Columbia University Press, 1985, p. 156.

25Joe Stephens, "The Body Hunters," *The Washington Post*, December 17, 2000, A01. This was the first of a six-part story that appeared between December 17 and December 22, 2000. The series is available at htsp://washingtonpost.com/wp-dyn/world/issues/bodyhunters/. Accessed December 22, 2000.

26P.M. McNeill, *The Ethics and Politics of Human Experimentation*. Oakley: Cambridge University Press, 1993.

27National Commission for the Protection of Human Subjects of Biomedical and Behavioral Research, *The Belmont Report: Ethical Principles and Guidelines for the Protection of Human Subjects of Research*. U.S. Government Printing Office,

Washington, D.C., 1979.

[28]Trials of War Criminals before the Nuremberg Military Tribunals under Control Council Law No. 10: Nuremberg, October 1946–1949, 2 vols. U.S. Government Printing Office, Washington, D.C.

[29]"World Medical Association Declaration of Helsinki, "Ethical Principles for Medical research Involved in Human Subjects," *JAMA*, December 20, 2000, Vol. 284 (23), pp 3043–3045. For other U.S.-focused principles, see especially the work of the National Bioethics Advisory Commission, including reports on Ethical and Policy Issues in research Involving Human Participants, and Ethical and Policy Issues in International Research Clinical Trials in Developing Countries, available at http://www.georgetown.edu/nbac. Accessed December 17, 2000.

[30]Ezekiel J. Emanuel, Dadid Wendler and Christine Grady, "What Makes Clinical Research Ethical?," *JAMA*, May 24/31, 2000, Vol. 283 (2), pp. 2701–2711.

[31]International Conference on Harmonization, Harmonized Tripartite Guideline and Guideline for Good Clinical Practice (1996). Information available at http://www.ifpma.org.

[32]T.L. Beauchamp and J.F. Childress, *Principles of Biomedical Ethics*. New York: Oxford University Press, 1986, pp. 30–34, 133–38.

[33]R.J. Boyle, *The Process of Informed Consent. Introduction to Clinical Ethics*, 2nd ed. University Publishing Group, 1997, pp. 91–93.

[34]Federal Policy for the Protection of Human Subjects, 45 CFR 46.116(a) 1–8.

[35]Marjorie A. Speers, Ph.D., *Basic Protections for Human Subjects in International Research*, Centers for Disease Control and Prevention (CDC).

[36]Ibid.

[37]Ibid.

[38]Multiple sources, but primary discussions on subjects contained in Council for International Organizations of Medical Sciences (CIMOS), International Ethical Guidelines for Biomedical Research Involving Human Subjects, WHO, Geneva, 1993.

[39]Speers, op. cit.

[40]Ibid.

[41]CIOMS,op. cit.

[42]N. Dickert and C. Grady, "What's the Price of a Research Subject? Approaches to Payment for Research Participation," *NEJM* 341(3) (1999): 198–203.

[43]L.M. Friedman, C.D. Furberg, and D.L. DeMets, *Fundamentals of Clinical Trials*, 3rd ed. New York: Springer Publishing, 1998.

[44]P.S. Appelbaum, L.H. Roth, and C.W. Lidz, "The Therapeutic Misconception: Informed Consent in Psychiatric Research," *International Journal of Law and Psychiatry* 4(3–4) (1982): 319–329.

[45]FDA regulation 45 CFR 46.111. Information available at http://www.fda.org.

[46]Ibid.

[47]N. Kass and A. Hyder, "Attitudes and Experiences of U.S. and Developing Country Investigators Regarding U.S. Human Subjects Regulations" (2000). Information available at http://www.NBAC.org.

[48]Emanuel, Wendler, and Grady, op. cit.

[49]CIOMS op. cit.

[50]Public Citizen's appeal to the Secretary, U.S. Department of Health and Human Services (Health Research Group Publication #1558) can be accessed at www.citizen.org/publications/release.cfm?ID=6761. Accessed January 7, 2002. Discovery Laboratories, Inc. response and research plans can be found at www.discoverylabs.com. Accessed January 7, 2002.

[51]P.S. Applebaum, L.H. Roth, and C.W. Lidz, "The Therapeutic Misconception:

Informed Consent in Psychiatric Research," *International Journal of Law and Psychiatry* 5(3–4) (1982): 412–419.

Chapter 8

1Genesis, 9:7.

2John Gannon, "The Global Infectious Disease Threat and its Implications for the United States." Available at http://www.odcl.gov/CIA/publications/nie/report/nie99-17d.html. Accessed October 10, 2001.

3Several novels have provided glimpses into the impact of infectious disease on a nation and the world: Alistair MacLean, *The Satan Bug*. New York: Fawcett Publications, 1962; Michael Crichton, *The Andromeda Strain*. New York: Knopf, 1969; Stephen King, *The Stand*. New York: Doubleday, 1978; and Frank Herbert, *The White Plague*. New York: Putnam, 1982.

4T. McKeown, *The Modern Rise of Population*. New York: Academic Press, 1976. G. Armelagos and N. Cohen, eds., *Paleopathology at the Origins of Agriculture*. New York: Academic Press, 1984. G. Armelagos, K. Barnes, J. Lin, "Disease in Human Evolution: The Re-emergence of Infectious Disease in the Third Epidemiological Transition," *National Museum of Natural History Bulletin for Teachers*, Vol. 18, No. 3, Fall 1996. Available at http://www.nmnh.si.edu/anthro/ outreach/anthnote/fall9/anthback.htm. David Satcher, "Emerging Infections: Getting Ahead of the Curve," Emerging Infectious Diseases, Vol.1, No.1, January–March 1995.

5Information available at http://www.doh.gov.uk/cjd. United Kingdom Department of Health. Accessed September 3, 2001.

6A. Kanabus and S. Allen, "The Origin of AIDS and HIV, and the First Cases of AIDS." Available at http://www.avert.org/origins.htm. Accessed December 1, 2001.

7E. Crubezy, et al, "Identification of mycobacterium DNA in an Egyptian," *C R Acad Sci* III 1998, Nov:321(11):942–51. Cockburn and Cockburn, eds., *Mummies, Diseases and Ancient Cultures*. New York: Cambridge University Press, 1995. D. Christensen, "Pre-Columbia mummy lays TB debate to rest," *Science News* 143:181 (March 19, 1994).

8Hippocrates, *Of the Epidemics, Book II* translated by Francis Adams. Available at http://classics.mit.edu/Hippocrates/epidemics.html. Accessed April 6, 2001.

9"T.B. Wars: Man's Ancient Struggle." Available at http://www.md.huji.ac.il/microbiology/bact330/lecturetb.html. Accessed April 6, 2001.

10K. Fackelmann, "Paleopathological Puzzles: Researchers unearth ancient medical secrets," *Science News Online*, August 30, 1997.

11"TB Wars: Man's Ancient Struggle." Available at http://www.md.huji.ac.il/microbiology/bact330/lecturetb.html. Accessed May 3, 2001.

12T. Dormandy, *The White Death: A History of Tuberculosis*. New York: New York University Press, 2000.

13Robert Desowitz, *The Malaria Capers (More Tales of Parasites and People, Research and Reality)*. New York: W. W. Norton & Company, 1991.

14Al-Ruzi (Rhazes) on Smallpox and Measles. Available at http://users.erols.com/gnqm/euromed3.html. Accessed May 3, 2001.

15David Satcher, Statement before the Committee on International Relations U.S. House of Representatives, June 29, 2000. Available at http://www.house/gov/international_relations/full/disease/satcher.html. Diseases of Entomological Importance. Available at http://www.entomology.unl.edu/history_bug. Accessed May 2, 2001.

16Suzanne Possehl, "The long reach of bugs without borders," *Hospital & Health*

Networks, Vol. 72, July 5, 1998.

[17]Leviticus, 14:37–53.

[18]Leviticus, 13:47–59, 14:8–9.

[19]Robert Mackey, "Ten diseases on the way out," *New York Times Magazine*, May 6, 2001, pp. 34–36.

[20]Information available at http://www.cartercenter.org. Accessed November 10, 2001.

[21]A. J. Cann, History of Smallpox. Available at http:/www.tulane.edu/~dmsander/Tutorials/pox. Accessed December 21, 2001.

[22]S. Fretwell and K. Winiarski, "Global warming could devastate human health," *The State*, April 7, 2001. Available at http://www.thestate.com. Accessed September 20, 2001.

[23]David Heymann, "The Urgency of a Massive Effort Against Infectious Diseases," June 29, 2000 Statement before the Committee on International Relations U.S. House of Representatives. Available at http://www.who.org. Accessed November 10, 2001.

[24]T. Dormandy, The White Death: A History of Tuberculosis. New York: New York University Press, 2000.

[25]Abigail Zuger, "Infectious Diseases Rising Again in Russia", *New York Times*, December 5, 2000. Available at http://www.nytimes.com. Accessed November 2, 2001.

[26]John Gannon, "The Global Infectious Disease Threat and its Implications for the United States". Available at http://www.odcl.gov/CIA/publications/nie/report/nie99-17d.html. Accessed November 2, 2001.

[27]G. Armelagos and N. Cohen, op. cit.

[28]Gro Harlam Brundtland, "Health and Population," BBC Reith Lectures 2000. Available at http://news.bbc.co.uk/hi/english/static/events/reith_200/lecture4.stm. Accessed May 18, 2001.

[29]Rebecca Voelker, "Travel Risk of HBV," *JAMA*, December 13, 2000, 284 (22), pp. 2863. This report describes a study of European travelers' knowledge of disease risks. Though nearly 75% were at risk for contracting HBV, only half understood the method of transmission and only 17% were vaccinated.

[30]Marilyn Chase, "New virulent forms of tuberculosis spur concerns world-wide," *Wall Street Journal*, December 17, 1999, p. B1.

[31]Personal Communication, Rick Glover, M.D. Air travel has been investigated as a source of infectious disease. See World Health Organization, Tuberculosis and air travel: guideline for prevention and control (Geneva, World Health Organization, 1998).

[32]P. Martens and L. Hall, "Malaria on the Move: Human Population Movement and Malaria Transmission," *Emerging Infectious Diseases*, Vol. 6, No. 2, March-April 2000. "Health: Malaria-Carrying Mosquitoes Hitch Rides on Airplanes," *Inter Press Service* English News Wire, August 23, 2000.

[33]John Gannon, "The Global Infectious Disease Threat and its Implications for the United States." Available at http://www.odcl.gov/CIA/publications/nie/report/nie99-17d.html. Accessed May 3, 2001.

[34]Pamela Constable, "For Nepali Girls, a Way Station to Dignity," *New York Times*, April 24, 2001, p. A14.

[35]*International Federation of Red Cross and Red Crescent Societies, World Disasters Report 2001*, International Federation of Red Cross and Red Crescent Societies, Geneva, p. 198.

[36]"Communicable diseases are main health threat to Kosovo refugees," April 6, 1999. Available at http://www.who.int/inf-pr-2q999/en/pr-18.html. Accessed May 6, 2001.

37Christopher Wren, "U.N. Council Addresses HIV/AIDS in its Focus," *New York Times*, January 20, 2001, p. A7. Alpha Nuhu, "Refugee Camps Attract Sex Workers and AIDS," *Panafrican News Agency*, January 5, 2001. Available at http://allafrica.com. Accessed May 3, 2001.

38"Defending National Borders." Available at http://www.who.org. Accessed May 3, 2001.

39Elizabeth Anne Fenn, *Pox Americana*. New York: Hill and Wang, 2001. See also: Gina Kolata, "New York was Bioterrorism Target, in 1864," *New York Times*, November 13, 2001, F7, col. 1; and Gina Kolata, "When Bioterror First Struck U.S. Capital," *New York Times*, November 6, 2001, p. F1, col. 4; and Mark Derr, "New Theories Link Black Death to Ebola-like Virus," *New York Times*, October 2, 2001, p. F4, col. 1.

401999 Country Reports on Human Rights Practices, Bureau of Democracy, Human Rights, and Labor, U.S. Department of State, February 25, 2000. Available at http://www.state.gov. Accessed May 6, 2001.

41Blaine Harden, "For Burmese, Repression, AIDS and Denial," *New York Times*, November 14, 2000. Available at http://www.nytimes.com. Accessed May 6, 2001.

42John Pomfret, "The High Cost of Selling Blood", *Washington Post*, January 11, 2001, p. A01.

43Denise Grady, "Drug Resistant Bacteria Still on the Rise," *New York Times*, December 28, 2000. Available at http://www.nytimes.com. Madeline Nash, "The Antibiotics Crisis," *Time.com*, January 10, 2001. Available at http://www.time.com.

44An unimmunized American child contracted measles and died after being exposed to the disease while standing in line next to a measles-infected Brazilian child at an amusement park in the U.S. Personal communication Robert Howard, Centers for Disease Control, 2002.

45F. Cox, Z.M. Khan, J.E. Schweinle, L. Okamoto, and T. McLaughlin, "Cost associated with the treatment of Influenza in a managed care setting," October 3, 2000. Available at http://www.medscape.com/medscape/GeneralMedicine/journal/2000/v02.n05/mgm1003.cox/pnt-mgm1003.cox.html. Accessed February 24, 2001. Centers for Disease Control and Prevention, "Prevention and control of influenza. Recommendations for the Advisory Committee on Immunization Practice (ACIP)," *Mortality and Morbidity Weekly Report (MMWR)* 1999; 48:1–28. K.L. Nichol, A. Lind, K.L. Margolis, M. Murdoch, R. McFadden, M. Hauge, S. Magnan, M. Drake, "The effectiveness of vaccination against influenza in healthy, working adults," *NEJM* 1995; 333:889–893.

46Guidelines for Prevention and Control of Pandemic Influenza in Healthcare Institutions Draft 03/23/2000. Available at http://www.ahcpub.com/ahc_root_html/hot/breakingnews/flue03232000.html. Accessed February 4, 2001.

47WHO Information Fact Sheet on Influenza. Posted February 1999. Available at http://www.who.int/inf-fs/en/fact211.html. Accessed February 4, 2001.

48Ibid.

49P.A. Patriarca and N.J. Cox, "Influenza pandemic preparedness plan for the United States" *Journal of Infectious Diseases* 1997; 176 Suppl 1:S4–7.

50S. Jones, "The Flu Hunters," *Time Magazine*, February 23, 1998, 151(7), p. 56.

51Centers for Disease Control and Prevention, Pandemic Influenza: A Planning Guide for State and Local Officials (Draft 2.1). Available at http://www.cdc.gov/nypo/pandemiclfu.htm. Accessed February 24, 2001. M.I. Meltzer, N.J. Cox, K. Fukuda, "The economic impact of pandemic influenza in the United States: priorities for intervention" *Emerging Infectious Disease* 1999; 5(5): 659–71.

[52]R. Snacken, A.P. Kendal, L.R. Haaheim, and J.M. Wood, "The Next Influenza Pandemic: Lessons from Hong Kong, 1997," *Emerg Infect Dis* 1999; 5(2): 195–203.

[53]FluNet: Global Influenza Surveillance Network. Available at http://oms2.b3e.jussieu.fr/fluenet. Accessed on March 2, 2001.

[54]D. Stamboulian, P.E. Bonvehi, F.M. Nacinovich and N. Cox, "Influenza," *Infect Dis Clin North Am 2000*; 14(1): 141–66. A. Flahault, V. Dias-Ferrao, P. Chaberty, K. Esteves, A. Valleron and D. Lavanchy, "FluNet as a Tool for Global Monitoring of Influenza on the Web," *JAMA* 1998; 280(15): 1330–2.

[55]Norman E. Cantor, *In the Wake of the Plague: The Black Death and the World It Made.* New York: The Free Press, 2001.

[56]Laurie Garrett, *Betrayal of Trust: The Collapse of Global Public Health.* New York: Hyperion, 2000.

[57]Elizabeth Anne Fenn, *Pox Americana.* See also: Gina Kolata, "New York Was Bioterrorism Target, in 1864," *New York Times*, November 13, 2001, F7, col. 1, and Gina Kolata, "When Bioterror First Struck U.S. Capital," *New York Times*, November 6, 2001, F1, col. 4.

[58]Jonathan Tucker, "Historical trends related to bioterrorism: An empirical analysis," *Emerg Infect Dis*, Vol. 5 (4). Available at www.cdc.gov/ncidod/eid/vol5no4/tucker.htm. Accessed May 6, 2001.

[59]Natalie Angier, "Together in sickness and in health," *New York Times Magazine*, May 6, 2001, pp. 67–69.

[60]James Hughes, Statement before the Subcommittee on National Security, Veterans Affairs, and International relations, Committee on Government Reform, U.S. House of Representatives, July 23, 2001. Available at http://www.bt.cdc/press/Hughes_072320001.asp. Accessed October 10, 2001. See also: Annie Fine and Marcelle Layton, "Lessons for the West Nile Viral Encephalitis Outbreak In New York City 1999: Implications for bioterrorism preparedness," *Clinical Infectious Diseases*, 2001:32:277–282.

[61]Joseph Barbera, et al., "Large-scale quarantine following bioterrorism in the United States: Scientific examination, logistic and legal limits, and possible consequences," *JAMA*, 2001:286: 2711–2717.

[62]Marilyn Werber Sheafini, "When quarantines are needed," *National Journal*, November 17, 2001, pp. 3612–3613.

[63]David Heymann, "The Urgency of a Massive Effort Against Infectious Diseases," Statement before the Committee on International Relations U.S. House of Representatives, June 29, 2000. Available at http://www.who.org. Accessed November 2001.

[64]"Resurgence of a killer," *National Journal*, April 28, 2001, p. 1241. Available at http://www2.exxonmobil.com/corporate/files/corporate/260401.pdf. Accessed January 16, 2002.

[65]Rebecca Voelker, "Mothers fight malaria," *JAMA*, September 13, 2000, Vol. 284 (10) p. 1235.

[66]Daren DeYoung, "Global AIDS Strategy May Prove Elusive," *Washington Post*, April 23, 2001, A01.

[67]Eric Schmitt, "Helms Urges Foreign Aids be Handled by Charities," *New York Times*, January 12, 2001. Transparency International 2000 Report on County Corruption. Available at http://www.transparency.org. Accessed May 3, 2001.

[68]Catherine Arnst and Kerry Capell, "Tuberculosis roars back," *Business Week*, October 2, 2000, p. 153.

[69]"Giving Something Back, A Survey of the New Rich," *The Economist*, June 18,

---

2001, pp. 15–17.

[70]Personal Communication with Jim Russo based on report of the World Bank pending publication.

[71]Gro Harlam Brundtland, "Health and Population." Available at http://news.bbc.co.uk/hi/english/static/events/reith_200/lecture4.stm. Accessed May 18, 2000.

Chapter 9

[1]Information at http://www.drini.com/mothertheresa/own_words/. Accessed March 18, 2000.

[2]Lawrence Altman, "U.N. issues grim report on the 11 million children orphaned by AIDS," New York Times, December 2, 1999, p. A12. See also United Nations Press Release PI/1205, "World AIDS Day held at headquarters, Focus on children orphaned by AIDS," December 1, 1999.

[3]Marilyn Chase, "New, virulent forms of tuberculosis spur concerns world-wide," Wall Street Journal, December 17, 1999, p. B1.

[4]David Satcher, "Tuberculosis-Battling an ancient scourge," JAMA, 1999, 282(21):1996.

[5]Judith Miller, "Study says new TB strains need an intensive strategy," New York Times, October 28, 1999, p. A6.

[6]Information available at http://www.worldbank.org. Accessed December 14, 1999.

[7]"Corporate hospitality," Economist, November 27, 1999, p. 71.

[8]Information available at http://www.gatesfoundation.org. Accessed December 14, 1999.

[9]Information available at http://www.capitalresearch.org. Accessed December 14, 1999.

[10]Information available at http://www.rotary.org. Accessed December 14, 1999.

[11]Information available at http://www.gatesfoundation.org. Accessed December 14, 1999.

[12]Information available at http://www.fdncenter.org. Accessed December 14, 1999.

[13]Gro Harlem Brundtland, "International Trade Agreements and Public Health: WHO's Role," presented by video at the Conference on Increasing Access to Essential Drugs in Globalized Economy, Amsterdam, November 25–26, 1999.

[14]"Lilly rushes antibiotic aid to more than one million Rwandan refugees," Lilly Press Release, July 27, 1994.

[15]"Lilly speeds needed drugs to Rwandan refugees," FDA Today, October 1994, pp. 4–5.

[16]"The goodwill pill mess," Time, 1996, 147(18):64.

[17]J.L. Zeballos, "Health aspects of the Mexico earthquake—19 September, 1985," Disasters, 1986, 10:141–149.

[18]P. Autier, M.C. Ferir and A. Hairapetiien, "Drug supply in the aftermath of the 1988 Armenian earthquake," Lancet, 1990; 335:1388–1390.

[19]H.M. Ali, M.M. Homeida and M.A. Abdeen, " 'Drug Dumping' in donations to the Sudan" (letter), Lancet, 1990, 336:745.

[20]L. Offerhaus, "Russia: Emergency drug goes awry," Lancet, 1990, 339:607.

[21]Personal communication, Hans Hogerziel, World Health Organization.

[22]Frank Greve, "Drug donations: A bitter pill?," Philadelphia Inquirer, June 16, 1999, p. 1.

[23]Department of Essential Drugs and Other Medicines, Guidelines for Drug Donations, Geneva: World Health Organization, 1999.

[24]Patrick Berckmans, Veronique Dawans, Gerard Schmets, Daniel Vandenbergh

and Philippe Autier, "Inappropriate drug-donotion practices in Bosnia and Herzegovina, 1992 to 1996," *New Engl J Med*, 337(25):1842–1845.

25Jacqueline Rieschick, "Drug donors get deductions for not-so-charitable contributions," *Tax Notes International*, January 13, 1999, 16:174–176.

26The Partnership for Quality Medical Donations (PQMD) is an alliance of 19 pharmaceutical companies and private voluntary organizations working to improve the quality of medicine donations around the world. Their domestic and international activities to facilitate the flow of medicines to the developing world have been significant, and they have emerged as the key voice representing the interests of their membership in continuing to donate medical products. Further information is available at http://www.pqmd.org.

27Personal communication, Sister Maura O'Donohue, M.D., Catholic Medical Mission Board.

28"Charitable giving: Will Americans be generous in the '90s?" *CQ Researcher*, 1993, 3(42):985–1008.

29Information available at http://www.merck.com. Accessed December 27, 1999.

30Information available at http://www.sb.com. Accessed December 27, 1999.

31Information available of http://www.glaxowellcome.com. Accessed December 27, 1999.

32Information available at http://www.iclinic.co.za/sept99/healthaid3.htm. Accessed December 29, 1999.

33Information available at http://inpma.org/ifpmaselectedprograms.htm. Accessed November 21, 2001.

34Personal communication, James Russo, Executive Director, PQMD.

35Michael R. Reich, ed., *An Assessment of U.S. Pharmaceutical Donations: Players, Processes and Products*, Boston: Harvard School of Public Health, 1999.

36"Corporate hospitality," *Economist*, November 17, 1999, p. 71.

37Personal communication, James Russo, Executive Director, PQMD. A final report of this joint study will be available in 2002. Additional information can be obtained through PQMD, which can be contacted at www.pqmd.org.

Chapter 10

1Claude Le Pen, "Innovation and Regulation in the Pharmaceutical Market," in Felix Lobo and German Velasquez, eds., *Medicines and the New Economic Environment*, World Health Organization, Editorial Civitas, Madrid, 1998, p. 213.

2Code of Hammurabi.

3M. Angell, "Is academic medicine for sale?," *N Engl J Med*, 2000, 342:1516.

4*Report of the Commission on Macroeconomics and Health, Microeconomics and Health: Investing in Health for Economic Development*. Available at http://www3.who.int/whosis/cmh/cmh_report/e/report.cfm?path=cmh. Accessed January 23, 2002.

5www.nih.gov, www.cdc.gov, www.dod.gov. Accessed January 30, 2002.

6Abraham Flexner, "Medical Education in the United States and Canada," *Carnegie Foundation Bulletin* 4, New York, 1990.

7Data provided by the Pennsylvania Biotechnology Association. See also www.pabiotech.org.

8Mark Hatfield, Hugo Sonnenschein, Leon Rosenberg, *Exceptional Returns: The Economic Value of America's Investment in Medical Research*, New York: Funding First, 1999. Available at www.fundingfirst.org.

9Fuchs, V. *Who Shall Live?* New York: Basic Books, 1974.

10Christopher Murray, Alan Lopez, *The Global Burden of Disease*, World Health Organization, Geneva, 1996.

[11] *Funding First, Exceptional Returns: The Economic Value of America's Investment in Medical Research*, available at www.fundingfirst.org. Accessed March 15, 2002.

[12] Michael Marmot, "Health and the psychosocial environment at work," in Michael Marmot, ed, *Social Determinants of Health*, Oxford: Oxford University Press, 1999. See also George Davey-Smith, "Socioconomic differentials in mortality risk among men screened for the Multiple Risk Factor Intervention Trial: White men," *American Journal of Public Health*, 86:489–496.

[13] *Report of the Commission on Macroeconomics and Health, Marcoeconomics and Health: Investing in Health for Economic Development*, World Health Organization, Geneva, 2001. Available at www3.who.int/whosis. Accessed January 23, 2002.

[14] D.E. Massing (Ed.), *USTM Licensing Survey: Fiscal Year 1998*. Norwalk, CT: Association of University Technology Managers, Inc., 1999.

[15] Kathleen Drennan, "Have the ultimate benefits of clinical trials been maligned beyond repair?," *Drug Discovery Today*, 6 (12):597–599.

[16] Medical devices represent 5% of all approved trials and non-drug therapies, such as surgical techniques or radiation, amount to 10%.

[17] *Agreement on the Trade-Related Aspects of Intellectual Property Rights*, WIPO, 1995. Available at www.wipo.org, Accessed March 18, 2001.

[18] Ibid.

[19] World Trade Organization, www.wto.org.

[20] Pharmaceutical Manufacturers' Association (PhRMA), "Chapter 8: Global Intellectual Property Protection," *Pharmaceutical Industry Profile 2001*. Available at www.phrma.org, Accessed March 17, 2001.

[21] The Drug Price Competition and Patent Term Restoration Act of 1984 recognizes that product testing, development, and compliance with federal marketing requirements can consume some of the patent term, thus reducing marketing time for recovery of research and development costs. The law restores time lost in government review. The law provides that only half of the development time can be restored, the extension can be no more than 5 years, and total patent life cannot exceed 14 years—that is, 14 years of marketing time. The Act also eased requirements and expedited approval of generic products by allowing manufacturers to use the safety and efficacy data from the developing company. In essence, the law balanced interests—offering innovators a longer period or protection, but providing generic companies with enhanced market access at the point of patent termination.

[22] F. Scherer, "The Pharmaceutical Industry and World Intellectual Property Standards," *Vanderbilt Law Review*, 53(6):2245–2254.

[23] Ibid.

[24] According to the Congressional Budget Office, in 1994, the pharmaceutical industry spent approximately 18% of sales on research and development. It is expected the industry will spend upwards of 20% in the coming years. Comparatively, other U.S. industries spend approximately 4% of sales in R&D. Among European Countries, 1993 figures reveal investment in R&D varies from 7% in Italy to 17% in the United Kingdom. S. Wolf, "Evaluating Damages in Patent Infringement Cases," *Pennsylvania CPA Journal*, 69(2): 9–12. Costs, according to the Boston Consulting Group, were estimated at $500 million in 1996. High R&D costs have been associated with a high attrition rate for what is termed "dry holes;" that is, compounds that have been investigated but abandoned during pre-clinical, phase I, and phase II stages for various reasons. TCSDD reports that of the 5,000 compounds in development, only 5 reach pre-clinical testing and, of those, only one may be approved for sale or become a "blockbuster." Innovative drugs cost more (in both time and money) to develop

than modifications to existing compounds. IPP is the means by which companies recover the dollars spent on R&D. In a survey of 100 U.S. firms in different industries, pharmaceutical industries indicated that 65% of medicines would not have been developed or commercially introduced without patent protection. High on the list as well were the Chemical and Petroleum industries, stating that 39% and 25% of their products, respectively, would not have been developed in the absence of IPP. The Boston Consulting Group, "Unleashing Managerial Advantage in Pharma R&D." Available at www.bcg.com. Accessed April 2, 2001. P. Danzon, "Pharmaceutical Price Regulation—National Policies versus Global Interests", Washington, D.C.: AEI Press, 1997. Pharmaceutical Manufacturers' Association (PhRMA), op. cit.

[25]P. Danzon, op. cit.

[26]*Tufts Center for the Study of Drug Development, Impact Report.* Available at www.tcsdd.edu. Accessed April 2, 2001.

[27]R. Rozek, R. Berkowitz, "The Effects of Patent Protection on the Prices of Pharmaceutical Products: Is Intellectual Property Protection Raising the Drug Bill in Developing Countries?," *The Journal of World Intellectual Property*, 1(2):179–243.

[28]K. Maskus, "Lesson from studying International Economics of Intellectual Property Rights," *Vanderbilt Law Review*, 53(6): 2219–2239.

[29]J. Revesz, *Trade-Related Aspects of Intellectual Property Rights.* Available at http://bilbo.indcom.gov.au/research/staffrcs/trips/index.html. Accessed April 25, 2001.

[30]USITC, *Prescription Drug Pricing Report.* Available at www.usitc.gov. Accessed April 26, 2001.

[31]H.E. Frech and R.D. Miller, *The Productivity of Health Care and Pharmaceuticals: An International Comparison*, Washington, D.C.: AEI Press, 1999.

[32]R. Dubois, et al. "Explaining drug spending trends: Does perception match reality?," *Health Affairs*, 2000: 19(2):231–239.

[33]F.R. Lichtenberg, *Pharmaceutical Innovation, Mortality Reduction and Economic Growth*, Cambridge, MA: National Bureau of Economic Research, May 1998. Working Paper W6569.

[34]The Boston Consulting Group, "The Contribution of Pharmaceutical Companies, What's At Stake for America," 1993.

[35]D.B. Audretsch and P.A. Stephan, "Company-scientist locational links," *American Economic Review*, 86: 641–652. See also: J. Meyer, "Assessing the Impact of Pharmaceutical Innovation: A Comprehensive Framework", New Directions for Policy, February 2000. Also available at www.npwnow.org. Accessed March 21, 2002.

[36]A. Holmer, "Industry strongly supports continuing medical education," *JAMA*, April 18, 2001, 285(15):2012–2014.

[37]M. Angell, "Is academic medicine for sale?," *N Engl J Med*, 2000; 342: 1516–1518. See also: C.D. DeAngelis, "Conflict of interest and the public trust," *JAMA* 2000, 284:2237–2238.

[38]H. Moses and J. Martin, "Academic relationships with industry: A new model for biomedical research," *JAMA*, Feb 21, 2001, 285(7):933–935.

[39]Branko Milanovic, "True world income distribution, 1998 and 1993: First calculation based on household surveys alone," *The Economic Journal*, 112:51–92.

[40]J. Cohen and J. Rogers, eds, Norman Daniels, *Is Inequality Bad for Our Health?* Boston, MA: Beacon Press, 2000.

[41]B. Pecoul, J. Orbinski, E. Torreele, eds. *Fatal Imbalance: The Crisis in Research and Development for Drugs for Neglected Diseases*, Geneva: Médecins Sans Frontières/Drugs for Neglected Diseases Working Group, 2001. Available at

http://www.accessmed-msf.org. Accessed January 30, 2002.

42M. Angell, "The pharmaceutical industry—to whom is it accountable?," *NEJM* 342:1902–1904.

43These government programs can be located at the website of the National Institute for Allergy and Infectious Disease (NIAID), Global Health Research. Available at http://niaid.nih.gov/dmid/global. Government and Industry Team up to Battle Infectious Diseases. Available at http://www.niaid.nih.gov/news-room/releases/challgrants.htm. Summit on Development of Infectious Disease Therapeutics (meeting summary). Available at http://www.niaid.nih.gov/dmid/drug/summit.htm.

Chapter 11

1Patch Adams, *Gesundheit! Bringing Good Health to You, the Medical System, and Society Through Physician Service, Complementary Therapies, Humor, and Joy*, Rochester, Vermont: Healing Arts Press, 1993, p. 51.

2In instances where there are no citations concerning the individual mentioned, it is because the biographical sketches are drawn from my discussions and experiences with the individuals themselves.

3E. Ransdell, "This 'killer app' saves money and lives," *Fast Company*, November 1999, pp. 112–113. See also www.diabeteswell.com.

4M. Patsos, "The internet and medicine: building a community for patients with rare diseases," *JAMA*, February 14, 2001, 285(6):805.

5Information on Completing a Life can be found at htpp://www.completingal-ife.msu.edu. Another related website can be found at htpp://www.promotingex-cellence.org. Accessed November 24, 2001.

6D.H. Freedman, "Intensive care," *Inc.*, February, 1999, pp. 72–80. See also http://www.griffinhealth.org.

7http://www.cvs.com.

8Personal communication with Robert Carr, M.D., Senior Vice President, GlaxoSmithKline.

9C. Gentry, "Doctor Yes, How is Merrill Lynch limiting health costs?, *Wall Street Journal*, May 23, 2000, p. A1.

10Information concerning the activities of Mayor John Street's Fitness Program can be found at http://www.phila.gov/fitandfun. Accessed November 20, 2001.

11A. Mokdad, B. Bowman, E. Ford, et al, "The continuing epidemics of obesity and diabetes in the United States," *JAMA*, September 12, 2001, 286(10):1195–1200.

12Information on Renew! can be obtained by contacting Ms. Kathleen Clark, Renew, 40 Tweed Terrace, San Rafael, CA 94901, 415-456-9727, woodskec@pacbellnet.

13U.E. Reinhardt, "Medicare can turn anyone into a crook," *Wall Street Journal*, January 21, 2000, p. A18.

14J. Scott, G. Gade, M. McKenzie and I. Venohr, "Cooperative health care clinics: A group approach to individual care," *Geriatrics*, 1998, 53(3):86–81. See also J. Scott and B.J. Robertson, "Kaiser Colorado's Cooperative Health Care Clinic: A group approach to patient care," *Managed Care Quart*, 1996, 4(3):41–45; A. Beck, J. Scott, P. Williams, B. Robertson, D. Jackson, G. Glade and P. Cowan, "A randomized trial of group outpatient visits for chronically ill older HMO members: The Cooperative Health Care Clinic," *J Amer Geriatr Soc*, 1997, 45(5):534–549.

15Center for Studying Health System Change, "Local Innovations Provide Managed Care for the Uninsured, Issue Brief Findings from HSC," *Mathematica*

Policy Research 25, January, 2000.

[16]H.D. Scott, J. Bell, S. Geller and M. Thomas, "Physicians helping the underserved: The Reach Out Program," *JAMA*, 2000, 283(1):99–104.

[17]"The Nursing Center in Concept and Practice: Delivery and Financing Issues in Serving Vulnerable People," *National Health Policy Forum, Issue Brief No. 746*, September 13, 1999.

[18]Personal communications with Brian Robinson, RTC Relationship Marketing and Rima Cohen, Greater New York Hospital Assocation.

[19]A. Sharpe. "Health care: Discounted fees cure headaches, some doctors find," *Wall Street Journal*, September 15, 1998, B1. See also http://www.simplecare.com.

[20]*Healthy People in Healthy Communities, A Dialogue Guide*, Chicago, IL: The Coalition for Healthier Cities and Communities, 1999. See also *Transforming Health Care: Lessons from Community Partnerships*, National Community Care Network Demonstration Program, Chicago, IL: Health Research and Education Trust, 1999; and C.F. Adams (ed.), *Voices from America: Ten Healthy Community Stories from across the Nation*, Chicago, IL: Coalition For Healthier Cities and Communities and the Health Research and Educational Trust, 1998.

[21]"What creates health? Individuals and communities respond," a national study conducted by DYG, Inc. for the Healthcare Forum, San Francisco, 1994. This study was conducted in partnership with the W.K. Kellogg Foundation, the Healthcare Forum, the Healthier Communities Partnership and the National Civic League (single copies are available free by calling 415-356-4317); See also *Leadership for a Healthy 21st Century*, Chicago, IL: The American Hospital Association, 1999 (single copies are available at no charge by calling 1-800-AHA-2626).

[22]D. Cummings, T. Hamilton, B. Crawford and B. Cherney, "Integrating Education, Technology, Wellness and Community with Traditional Medicine: A View of the Future." Paper presented at the Ninth National CEO Summit, Atlanta, March 29–30, 1999.

[23]Information concerning Celebration Health is based on personal communications with Des Cummings, Florida Hospital Health Systems.

[24]Information concerning the ACT Project is based on personal communications with Brian Crawford, Center for Health Futures at Celebration Health; Kathryn Johnson, Wynne Grossman, and Michael Bilton of the Health Forum; and Robert Gold, Macro International.

[25]"Outcomes Toolkit: The Results-Oriented System for Community Improvement," Healthcare Forum of the American Hospital Association and Macro International. Further information is available by contacting the Health Forum Customer Service Department at 1-800-821-2039.

Chapter 12

[1]John H. Bryant, and Zbigniew Bankowski, "Health Policy, Ethics and Human Values—An International Dialogue," XVIIIth Council for International Organizations of Medical Sciences (CIOMS), Switzerland: CIOMS, 1984, p. 7.

[2]D. Berwick, Janeway, P. Hiatt, and R. Smith, "An ethical code for everybody in healthcare." *Brit Med J*, 1997, 315:1633–1634.

[3]In one study of routine neonatal circumcision, 63% of parents did not discuss the procedure with any medical professional prior to admission to the hospital for childbirth and 20% were confronted with the decision at that time. Of those parents delivering male children, 37% discussed circumcision with a medical professional, 9% with friends, 20% with the hospital admissions clerk, and 34% discussed it with no one. A.J. Herrera and J.B. Trouern-Trend, "Routine neonatal

circumcision," *Am J Dis Child*, 1979, 133:1069–1070.

4Lynn Clothier, personal communication.

5J.A. Benson, "Contemporary Use of Oaths and Covenants." Paper presented at the Institute of Medicine, Washington, D.C., October 13, 1998.

6L. Foster, "The Johnson & Johnson Credo and the Tylenol Crisis," New Jersey Bell Journal Reprint. Copies of this reprint, as well as a copy of the Credo may be obtained through the Johnson & Johnson Corporate Communications Department at 732-524-0400.

7*Putting Patients First®: Patient Rights and Responsibilities*, Washington, D.C.: National Health Council, 1995.

8Martin Wasserman, M.D., personal communication.

Epilogue

1PMPM refers to "per member per month" and is the payment made to a plan or physician provider to care for the patients in the plan each month of the patient enrollment.

2S. Covey, *The 7 Habits of Highly Effective People: Restoring the Character Ethic*, New York, NY: Simon & Schuster, 1989.

Index

Hygeia, 14
hypertension, 85–86

I

ideas, protecting, 275–278
idiopathic respiratory distress syndrome
(IRDS), clinical trial, 194–195
immanent justice, 8, 9, 10
incubational model, 26
independent covenants, 34
independent review, 194
industry
academia and, 280–281
research and, 271–274
infectious disease, 201–213, 221–225
origin, 203
transmission, 218
influenza, 84, 91, 102–103, 214–217
history, 205
mortality, 215–216
types, 214
informed consent, 145, 146, 188–190
challenges, 190–193
elements, 189–190
Tuskegee study, 186–187
injuries, 92
Inlander, Charles B., 296
innovation, 257
pharmaceutical companies, 276
innovation sector, 261–264, 266–270
crafting a covenant, 270–271
funding, 267–268
resources, 271–275
Institutional Review Boards (IRBs), 188, 193
insurance, xxix–xxx, 75–77
companies, xxiv
group plans, xxxiv
health, 302–305
intellectual property, 275–278
protection, 277
intercessory model, 26
interdependence, 71, 75–107
Internal Revenue Service (IRS), 241–242
international aid, 229–231
international issues, xxv, 345–346
investors, 284, 285–286
Islamic Code of Medical Ethics, 44
Islamic Medical Oath, research and, 180
isolation, 293–294, 295–296
Israelites, 37–38

J

Jeffcoat, Sally, 315–316
Jenner, Edward, 206
Jesus, 15
Job, 7, 8
Johnson, Lyndon B., xxxi, 3
Johnson, Robert Wood, 336
Johnson & Johnson Company, 309
Credo, 335–336
Joint Commission for the Accreditation of
Health Care Organizations (JCAHO),
76
pain relief, 161–162
Jones, Judy Miller, 296–297
Judaism, 10–12, 40

K

Kaiser, Leland, i–iii
Kateri Tekakwitha, 22
Kessler, David, 232
Kevorkian, Jack, 166
Ko Hung, 13
Kosovo, 236
Kucinich, Dennis J., 241, 242
Kydd, Ronald, 26–27

L

Lamaze Method, 10
law, 5–6
law enforcement
medicine and, 165–166, 168
pain relief, 172
Le Pen, Claude, 257
legislation, pain relief, 172
legislative autonomy, federal and state,
147–148
leprosy, 205
Lerner, Julie and Paul, 293
Lethal Drug Abuse Prevention Act, 166
licensing income, 273
Life-Science Greenhouses, 266–267
life science companies, 266–267
lifestyle, 84, 88–89, 94, 106–107, 306
high-risk behavior, 95–96
literacy and language, informed consent,
191–192
litigation, animal rights groups, 121–122
Luke, 16

M

MacArthur, Douglas, 204
Mack, Connie, 167
Maimonides, 40–41, 63
    Prayer of, 41–43
    research and, 179–180
malaria, 204, 206, 207
Malarone®, 249
malevolence, 8
Mammotome Breast Biopsy System,
    309–310
Managed Care Consumer Bill of Rights, 99
managed care, xxviii–xxix, xxxi, xxxiii, xxxiv,
    260
March of Dimes, animal activists, 122–123
market, 52
Martin, Howard, 24
Maryland, 337–338
May, William, 35, 38, 51
measles, 204, 205, 206, 207
Measles-Mumps-Rubella vaccine, 298
Mectizan®, 249
medical devices, 111–112
medical education, 265–266
medical records, 135–136
medical school, 45–48
Medicare, xxvi, xxix, xxxi, 4
medication
    access to, 230–231
    pain relief, 157–158, 162
    see also access to care; drugs
Merck, 249
Merck, George, xxxii–xxxiii
Meyers, Abbey, 296
microbes, 220
Middle Ages, 8–9, 18
midwifery, 304
migration, infectious disease and,
    210–211
mildew, 205
Milnovic, Branka, 281–282, 283
miracle-focused healing, 26–27
models
    healers, 289–300
    health insurance, 303–305
modern mystery and medicine, 23–27
morphine, 159
Morris, Charles, xxxix
Mosaic Law, 10–11
Moses, 37
Muhammad, 15

mutual covenants, 34
Myss, Carolyn, 24–25

N

National Association for Biomedical
    Research (NABR), 125
National Chimpanzee Research Retirement
    Act, 123
National Committee for Quality Assurance
    (NCQA), 76
National Committee for the Treatment of
    Intractable Pain, 159
National Health Council, 336–337
National Institutes of Health (NIH), xxvi,
    265
National Provider Data Bank (NPDB), 76
Nergal, 8
New Age, 23–24
new ideas, 31–32
New Zealand, Great Apes Project, 122
Newkirk, Ingrid, 114, 118
news media, xxii, 60–61, 137–138, 139,
    233–234, 319
    pain relief, 172
Nightingale Pledge, 56
Noah, 36, 37
North American tribes, 22
Notre Dame conference, 240–241, 248
nurses, oath, 56
Nursing Center concepts, 304

O

oaths, 39–48
obesity, 89
obligation, 325
    see also covenants of obligation
Ocycontin®, 168
O'Donohue, Maura, 299
on call, 51
O'Neil, Michael, 293–294
opportunities, 73–74
Orlando Convention Center, 311
Ornish, Dean, 24
Outcomes Toolkit, 313–315
outdated supplies, 236, 241, 245
oversight, 198–199
    clinical trials, 198–199

P

pain, 18, 153–176
 addressing, 155–156
 chronic, 154
 cost, 154
 intractable, 157–159
 management, 161
 terminal illness, 154–155
 see also suffering
pain relief, 157–158, 161
 dilemma, 160
 law enforcement and, 162
 end of life, 170–174
Pain Relief Promotion Act of 1999, 167
palliative care, 171
Palmer, Robert, 28
Panacea, 14
partners in care, 45–48
Partnership for Quality Medical Donations,
 244
Pascal, Blaise, 9
patents, 243, 275–276
patient-community relationship, 339
Patient Protection Act, 98–99
patients, 292, 320, 343
 consent and authorization, 145, 146
 covenants and, 62–65
 dependency, 69
 healing and, 49
 health care data and privacy,
  140–142
 responsibility, 94–97
 rights, 147, 337
 role, 69
 vocal, 99–101
 see also informed consent
patients' bill of rights, 97–99
Peer Review Organizations (PROs), 77
Pellegrino, Edmund, 317
Pennsylvania, 266–267
People for the Ethical Treatment of Animals
 (PETA), 114
Person, Judi Lund, 162
personal rights, 221
pets, 117
peyotl, 23
pharmaceutical industry, 59, 258,
 260–261, 266
 clinical studies, 182, 183–184
 clinical trials, 274
 innovative drugs, 276

 see also drug donations; drugs
pharmacists, 57
 oath, 55–56
pharmacopoeia, 13
Philadelphia, 266–267
Physician Based Research Networks (PBRN),
 274
physician-patient relationship, 49–50
physicians, xxxvi–xxxvii
 contracts and, 51
Picture Archival Communications System
 (PACS), 309
Pius XII, 10
plague, 12, 17, 211–212, 218
pneumonia, 205
policy, 260
policy analysis, xxiv–xxv, xxvi, 296–297
policy making, 263, 350–351
 pain relief, 172
polio, 205
politics, xxii, xxxvii–xxxviii
 animal rights, 124
 informed consent, 192–193
population, infectious disease and,
 208–209
poverty
 infectious disease and, 210
 innovation and, 281–282, 283
prayer, 25–26
Prendergast, Joe, 294
prevention, 81, 84–86, 88, 102–103
primates, 118, 122
privacy, 136
 covenant, 148–151
 covenants and, 143–145
 debate, 145–148
 defined, 142
 efficiency and effectiveness vs.,
  131–152
 penalties for violations, 147
 principles, 144
 public awareness, 137–140
 regulations, 139–140, 142
 tradeoffs, 150, 151
 see also confidentiality
profit, xxv
Protestant Reformation, 20
psychotherapy, privacy, 138
public demand, xxi–xxii
public health, xxviii, 12, 60–62, 66–67,
 90, 205, 222
 developing world, 228–229

About the Author

Glenna M. Crooks, Ph.D. is President and CEO of Strategic Health Policy International, Inc. (SHPI), a firm that assists governments and businesses solve health care problems. She calls it "organizing chaos and charting a course through it."

Usually behind the scenes, she has worked for more than 20 years to solve major problems facing health care, both in the U.S. and overseas, and offers the unique perspective of having held senior executive positions in both government and the pharmaceutical industry.

After her tenure as a Reagan Appointee, she developed and managed policy operations for domestic and international markets at Merck&Co., Inc, and was recognized by her peers when the company's policy group was judged best of the Fortune 500. Later, she became Vice President for Worldwide Operations of Merck's Vaccine Business.

She serves on the Board of Directors of several health organizations, including Partnership for Prevention, and is Adjunct Professor of Health Policy at the University of the Sciences in Philadelphia. She was a member of the National Council of the Institute for Child Health and Human Development at the National Institutes of Health, Chairman of the National Commission on Rare Diseases, and received the Congressional Exemplary Service Award for Orphan Products Development. She is a recipient of the highest award in public health, the Surgeon General's Medallion, awarded by C. Everett Koop. Dr. Crooks holds a Ph.D. from Indiana University, awarded in 1977.

Since authoring *Creating Covenants: Healing Health Care in the New Millennium*, she speaks frequently at national medical and health care meetings and conducts workshops to assist those in health care who want to create covenants to improve their healing enterprises. Her next book, already underway, is entitled *The Yoga of Healing*.

To learn more about SHPI see www.strategichealthpolicy.com. Information about Dr. Crooks' work on healing covenants can be found at www.createcovenants.com. She can be reached through both websites.

3140021